Understanding and Managing Allergies

Understanding and Managing Allergies

Editor: Trisha Coppola

FOSTER ACADEMICS
www.fosteracademics.com

www.fosteracademics.com

FOSTER ACADEMICS

Cataloging-in-Publication Data

Understanding and managing allergies / edited by Trisha Coppola.
p. cm.
Includes bibliographical references and index.
ISBN 978-1-63242-865-3
1. Allergy. 2. Allergy--Diagnosis. 3. Allergy--Treatment. 4. Immunologic diseases. I. Coppola, Trisha.
QR188 .U53 2019
616.97--dc23

Foster Academics,
118-35 Queens Blvd., Suite 400,
Forest Hills, NY 11375, USA

ISBN 978-1-63242-865-3 (Hardback)

Printed and bound in China.

Contents

Preface

The conditions caused due to the hypersensitivity of the immune system to the substances present in the environment that are generally harmless for people are called allergies. Some common allergies are food allergies, hay fever, allergic asthma, atopic dermatitis and anaphylaxis. Symptoms include itchy rashes, runny nose, swelling, red eyes and shortness of breath. Some specific foods, medications, metal and pollen insect stings are some common causes of allergy. Blood tests, skin prick tests, patch tests, enzyme-linked immunosorbent assay and radioallergosorbent test (RAST) are the main diagnostic techniques. Treatment methods include allergen immunotherapy and enzyme potentiated desensitization. The topics included in this book on allergies are of utmost significance and bound to provide incredible insights to readers. It aims to shed light on some of the unexplored aspects of allergies and the recent researches related to such medical conditions. Those in search of information to further their knowledge will be greatly assisted by this book.

Significant researches are present in this book. Intensive efforts have been employed by authors to make this book an outstanding discourse. This book contains the enlightening chapters which have been written on the basis of significant researches done by the experts.

Finally, I would also like to thank all the members involved in this book for being a team and meeting all the deadlines for the submission of their respective works. I would also like to thank my friends and family for being supportive in my efforts.

Editor

1

360 degree perspective on allergic rhinitis management in Italy: a survey of GPs, pharmacists and patients

G. Walter Canonica[1*], Massimo Triggiani[2] and GianEnrico Senna[3]

Abstract

Background: General practitioners (GPs), community pharmacists and allergic rhinitis (AR) patients in Italy were surveyed in order to gain insight from all three perspectives into the diagnosis, management and burden of AR in Italy.

Methods: General practitioners and pharmacists (n = 100 for each) were surveyed by telephone; questions related to overall practice and to last AR patient seen. Patients (n = 552) completed a questionnaire after visiting specialist allergy centres. Questions related to diagnosis and treatment, degree of everyday limitation from AR, and satisfaction with treatment. The data were analysed descriptively.

Results: Allergic rhinitis was managed mainly by GPs, who reported making the diagnosis themselves in 68 % of cases; rhinorrhea (64 %), sneezing (57 %) and congestion (49 %) were the symptoms most frequently taken into account. Limitation from AR on everyday life was rated 6.2 out of 10 by GPs. Pharmacists most often considered eye tearing (54 %) in their diagnosis. Almost half of GPs (49 %) and 87 % of pharmacists were unaware of the Allergic Rhinitis and its Impact on Asthma (ARIA) guidelines. The most commonly reported prescribed treatments by GPs were branded mometasone furoate, desloratadine, ebastine and generic mometasone; 21 % prescribed homeopathic products occasionally. On average, GPs remembered that their last patient case had moderate/severe disease, was prescribed anti-histamine monotherapy (37 % of cases), and did not change prescription (78 %). Pharmacists recommended an antihistamine for 56 % of clients who asked for advice, and a nasal decongestant for 21 %. Patients rated limitation from AR on everyday life as 5.7/10. 55 % reported using multiple therapies, and 43 % were not satisfied or weakly satisfied with their current treatment. Patients' main expectation for the future was to succeed in managing their AR symptoms (45 %), while 22 % hoped for a definitive cure. Many patients (61 %) were concerned their health would deteriorate.

Conclusions: Allergic rhinitis is largely managed by GPs in Italy, with pharmacists also playing a role, yet awareness of the ARIA guidelines among these groups is low. Patient satisfaction with treatment is moderate or low. New more effective treatments are needed to improve AR management in Italy. Allergy education programs need to be better targeted to GPs and pharmacists, and communication with patients regarding symptom control must be improved.

Keywords: Allergic rhinitis, Burden, Italy, Physician, Pharmacist, Patient, Treatment, Survey

Background

Allergic rhinitis (AR) is the 'poor relation' of the allergy world, firmly placed behind asthma and atopic dermatitis in order of importance. The burden of AR is often ignored, but it is associated with a significant negative impact on productivity (comparable with that of heart disease and diabetes) [1] and high costs; estimated in Italy at €210.43/patient/year, a total cost to the Italian economy of approximately €2.4 billion/year [2–4]. AR has even been associated with an increased risk of having a road traffic accident (similar to that associated with

*Correspondence: canonica@unige.it
[1] Respiratory and Allergy Clinic, DIMI-Department of Internal Medicine, University of Genoa, IRCCS Aou San Martino, Largo Rosanna Benzi 10, 16132 Genoa, Italy
Full list of author information is available at the end of the article

having a blood alcohol concentration of 0.05 %, the legal limit in many countries) [5]. The Allergic Rhinitis and its Impact on Asthma (ARIA) guidelines are the recognised worldwide authority on AR diagnosis and management [6, 7]. The ultimate aim of the guidelines is to achieve AR control. However, disease control in AR remains an elusive concept, and indeed has not been fully defined.

There are several reasons why AR remains poorly controlled for many patients, including the complexity of its underlying pathology, lack of a universally accepted 'control-concept' and control language [8], a shifting landscape of severity [9, 10], sensitisation patterns [11, 12] and phenotypes [13, 14], and insufficiently effective and fast-acting treatments [15, 16]. Currently considered first-line therapies (even multiple therapies) do not consistently offer optimal symptomatic relief for many AR patients [17, 18]. Factors relating to patients and healthcare providers (HCPs) also contribute, and it is these factors that we examine in the current survey, specifically from the Italian viewpoint.

In Italy the prevalence of AR is high, estimated at 18.9 % of the population and rising [2, 3]. As in most jurisdictions, treatment patterns may be influenced by reimbursement regulations. Antihistamines are reimbursed in all regions of Italy for chronic (>3 months) treatment of AR but not for on-demand therapy. Nasal corticosteroids are not reimbursed, except in Tuscany.

The burden of AR in Italy has been assessed in the past, but these surveys have focused on a particular patient population (e.g. children) [19] or else the data from Italy has been combined with that of other European countries [9] and the United States [20]. However, in order to assess the true burden of AR in Italy and describe the current AR landscape, a '360-degree' perspective should be employed. Such a perspective includes the viewpoint of the general practitioner (GP) who diagnoses AR and prescribes medication, that of the pharmacist who dispenses medication and advises on AR treatments and referrals, and that of the patient who lives with the symptomatic burden and the consequences of medication and referral choices.

The aim of the current survey was to fill gaps in our knowledge on the burden and management of AR in Italy. We sought to collect a global perspective on AR management in Italy for the first time, by surveying GPs, pharmacists and patients from diagnosis to treatment and beyond. Specifically, the survey aimed to compose a picture of how AR is diagnosed and treated by GPs and pharmacists and to assess concerns and expectations for the future from the patient perspective.

Methods

Separate surveys were conducted of GPs, community pharmacists and AR patients. Survey questions are listed in Additional file 1. The GP and pharmacist surveys were carried out using computer-assisted telephone interviews, with a sample of 100 individuals from each category. The GPs and pharmacists participating in the study were randomly selected from a national database and were considered representative of their professional group working within the different geographical regions of Italy. Any GPs or pharmacists who had participated in market research within the previous 6 months were not enrolled. Interviews were carried out between 4th September 2013 and 24th September 2013.

GP survey

Information was collected on participant demographics, length of practice, number of patients with AR seen each month, practice in relation to diagnosis and referral of AR, symptoms considered when diagnosing AR, pathologies and comorbidities associated with AR, practice relating to the treatment of AR patients (including most frequently prescribed treatments and modalities), and awareness of the ARIA guidelines. GPs were also asked how much AR limited their patients' everyday life (on a scale from 1 to 10 where 1 = not at all and 10 = very limiting).

Pharmacist survey

The information collected from pharmacists was similar to that described above for GPs, except that beliefs about underlying inflammation and relationship to asthma were surveyed instead of more open questions on pathology and comorbidity, and questions on treatment patterns were broken down into doctors' prescriptions, cases where the patient asked for a recommendation, and cases where the patient chose their own treatment. Pharmacists were not questioned on the degree of limitation suffered by patients.

The GP and pharmacist surveys referred to participants' practice in general, except for a section that questioned them specifically on the last AR patient seen. This 'last patient case' approach enabled more specific questions to be asked about the case severity and treatment approach, and was also expected to provide a greater degree and accuracy of memory recall.

Patient survey

Patients were recruited from multiple specialist allergy centres throughout Italy. Eligible patients were those with AR attending participating centres for the first time. Patients were surveyed via a self-completed written questionnaire, which was completed by a total of 552 individuals. Questions covered duration of symptoms, time since diagnosis, role of different categories of HCP in patient's diagnosis and treatment, sources of information

Table 1 Participant characteristics

	General practitioners (n = 100)	Pharmacists (n = 100)	Patients (n = 552)
Age, years mean (SD)	57 (4.85)	55 (9.34)	32 (14.63)
Gender (% male)	75	54	52
Years of practice	78 % had ≥25 years' practice	67 % had ≥25 years' practice	N/A
Duration of AR symptoms	N/A	N/A	Mean (SD): 5.4 (8.19) years; 47 % were diagnosed with AR over 1 year ago
Mean no. of patients (SD)[a]	1287 (316) registered	3227 (2272) seen/month	N/A
Mean no. of patients with AR[a]	46 seen/month	20 % (17.95) of pts have AR	N/A

N/A not applicable

[a] Estimated

about AR, treatments used, satisfaction with treatment, degree of limitation from AR in everyday life (1–10 scale as for GP survey), beliefs on links with other pathologies, chief concerns relating to AR, and expectations of future treatment.

Statistical analysis

Statistical analysis of responses was descriptive only, and presented as mean, standard deviation, median and range.

Results

Tables showing detailed summary statistics for the responses from each group (GPs, pharmacists and patients) are available in Additional file 2.

Participant characteristics

Participant characteristics are summarised in Table 1. GPs were predominantly male and of older age, with only 10 % of respondents aged ≤50 years. Of the pharmacists, 73 % were aged ≥50 years. The mean age of patients was 32 years, with participants approximately equally split between age categories (≤20, 21–30, 31–40, over 40). The majority were office workers, students or unemployed.

Associated burden of AR

The average rating for limitation from AR on daily life given by GPs was 6.2 out of a maximum of 10, but 50 % gave a rating of 7 or 8 and 4 % a rating of 9 or 10. The average rating of limitation among patients themselves was slightly lower, at 5.7, but 30 % gave a rating of 7 or 8 and 15 % a rating of 9 or 10. When GPs were asked to rate the severity of AR in their last patient seen (on a scale of 1–10 where 1 = not at all severe and 10 = extremely severe), the average rating was 6.03 and 38 % gave a rating of 7–8, indicating that on average the last patient seen had moderate-to-severe AR.

When asked to choose which of three options was their main concern for the future with respect to AR, 61 % of patients chose 'my health getting worse', 28 % chose 'limitations on my everyday life', and 7 % chose 'cost of treatment' (5 % did not record a choice). This indicates that AR is a source of anxiety or concern for many patients. Fifty-nine per cent thought that AR could lead to the onset of other diseases, most notably asthma, which was mentioned by 81 % of patients who thought other diseases could develop.

Diagnosis and symptoms

In Italy, AR appears to be diagnosed and managed mainly by GPs (in those patients who are under medical care). On average GPs estimated that they made the diagnosis personally in 68 % of cases, referred 17 % to another doctor [of whom 54 % were referred to an allergist and 39 % to an ear, nose and throat (ENT) specialist], and referred 15 % to a specialist allergy centre. Most GPs said that some patients prefer not to go a specialist centre, mainly for reasons of convenience, trust in the GP or the desire for immediate diagnosis and treatment. Of the patients surveyed, 79 % said a specialist had made the diagnosis, which was not unexpected given that participating patients were all under the care of specialist centres. Only 30 % had independently sought information on AR before diagnosis. General practitioners and internet sites were the most frequent sources of such information.

When making the diagnosis of AR, 18 % of GPs said they did not use diagnostic tests. Those who did use tests were most likely to use total serum IgE (paper radioimmunosorbent test; PRIST), specific serum IgE measurement (radioallergosorbent test: RAST) or skin prick tests; usage of other tests was negligible.

The symptoms most frequently taken into account by GPs when diagnosing AR were nasal secretion, fits of sneezing and nasal obstruction. Ocular symptoms were given substantially less significance in the diagnosis (Table 2). In contrast, tearing of the eyes was considered by pharmacists as the chief symptom that made them suspect AR, followed by the aforementioned nasal

Table 2 Symptoms considered by GPs and pharmacists when diagnosing AR, and symptoms first experienced by patients

Symptom	% citing as chief symptom		Total number of mentions		Symptoms at 1st emergence of AR (% citing)
	GPs	Pharmacists	GPs	Pharmacists	Patients
Nasal symptoms					
Nasal secretion	28	12	64	35	68
Fits of sneezing	28	24	57	41	73
Nasal obstruction	22	19	49	38	63
Itchy nose	7	9	36	29	56
Rhinorrhoea	1	5	7	8	–
Ocular symptoms					
Tearing	8	19	42	54	55
Redness of eyes	–	9	20	29	49
Conjunctivitis	–		4	–	–
Other symptoms					
Cough	1		7	3	25
Itchy palate	–	2	8	11	33
Headache	–		3		–
Respiratory problems	–	1	–	4	–
Other	2		2	4	4

symptoms. They also cited tearing of the eyes as the most frequent symptom seen in the AR patients who consulted them. The same nasal symptoms mentioned by GPs were also most frequently mentioned by patients when asked which symptoms of AR they first experienced. Patients mentioned ocular symptoms less frequently than nasal symptoms.

Asthma was by far the most likely comorbidity to be taken into account by GPs when diagnosing AR. Of pharmacists, 8 out of 10 believed that AR is associated with underlying inflammation, and three-quarters believed that AR can cause asthma if not treated in a timely manner.

Treatment decision-making

The GPs estimated that for 69 % of their patients they decided on the treatment themselves, while a specialist decided the treatment for 20 % and an allergy centre for 11 %. The average duration of a consultation in which a treatment was formulated for the first time was 16 min, while consultation times for patients whose treatment was already formulated were reduced to 9 min on average. In consultations involving new treatments, an average of 38 % of the time was spent framing the pathology, 23 % was spent detailing the administration method, 21 % giving reasons for proper treatment compliance, and 18 % educating the patient about any risk linked to comorbidity.

Of the patients, just over half had their current treatment prescribed by a specialist (again, to be expected given the population surveyed) and a third were using treatment prescribed by a GP. Only 4 % had their treatment recommended by a pharmacist and 4 % had chosen their own. However, pharmacists appear to play an important role in treatment decisions in the wider patient population: pharmacist respondents estimated that a third of patients they saw asked the pharmacist for a treatment recommendation. A quarter asked for a specific treatment without a prescription, and 40 % presented a doctor's prescription.

Treatment patterns

Almost half of GPs (49 %) and the great majority of pharmacists (87 %) were unaware of the ARIA guidelines (Fig. 1). Of all treatments prescribed by GPs, 57 % were oral medications and 46 % nasal medications. About half were ongoing treatments and half were for use as needed. When asked which three products they prescribed most frequently for AR, GPs mentioned branded mometasone furoate most frequently, followed by desloratadine, ebastine and generic mometasone (Fig. 2). Antihistamines were mentioned more frequently than intranasal steroids (INSs). Twenty-one percent of GPs said they sometimes prescribed homeopathic products.

For the 'last patient' case, which had moderate-to-severe AR on average, 37 % of GPs reported prescribing antihistamine alone and 27 % prescribed two products, most commonly an antihistamine and an INS (Fig. 3). For 'last patient' cases who were already on treatment, GPs reported that in 78 % of cases they did not change the

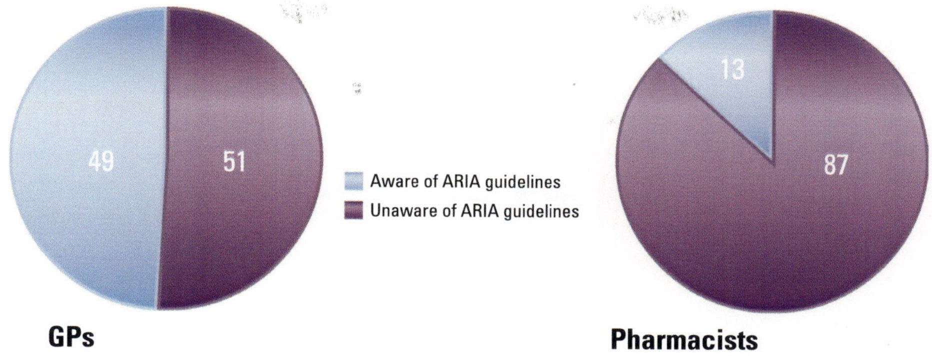

Fig. 1 Awareness of the ARIA guidelines among GPs and pharmacists

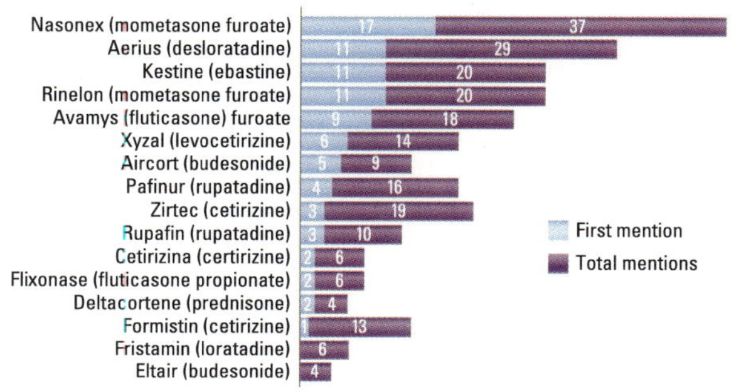

Fig. 2 Most frequent prescribing by GPs (% mentioning product in their 3 most frequently prescribed treatments). 'First mention' denotes percentage who mentioned it as the product they most frequently prescribe; 'other mentions' denotes percentage mentioning the product as being one of the three they prescribe most frequently

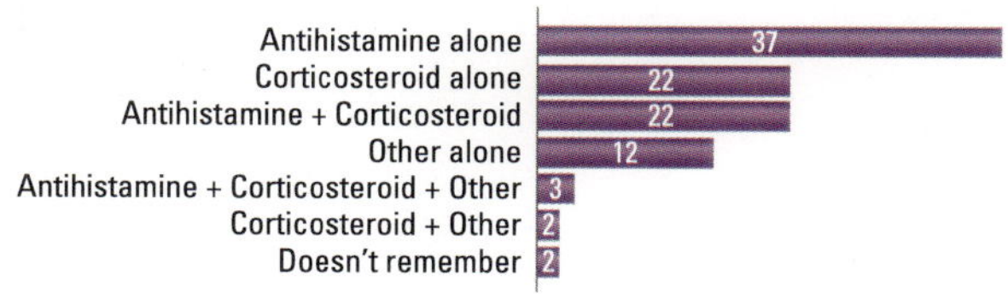

Fig. 3 Prescribing by GPs for last AR patient seen (% prescribing product)

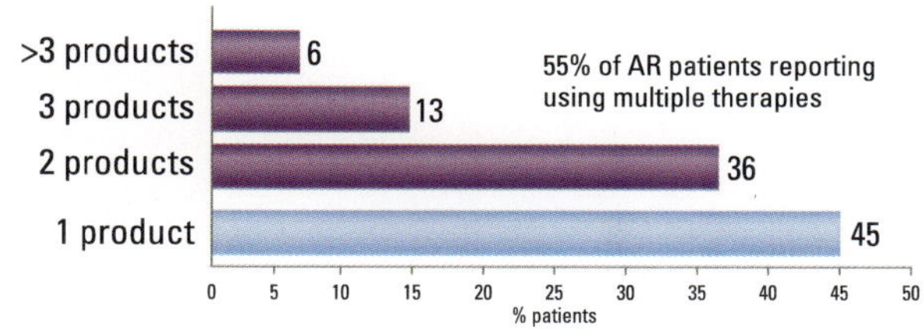

Fig. 4 Proportion of patients using multiple therapies

prescription, which was an antihistamine in the majority of cases.

The pharmacist and patient surveys provided additional perspectives on treatment patterns. Pharmacists reported recommending an antihistamine for most cases (56 %) who asked for a recommendation, followed by a vasoconstrictor (21 %), homeopathic therapy (12 %) or an intranasal/oral corticosteroid (12 %). They estimated that 55 % of doctors' prescriptions they dealt with were for antihistamines, 37 % for intranasal or oral corticosteroids, and 15 % for vasoconstrictors. Half of independent requests by patients were estimated to be for antihistamines, and a quarter each for INS and vasoconstrictors. These trends were broadly reflected in the 'last patient' case responses (data not shown).

When patients were asked what products they currently used to control their AR, 69 % said they used an antihistamine and 25 % an INS, which was in agreement with the GP and pharmacist surveys. However, only 4 % used vasoconstrictors and 3 % homeopathy. Nine per cent used other remedies and 17 % were not using any treatment. A quarter said they would consider using homeopathy. On average, patients were using 1.7 products, and 55 % reported using multiple therapies (Fig. 4). The most common combination was an antihistamine and an INS.

Satisfaction with treatment

Just over 40 % of patients were either not satisfied or weakly satisfied with their current treatment (satisfaction rating of $\leq$6 out of 10), with an average rating of 6.47 (Fig. 5). Satisfaction with the way healthcare professionals had managed their AR to date was somewhat higher (average rating 7.25). Patients' main expectation for the future was to succeed in managing or easing their AR symptoms (45 %), while 22 % hoped for a definitive cure.

Discussion

This survey details for the first time the practices of GPs and pharmacists in relation to diagnosis and treatment of

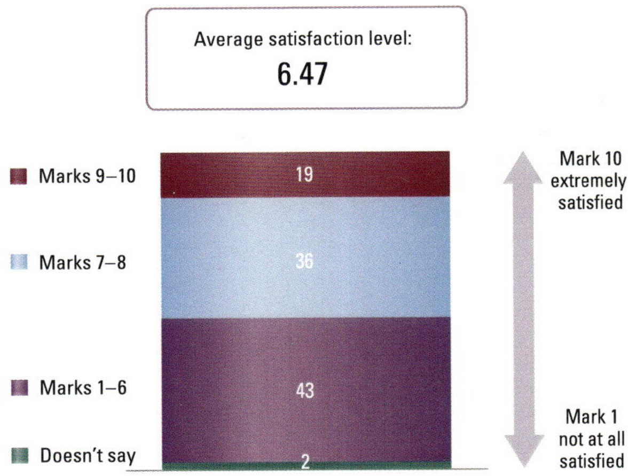

Fig. 5 Patient satisfaction with current AR treatment

AR in Italy. It also gives significant insight into patients' behaviours and attitudes to this prevalent condition and its treatment.

Allergic rhinitis is on the increase [21] and becoming ever more challenging to treat so it is more important than ever that HCPs have the most up-to-date evidence on the best treatments. The ARIA guidelines [7] set out evidence-based standards of best practice for diagnosis and treatment of AR. However, the current survey suggested that only half of GPs in Italy are aware of these guidelines, despite seeing an average of 46 AR patients a month. Awareness is even lower among community pharmacists, at just 13 %, even though participating pharmacists estimated that 20 % of their clients had AR. There are specific ARIA guidelines for pharmacists detailing all aspects of AR diagnosis and treatment, with advice given on when referral to a physician is appropriate [22]. Clearly, more needs to be done to make HCPs aware of the guidelines for diagnosing and treating this extremely common condition.

Allergic Rhinitis and its Impact on Asthma recommends that patients who present with two or more symptoms of AR (rhinorrhoea, sneezing, nasal obstruction/pruritus ± conjunctivitis) for >1 h a day, and who have a positive allergen test, should be referred to a specialist for diagnosis and disease classification (e.g. intermittent, persistent, non-allergic) [6, 23]. However, the survey showed that in Italy it is GPs, not allergy specialists, who are making the majority of AR diagnoses and formulating the treatment plan, either when the patient presents directly or is referred by a pharmacist. Only a third of patients presenting to GPs with possible AR were referred to specialist doctor or allergy centres. One reason for this referral deficit is that some patients prefer the convenience and immediacy of diagnosis and treatment by their GP and do not wish to visit a specialist.

With regard to treatment, the ARIA algorithm recommends a step-up, step-down approach depending on whether the symptoms are intermittent or persistent. Antihistamines and leukotriene-receptor antagonists (LTRA) are recommended as first-line for patients with mild symptoms, while INSs are considered first-line for patients with moderate-to-severe AR [7, 23]. This survey revealed a significant mismatch between treatment patterns among Italian GPs and pharmacists and the ARIA recommendations. GPs perceived that the average patient presenting to them had moderate-to-severe AR, yet the most frequently prescribed AR treatment was an antihistamine alone, which is not concordant with the ARIA guidelines. Judging by the fact that 69 % of patients reported using an antihistamine and 25 % an INS, and just over half said their treatment had been prescribed by a specialist, there also appears to be some deviation from the ARIA guidelines among specialists, although the prescribing patterns of specialists were not surveyed directly, and neither was the AR severity of the patients. There was also a reluctance by GPs to change AR treatment even if the patient had moderate-to-severe symptoms remaining. This may reflect the fact that oral antihistamines are reimbursed for chronic AR throughout Italy, whereas only one region (Tuscany) currently reimburses nasal corticosteroids. Nasal antihistamines are not reimbursed so are not widely used in Italy. Pharmacists too recommended antihistamines most frequently, although this may reflect a milder degree of symptoms in those patients seeking treatment without a doctor's prescription. There was also some confusion among pharmacists about the principal symptoms of AR. Eye watering was cited above nasal symptoms as the main symptom leading to suspicion of AR, even though it is not classified as a major indicator of AR in the guidelines. Pharmacists reported that they referred just under half of patients to a doctor.

Despite reporting satisfaction with the management of their AR by doctors and pharmacists, patients in Italy are less happy with AR treatments. The average satisfaction rating was reported as 6.4 out of 10, with 43 % of patients reporting a rating of 6 or below. One reason for the low satisfaction may be the knowledge base from which GPs and pharmacists are working, and therefore prescribing. However, AR is known to be a difficult condition to treat. It is likely that patients' dissatisfaction also stems from the therapeutic deficits of commonly prescribed therapies; participating patients were using an average of 1.7 therapies and 55 % of patients were on more than one treatment. Adding an oral antihistamine or LTRA to an INS is neither officially recommended by the guidelines [7] nor is it supported by the scientific evidence [24, 25].

Patients have a significant impact on their own AR management. Many AR medications are over the counter and patients frequently self-diagnose. Pharmacists reported that 1 in 4 patients asked for a specific treatment, and that it was most often an antihistamine. Patients also decide whether or not to adhere to prescribed medication. Perhaps surprisingly, GPs and pharmacists on average perceived a slightly greater degree of limitation to daily life from AR symptoms than was reported by patients themselves, even though the patients recruited were under the care of specialist centres. This suggests that failure by HCPs to take AR seriously is not a major issue in Italy. However, 15 % of patients gave a limitation rating of 9 or 10, showing that for a minority of sufferers AR imposes a very severe limitation on everyday activities.

What can be done to improve the management of AR in Italy and elsewhere? It is clear that a greater awareness of formal guidelines for treatment would be beneficial for all parties. It would enable GPs to assess disease severity with greater accuracy and to prescribe the most effective treatment options for individual patients. For pharmacists, it is important to be able to accurately recognise AR and assess its severity, and make a guideline-informed treatment recommendation, whether it is medication or referral to a physician.

To close the gap between current practices and the most up-to-date evidence-based treatment strategies, allergy societies and guidelines need to adapt to the reality that AR is diagnosed and managed by generalist physicians in the majority of cases. Assessment of AR needs to be standardised and simplified, for example by using a visual analogue scale (VAS). This would likely lead to improved prescribing for moderate-to-severe disease. Patients on multiple therapies and those whose symptoms are insufficiently controlled on INS or intranasal antihistamine monotherapy could benefit from increased awareness of new and more effective AR treatments, which could potentially increase treatment satisfaction through improved convenience and more efficient drug delivery [26]. For example, an advanced intranasal delivery system of azelastine hydrochloride and fluticasone propionate (Dymista®, Meda, Solna, Sweden) is now available in Italy which is twice as effective as an INS and provides rapid symptom control in real-life [27–31]. Improved communication between HCPs and patients regarding degree of symptom control is also needed, so that GPs can more easily recognise dissatisfaction with treatment and are encouraged to change a patients' treatment if it is not providing adequate control. Progress is being made in this direction: for example, ARIA in collaboration with MACVIA-LR (a reference site of the European Innovation Partnership on Active and Health Aging) is currently developing a digital VAS-based app for patients to document AR symptom control on therapy [32]. Companion apps for pharmacists and GPs are also planned with the aim of introducing a common language of AR control for all stakeholders and ultimately improving inter-discipline and patient communication and the way AR is assessed and treated.

Conclusion

Allergic rhinitis is largely managed by GPs in Italy. Pharmacists are also important, acting as gatekeepers to treatment. Awareness of the ARIA guidelines among GPs and pharmacists is low, and treatment is not always in accordance with evidence-based best practice. Patient satisfaction with treatment is moderate or low. Allergy education programs need to be targeted at GPs and pharmacists, and communication with patients regarding symptom control needs to be improved.

Abbreviations

AR: allergic rhinitis; ARIA: Allergic Rhinitis and its Impact on Asthma; ENT: ear, nose and throat; GP: general practitioner; HCP: healthcare provider; INS: intranasal steroid; OTC: over the counter; PRIST: paper radioimmunosorbent test; RAST: radioallergosorbent test; VAS: visual analogue scale.

Authors' contributions

GWC, MT, GS: study design, analysis of data, manuscript reviewing. All authors read and approved the final manuscript.

Author details

[1] Respiratory and Allergy Clinic, DIMI-Department of Internal Medicine, University of Genoa, IRCCS Aou San Martino, Largo Rosanna Benzi 10, 16132 Genoa, Italy. [2] Division of Allergy and Clinical Immunology, University of Salerno, Salerno, Italy. [3] Allergy Unit, University Hospital Verona, Verona, Italy.

Acknowledgements

The study was partially supported by Meda pharma. Medical writing assistance was provided by Dr Ruth B Murray and Ms Jo Whelan (Medscript Ltd). The survey was conducted and analysed by Doxa (Italy).

Competing interests

G Walter Canonica: Research Grant, Consultanion fee, Speaker fee: A.Menarini, Alk-Abello', Allergy Therapeutics, Anallergo, AstraZeneca, Boeringher Ingelheim, Boston Scientific, Chiesi, Circassia, Faes, Glaxo Smith Kline, Lofarma, Malesci, Meda Pharma, Mundifarma, Novartis, Pfizer, Roche, Sanofi, Stallergenes, Thermo Fisher, Uriach, Teva, Valeas. Massimo Triggiani: Research grant from Shire, CSL Behring; Consultation fees: Novartis, Meda Pharma, Rottapharm. GianEnrico Senna: Consultanion fee, Speaker fee: A.Menarini, Alk-Abello', Glaxo SmithKline, Malesci, Meda Pharma, Novartis, Stallergenes.

References

1. Lamb CE, Ratner PH, Johnson CE, Ambegaonkar AJ, Joshi AV, Day D, et al. Economic impact of workplace productivity losses due to allergic rhinitis compared with select medical conditions in the United States from an employer perspective. Curr Med Res Opin. 2006;22(6):1203–10.
2. Zanolin ME, Pattaro C, Corsico A, Bugiani M, Carrozzi L, Casali L, et al. The role of climate on the geographic variability of asthma, allergic rhinitis and respiratory symptoms: results from the Italian study of asthma in young adults. Allergy. 2004;59(3):306–14.
3. Bugiani M, Carosso A, Migliore E, Piccioni P, Corsico A, Olivieri M, et al. Allergic rhinitis and asthma comorbidity in a survey of young adults in Italy. Allergy. 2005;60(2):165–70.
4. Italian National Institute of Statistics. 2011. Accessed Mar 2015.
5. Vuurman EF, Vuurman LL, Lutgens I, Kremer B. Allergic rhinitis is a risk factor for traffic safety. Allergy. 2014;69(7):906–12.
6. Bousquet J, Khaltaev N, Cruz AA, Denburg J, Fokkens WJ, Togias A, et al. Allergic Rhinitis and its Impact on Asthma (ARIA) 2008 update (in collaboration with the World Health Organization, GA(2)LEN and AllerGen). Allergy. 2008;63(Suppl 86):8–160.
7. Brozek JL, Bousquet J, Baena-Cagnani CE, Bonini S, Canonica GW, Casale TB, et al. Allergic Rhinitis and its Impact on Asthma (ARIA) guidelines: 2010 revision. J Allergy Clin Immunol. 2010;126(3):466–76.
8. Demoly P, Calderon MA, Casale T, Scadding G, Annesi-Maesano I, Braun JJ, et al. Assessment of disease control in allergic rhinitis. Clin Transl Allergy. 2013;3(1):7.
9. Canonica GW, Bousquet J, Mullol J, Scadding GK, Virchow JC. A survey of the burden of allergic rhinitis in Europe. Allergy. 2007;62(Suppl 85):17–25.
10. Schatz M. A survey of the burden of allergic rhinitis in the USA. Allergy. 2007;62(Suppl 85):9–16.
11. Mosges R, Klimek L. Today's allergic rhinitis patients are different: new factors that may play a role. Allergy. 2007;62(9):969–75.
12. Valovirta E, Myrseth SE, Palkonen S. The voice of the patients: allergic rhinitis is not a trivial disease. Curr Opin Allergy Clin Immunol. 2008;8:1–9.
13. Bousquet PJ, Castelli C, Daures JP, Heinrich J, Hooper R, Sunyer J, et al. Assessment of allergen sensitization in a general population-based survey (European Community Respiratory Health Survey I). Ann Epidemiol. 2010;20(11):797–803.
14. Settipane RA, Lieberman P. Update on nonallergic rhinitis. Ann Allergy Asthma Immunol. 2001;86(5):494–507.
15. Pitman R, Paracha N, Parker C, Acaster S, Bachert C, Bousquet J. Episode pattern and healthcare utilisation in patients with seasonal allergic rhinitis. Allergy. 2012;67(Suppl 96):1–687.
16. Acaster S, Shehzed A, Breheny K, Bachert C, Bousquet J, Price D. Treatment preferences in patients with moderate/severe seasonal allergic rhinitis: findings of a discrete choice experiment. Allergy. 2012;67(Suppl 96):344.
17. Price D, Bousquet J, Pitman D, Lieberman P, Munzel U, Meltzer E. Sub-optimal control of allergic rhinitis: the need for a new and more effective treatment option. Allergy. 2013;68(Suppl 97):1–744.
18. Bousquet PJ, Demoly P, Devillier P, Mesbah K, Bousquet J. Impact of allergic rhinitis symptoms on quality of life in primary care. Int Arch Allergy Immunol. 2013;160(4):393–400.
19. Zicari AM, Indinnimeo L, De Castro G, Incorvaia C, Frati F, Dell'Albani I, et al. A survey on features of allergic rhinitis in children. Curr Med Res Opin. 2013;29(5):415–20.
20. Canonica GW, Mullol J, Pradalier A, Didier A. Patient perceptions of allergic rhinitis and quality of life: findings from a survey conducted in Europe and the United States. World Allergy Organ J. 2008;1(9):138–44.
21. de Marco R, Cappa V, Accordini S, Rava M, Antonicelli L, Bortolami O, et al. Trends in the prevalence of asthma and allergic rhinitis in Italy between 1991 and 2010. Eur Respir J. 2012;39(4):883–92.
22. MotA Workshops. ARIA in the pharmacy: management of allergic rhinitis symptoms in the pharmacy. Allergic rhinitis and its impact on asthma. Allergy. 2004;59(4):373–87.
23. Bousquet J, Reid J, van Weel C, Baena Cagnani C, Canonica GW, Demoly P, et al. Allergic rhinitis management pocket reference 2008. Allergy. 2008;63(8):990–6.
24. Anolik R. Clinical benefits of combination treatment with mometasone furoate nasal spray and loratadine vs monotherapy with mometasone furoate in the treatment of seasonal allergic rhinitis. Ann Allergy Asthma Immunol. 2008;100(3):264–71.
25. Esteitie R, deTineo M, Naclerio RM, Baroody FM. Effect of the addition of montelukast to fluticasone propionate for the treatment of perennial allergic rhinitis. Ann Allergy Asthma Immunol. 2010;105(2):155–61.
26. Derendorf H, Munzel U, Petzold U, Maus J, Mascher H, Hermann R, et al. Bioavailability and disposition of azelastine and fluticasone propionate when delivered by MP29-02, a novel aqueous nasal spray. Br J Clin Pharmacol. 2012;74(1):125–33.
27. Dymista® Nasal Spray Summary of Product Characteristics. Last updated on eMC 13-Jan-2015. http://www.medicines.org.uk/emc/medicine/27579. 2015. Accessed 3 Aug 2015.
28. Meltzer E, Ratner P, Bachert C, Carr W, Berger W, Canonica GW, et al. Clinically relevant effect of a new intranasal therapy (MP29-02) in allergic rhinitis assessed by responder analysis. Int Arch Allergy Immunol. 2013;161(4):369–77.
29. Carr W, Bernstein J, Lieberman P, Meltzer E, Bachert C, Price D, et al. A novel intranasal therapy of azelastine with fluticasone for the treatment of allergic rhinitis. J Allergy Clin Immunol. 2012;129(5):1282–9.
30. Price D, Shah S, Bhatia S, Bachert C, Berger W, Bousquet J, et al. A new therapy (MP29-02) is effective for the long-term treatment of chronic rhinitis. J Investig Allergol Clin Immunol. 2013;23(7):495–503.
31. Klimek L, Grevers G. Pharmacotherapy and diagnosis of allergic rhinitis. MMW Fortschritte der Medizin. 2014;156(4):48–52.
32. Bousquet J, Bachert C, Price D, Acaster S, Demoly P. Assessing allergic rhinitis symptom control using a simple visual analogue scale: the digital solution (MACVIA-ARIA). Allergy. 2014;69(Suppl 99):1–646.

2

Asthma management among allergists in Italy: results from a survey

M. S. Magnoni[1*], M. Caminati[2], G. W. Canonica[3], F. Arpinelli[1], A. Rizzi[1] and G. Senna[2]

Abstract

Background: In Europe more than 50% of asthmatic treated patients have not well-controlled asthma. Asthma affects about 2.5 million of patients in Italy.

Aims and objectives: The present survey aims at investigating how Italian allergists approach asthmatic patients, in order to highlight pitfalls and unmet needs concerning real-life asthma management.

Methods: An anonymous 16 item web questionnaire was available (April–October 2015) to all allergists who visited the web site of SIAAIC (Società Italiana di Allergologia, Asma Immunologia Clinica). Those who wished to give their contribution had the opportunity to answer about epidemiology, risk factors, treatment approaches, and adherence to therapy.

Results: One hundred and seventy four allergists answered the survey. 54% of them reported up to 10 patient visits per week and 35.3% between 10 and 30. The most frequent reasons of follow up visits are routine check-up (56.5% of allergists). and worsening of symptoms (41% of allergists). Nocturnal apnoeas, gastro-esophageal reflux and obesity are the most important comorbidities/risk factors of poorly controlled asthma. Bronchial hyper-responsiveness, increased NO levels and reduced exercise tolerance are the most important indicators of asthma severity. Concerning therapy, ICS combined with LABA is the treatment of choice suitable for the majority of patients. A rapid onset of action and a flexible ICS dosage are indicated as the optimal characteristics for achieving the therapeutic goals. Poor adherence to therapy is an important reason for symptom worsening for the majority of allergists. Complex dosage regimens and economic aspects are considered the most important factors impacting on adherence.

Conclusions: Allergists are involved in the management of asthma, regularly seeing their patients. Co-morbidities are frequent in asthmatic patients and may impact negatively on disease control, thus identifying patients who need a more careful and strict monitoring. Airway hyper-responsiveness to methacholine challenge test and nitric oxide are considered important indicators of asthma severity. The combination of LABA and inhaled steroids is considered the treatment of choice for most asthmatic patients, in keeping with broad evidence indicating that the combination therapy is more effective and rapid in gaining asthma control than inhaled corticosteroids alone. Adherence to medication regimens is considered of essence to achieve the therapeutic goals.

Keywords: Asthma, Online survey, Follow-up and monitoring tools, Treatment, Adherence

Background

Asthma is one of the most prevalent chronic conditions, affecting approximately 300 million people worldwide [1]. In developed countries its prevalence is estimated to be between 4 and 12% in adults and 10–15% in children [2]. In Italy the overall estimate is 5% [3], corresponding to around 2.5 million patients.

Asthma cannot be cured, but appropriate management can control the disorder and enable people to enjoy a good quality of life. However, despite the advances in therapeutic approaches and the dissemination of guidelines [4], observational studies have shown that in Europe more than 50% of treated patients report not well-controlled asthma [5], causing substantial

*Correspondence: maria-sandra.s.magnoni@gsk.com
[1] Medical and Scientific Department, GlaxoSmithKline, Verona, Italy
Full list of author information is available at the end of the article

limitations in daily life, in terms of reduced productivity at work or school and frequent inability to perform normal activities.

The cornerstone of asthma management is to achieve and maintain the control of the disease [4] and several specialists, including allergists, should contribute to this goal. The present survey aims at investigating how Italian allergists approach patients with asthma, in order to point out pitfalls and unmet needs concerning real-life management of the disease.

Methods

A board of experts belonging to Società Italiana di Allergologia, Asma Immunologia Clinica (SIAAIC) developed a questionnaire composed of 16 multiple choice questions covering epidemiological (number of patients assisted) and clinical (presence of co-morbidities or risk factors) aspects about asthma, and exploring the overall management strategies (follow up, treatments, adherence) adopted by the Italian allergists (see Additional file 1: Appendix S1).

All the SIAAIC members were invited to complete the survey through an email invitation letter. Between April and October 2015 the questionnaire was available to all allergists who visited the web site of SIAAIC. The questionnaire was anonymous. All the data and answers entered into the system were checked for consistency and completeness and each respondent could only complete the questionnaire once.

In this paper we report a descriptive analysis of the data.

Results

A total of 174 questionnaires have been analyzed; this sample represents 25% of SIAAIC Allergists (SIAAIC is the scientific society that collects the highest number of Italian allergists).

Number of visits

Ninety allergists (54%) reported to see up to 10 asthma patients per week and 60 (35.3%) between 10 and 30 patients (Fig. 1). During the pollen season, the number of visits increased for 87 allergists (51%), whereas for 43 (25%) it remained constant over the year (Fig. 2).

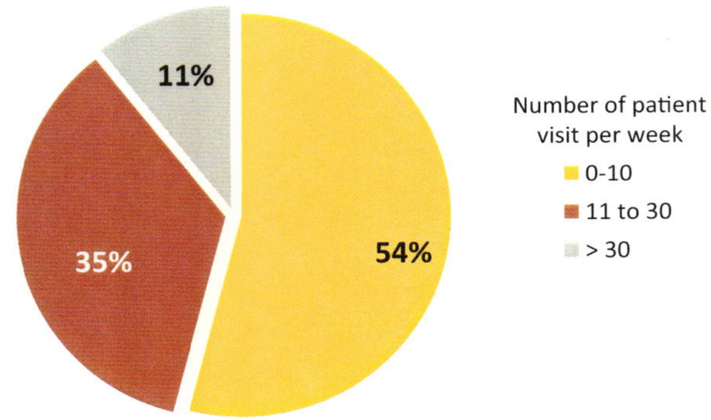

Fig. 1 Percentage of allergists according to the number of patient visits per week

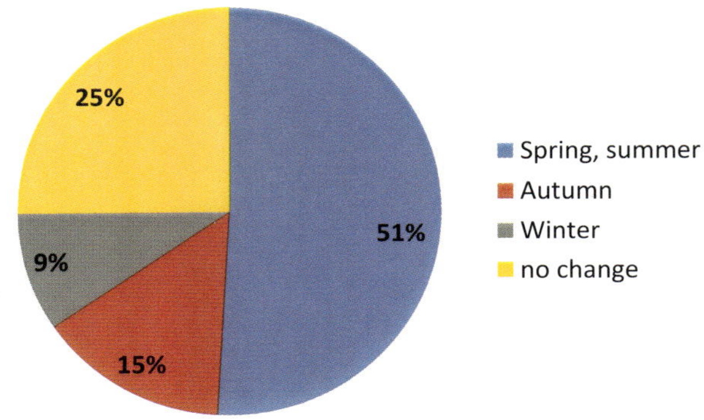

Fig. 2 Percentage of allergists reporting the period of the year with increased number of patients with respiratory symptoms

Follow-up and risk factors for poorly controlled asthma

The most frequent reasons of follow up visits were routine checkup for 91 allergists (56.5%), and worsening of symptoms for 66 allergists (41%), whereas the percentage of visits due to drug adverse effects was negligible (3%).

Around 70% of allergists declared to assess their patients regularly with scheduled follow up visits: 25–50% of patients according to 54 allergists (35.5%) and >50–75% of patients according to 50 allergists (33.8%).

For the assessment of patient's condition in the follow up, airway hyper-responsiveness by methacholine challenge testing was considered the most important indicator, followed by nitric oxide (NO) levels and home PEF monitoring (Fig. 3a). Accordingly, airway hyper-responsiveness and NO levels were also rated as the most important indicators of asthma severity, together with exercise tolerance and lung volumes (residual volume, inspiratory capacity), whereas severe exacerbations had the lowest rate (Fig. 3b).

Nocturnal apneas and obesity were rated as the most important co-morbidities/risk factors of poorly controlled asthma, followed by gastro-esophageal reflux and smoking habits and lastly by rhinitis and rhino-sinusitis (Fig. 4).

Treatment and adherence

Concerning therapy, regular use of inhaled corticosteroids (ICS) combined with long acting beta agonists (LABA) was considered the treatment of choice suitable for the majority of patients (Fig. 5). A rapid onset of action and a good safety profile were rated as most important

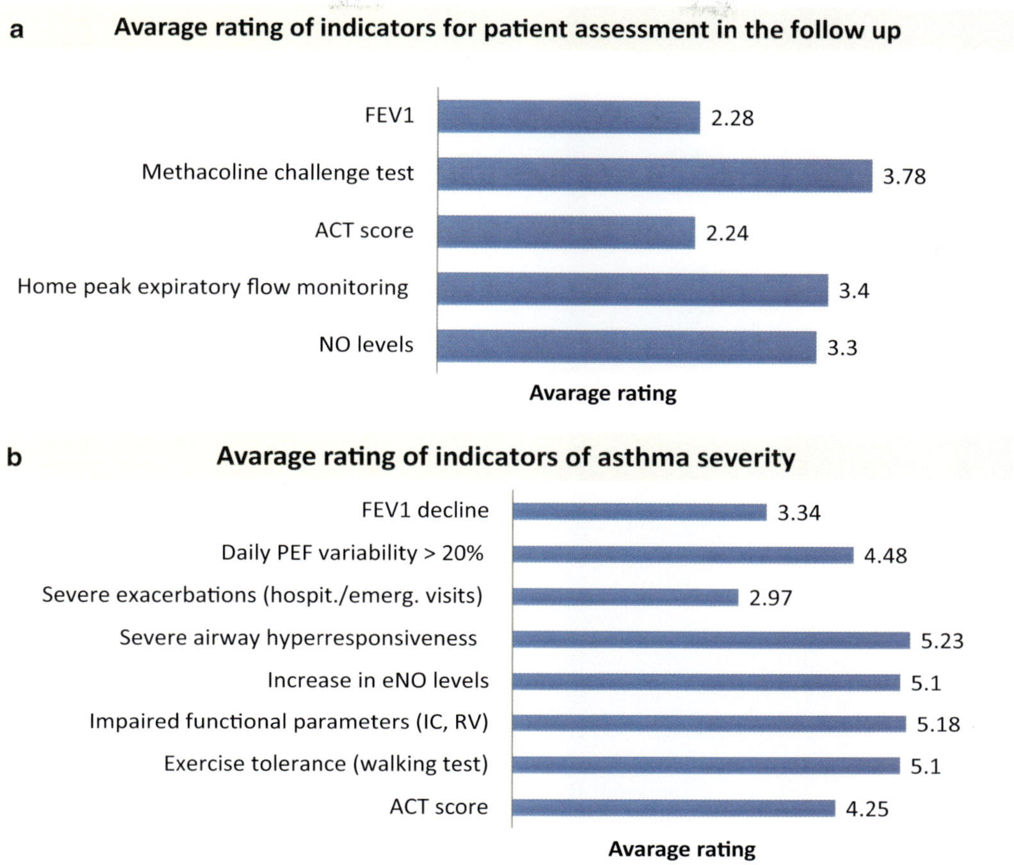

Fig. 3 Avarage rating of indicators (in order of importance) for the assessment of asthmatic patients during the follow up (**a**) and for staging of asthma severity (**b**)

therapeutic goals than the prevention of exacerbations and rescue medication use (Fig. 6). A flexible ICS dosage and a rapid onset of action were indicated as optimal characteristics for achieving the therapeutic goals (Fig. 7).

Poor adherence to therapy was considered an important cause of symptom worsening for the majority of allergists, and 37% of them (n. 56) believed that it was the prevalent cause. Notably, complex dosing regimens and cost of therapy were rated as the most important factors impacting on adherence (Fig. 8a).

As regards the inhaler, consistency of the released dose and low number of critical errors were considered the most important characteristics impacting on adherence (Fig. 8b).

Discussion

Allergists are involved in the management of asthma, seeing their patients more frequently, but not exclusively, in the pollen season. Interestingly, they rely on airway hyper-responsiveness and inflammation for classification of asthma severity and monitoring of asthma control during follow-up visits, as indicated by the high rate attributed to methacholine challenge testing and NO levels. Indeed, the degree of airway hyper-responsiveness and inflammation are usually in proportion to the severity of the underlying asthma and may reflect the response to the treatment [6]. Of note, also changes in lung volumes, indicators of pulmonary hyperinflation, which is responsible for low tolerance to physical efforts, are rated as important markers of asthma severity, whereas severe exacerbations seem to be less relevant. Allergists mostly manage mild to moderate allergic asthma and their patients are regularly followed up in order to prevent exacerbations triggered by allergen exposure. Thus, in comparison with respiratory medicine specialists who usually deal with severe non-allergic refractory asthma, allergists are probably less involved in the management of severe exacerbations. This may account for the low rate attributed to asthma exacerbations as a marker of control.

Consistently with international reports [7–10], allergists are aware that risk factors and co-morbidities may impact on the natural history of asthma, leading to

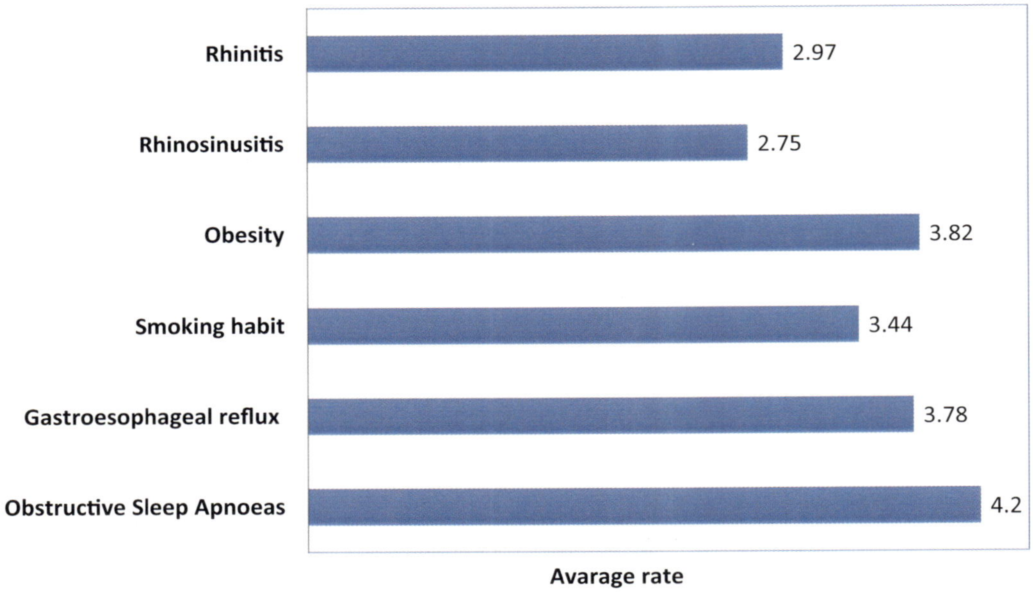

Fig. 4 Avarage rating of co-morbidities/risk factors impacting on asthma control (in order of importance)

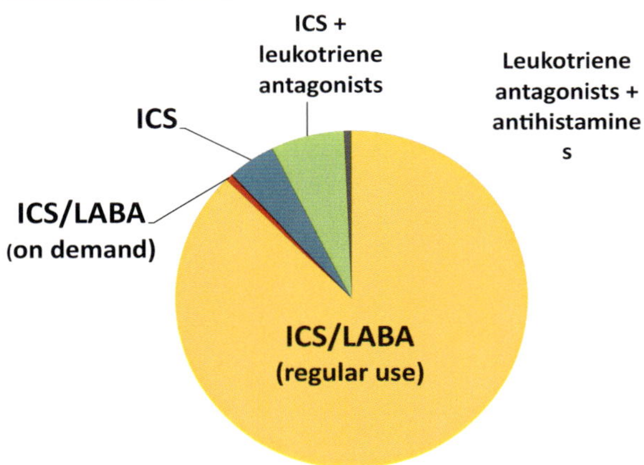

Fig. 5 Asthma treatment according to Italian allergists (% of allergists)

symptoms worsening and reduced treatment efficacy, thus identifying patients who need a more careful and strict monitoring to maintain control. It is intriguing that rhinitis and smoking habits are considered less impactful on asthma control than nocturnal apneas and obesity: possibly, the latters are regarded as risk factors/comorbidities which are more difficult to control or cure.

For allergists the combination of LABA and ICS is the treatment of choice for most asthmatic patients. This is consistent with broad literature evidence indicating that that combination therapy is the most effective strategy in preventing clinical manifestations and gaining rapid asthma control than ICS alone [11]. Furthermore, a flexible ICS dosage is considered a key point in the management of asthma, allowing titration according to the level of clinical manifestation and airway inflammation, which is the dominant process in asthma. On the other hand, a high percentage of allergists rate a rapid onset of action as a more important therapeutic goal than the reduction of exacerbations and the prevention of symptoms and use of rescue medication, which are sensitive markers of poorly controlled asthma according to international guidelines. This was an unexpected finding. Clearly, a rapid onset of action is essential in the management of acute asthma but less critical for chronic therapy. We speculate that this finding could be attributed to the fact that allergists generally manage mild to moderate allergic asthma, mostly characterized by seasonal symptoms, and therapeutic strategies are often tailored accordingly. Under this perspective, a rapid onset of action might be considered as an added value of the treatment.

Like in every chronic disease, adherence to medication regimens is considered of essence to achieve and maintain asthma control [12]. Indeed, there is no doubt that poor adherence to medication regimens represents a significant barrier to optimal management of chronic respiratory diseases, contributing to a substantial worsening of symptoms, reduction in health-related quality of life and increase in healthcare costs [12, 13]. Complex dosing regimens have been rated are rated as major factors impacting on adherence to medication, as suggested by several studies [14, 15]. Indeed, multiple-inhaler use has

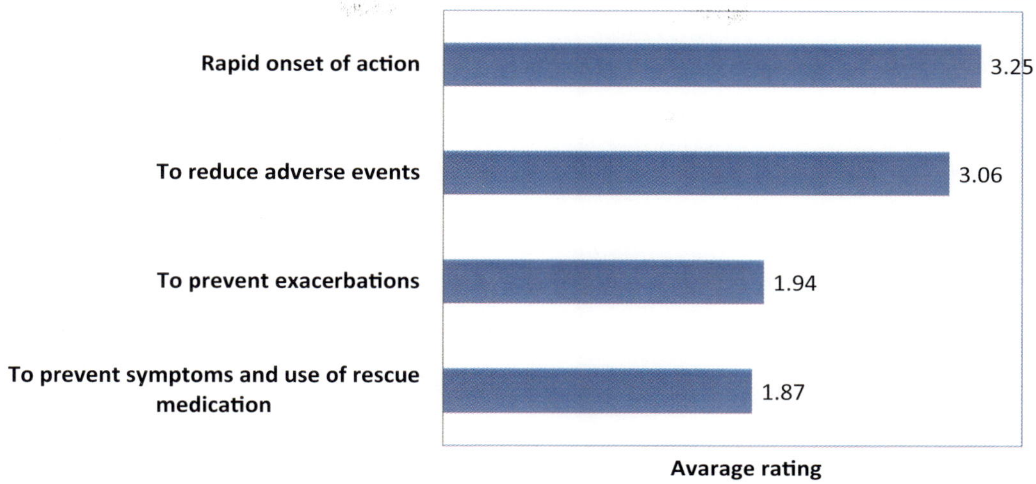

Fig. 6 Main therapeutic goals for the asthmatic patient (in order of importance)

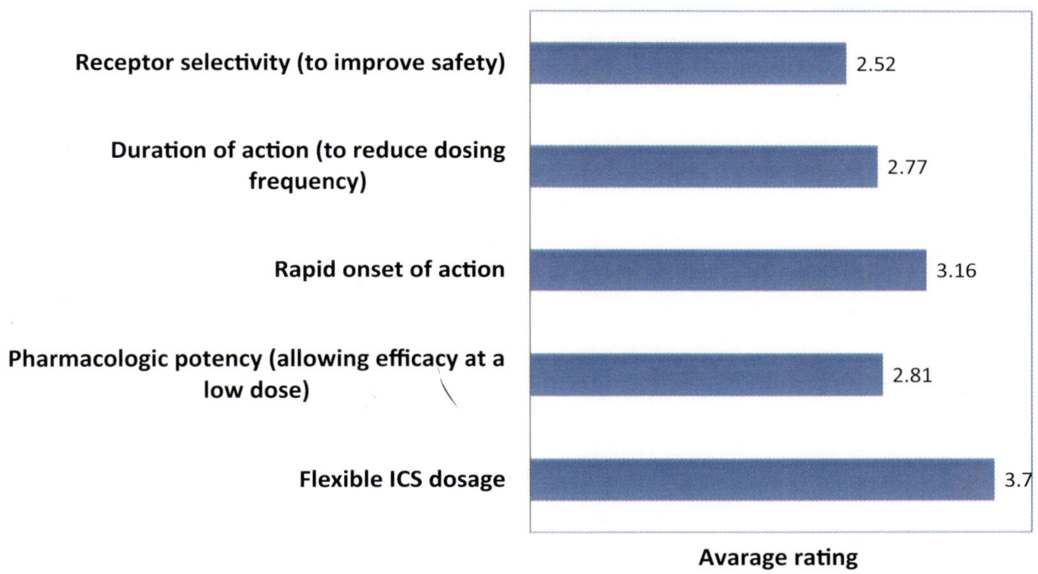

Fig. 7 Optimal drug features to achieve therapeutic goals (in order of importance)

been associated with higher rates of non-adherence than single-inhaler use in both asthma and COPD patients, potentially because of the increased complexity introduced by the additional inhaler(s). Also medication dosing frequency has important effects on adherence: the simplification of medication dosing seems to be the single intervention with the strongest impact on adherence, with once-daily regimes resulting in up to twice as many adherent days as more frequent dosing regimens [16]. Interestingly, also economic aspects have been considered important for adherence, possibly with reference to intranasal steroids for the treatment of comorbid rhinitis. Since only a small proportion of follow up visits was due to drug related side effects, they do not seem to be one of the drivers for poor adherence.

In regards to inhaler preferred features, allergists give high importance to inhaler efficiency in terms of consistency in dose delivery across different flow rates, making the device suitable and reliable also in patients with severe airflow limitation. Another important feature is the low risk of critical errors that impair the delivery of medication to the lung.

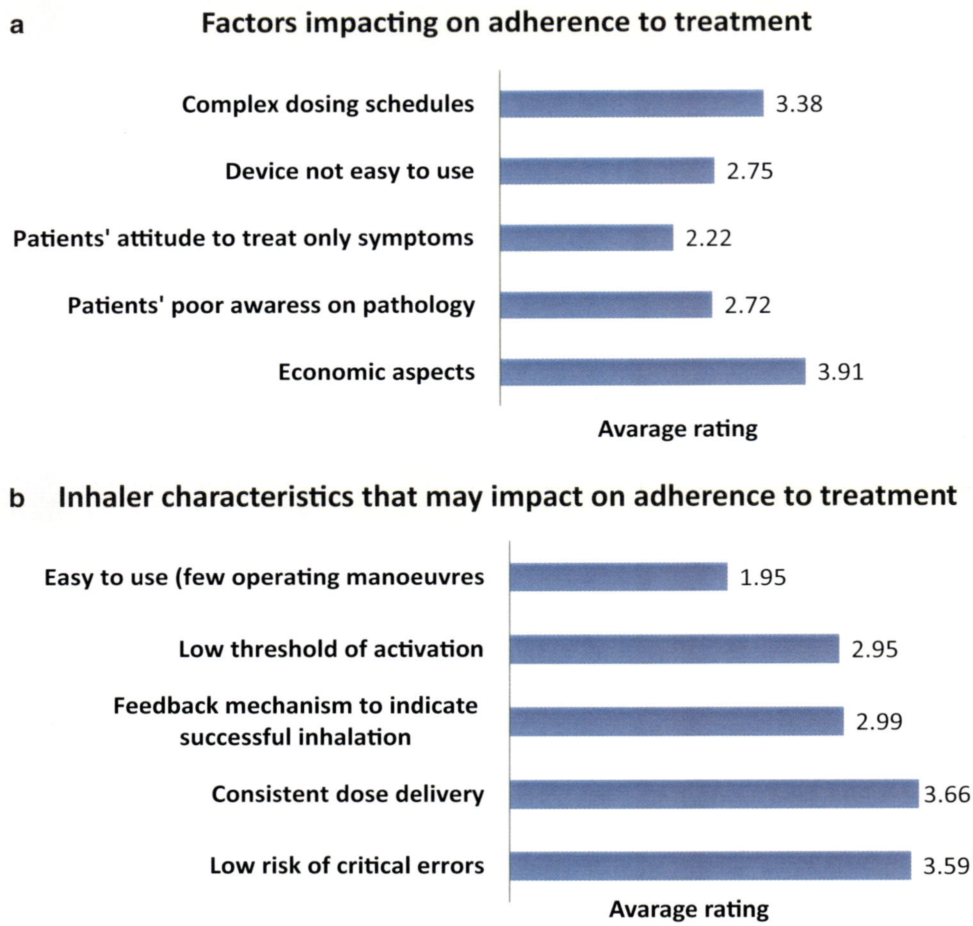

Fig. 8 Factors impacting on adherence (**a**) and inhaler characteristics that may impact on adherence (**b**)

Our survey has some limitations: (1) it has been addressed only to allergists, and we are aware that it would be of interest to compare the responses of different kinds of specialists (pneumologists, general practitioners) on the management of asthma; (2) the questionnaire did not investigate the knowledge of severe asthma, thus information is missing about the management of this kind of patients by allergists; (3) like in all surveys, the responses from physicians may not always correspond to their daily clinical practice, but rather reflect their opinions and insights on optimal disease management.

Conclusions

Allergists are involved in the management of asthma, regularly seeing their patients. Co-morbidities may identify patients who need a more careful and strict monitoring to achieve asthma control. The combination of LABA and inhaled steroids is considered the treatment of choice for most asthmatic patients, in keeping with broad literature evidence indicating that the combination therapy is more effective and rapid in gaining asthma control than inhaled corticosteroids alone. Adherence to medication regimens is considered of essence to achieve the therapeutic goals. Complex dosing regimens and poor inhalation technique may negatively impact on adherence.

Abbreviations

ICS: inhaled corticosteroids; LABA: long acting beta agonists; NO: nitric oxide; SIAAIC: Società Italiana di Allergologia, Asma Immunologia Clinica.

Authors' contributions

The contribution of the authors to the manuscript is as follows: MSM: study design, data analysis, and manuscript preparation; MC: data collection and analysis; GS: study design, data collection and analysis; GWC: data analysis; FA: data analysis; AR: data analysis. All authors read and approved the final manuscript.

Author details
[1] Medical and Scientific Department, GlaxoSmithKline, Verona, Italy. [2] Asthma Center and Allergy Unit, Verona University Hospital, Verona, Italy. [3] Personalized Medicine Asthma & Allergy Clinic, Humanitas University-Research Hospital, Rozzano, Milano, Italy.

Funding
The study was supported by GlaxoSmithKline.

References

1. World Health Organization. Global surveillance, prevention and control of chronic respiratory diseases: a comprehensive approach. Geneva: World Health Organization; 2007.
2. Baiz N, Annesi-Maesano I. Is the asthma epidemic still ascending? Clin Chest Med. 2012;33(3):419–29.
3. ISTAT. Annuario statistico italiano edizione 2015. (http://www.istat.it/it/files/2015/12/ASI_2015_nota-stampa.pdf). Accessed 20 Oct 2016.
4. Global Initiative for Asthma (GINA). Global strategy for asthma management and prevention. http://www.ginasthma.org. Update 2016.
5. Demoly P, Annunziata K, Gubba E, Adamek L. Repeated cross-sectional survey of patient-reported asthma control in Europe in the past 5 years. Eur Respir Rev. 2012;21(123):66–74.
6. Busse WW. The relationship of airway hyperresponsiveness and airway inflammation. Chest. 2010;138(2_Suppl):4S–10S.
7. Boulet LP, Boulay ME. Asthma-related comorbidities. Expert Rev Respir Med. 2011;5(3):377–93.
8. Gershon AS, Guan J, Wang C, Victor JC, To T. Describing and quantifying asthma comorbidity: a population study. PLoS ONE. 2012;7(5):e34967.
9. Braido F, Baiardini I, Menoni S, et al. Patients with asthma and comorbid allergic rhinitis: is optimal quality of life achievable in real life? PLoS ONE. 2012;7(2):e31178.
10. Cazzola M, Calzetta L, Bettoncelli G, et al. Asthma and comorbid medical illness. Eur Respir J. 2011;38(1):42–9.
11. Bateman ED, Boushey HA, Bousquet J, GOAL Investigators Group, et al. Can guideline-defined asthma control be achieved? The Gaining Optimal Asthma ControL study. Am J Respir Crit Care Med. 2004;170(8):836–44.
12. Engelkes M, et al. Medication adherence and the risk of severe asthma exacerbations: a systematic review. Eur Respir J. 2015;45(2):396–407.
13. Castro M, Zimmermann NA, Crocker S, et al. Asthma intervention program prevents readmissions in high healthcare users. Am J Respir Crit Care Med. 2003;168:1095–9.
14. Makela MJ, Backer V, Hedegaard M, Larsson K. Adherence to inhaled therapies, health outcomes and costs in patients with asthma and COPD. Respir Med. 2013;107:1481–90.
15. Yu AP, Guerin A, Ponce de Leon D, Ramakrishnan K, Wu EQ, Mocarski M, et al. Therapy persistence and adherence in patients with chronic obstructive pulmonary disease: multiple versus single long-acting maintenance inhalers. J Med Econ. 2011;14:486e96.
16. Saini SD, Kaulback K, Dubinsky MC. Effect of medication dosing on adherence on chronic disease. Am J Manag Care. 2009;15(6):e22–33.

3

Burden of allergic respiratory disease

A. Linneberg[1,2,3*], K. Dam Petersen[4], J. Hahn-Pedersen[5], E. Hammerby[5], N. Serup-Hansen[5] and N. Boxall[6]

Abstract

This meta-analysis compared the health-related quality of life (HRQL) of patients with allergic rhinitis (AR) and/or allergic asthma (AA) caused by perennial house dust mite (HDM) versus AR and/or AA caused by seasonal pollen allergy. Following a systematic search, the identified studies used the disease-specific rhinitis quality of life questionnaire or generic instruments (SF-36 and SF-12). Summary estimates obtained by meta-analysis showed that HRQL in patients with perennial HDM allergy was significantly worse than that of patients with seasonal pollen allergy, when measured by both disease-specific and generic HRQL instruments, and was reflected by an impact on both physical and mental health. A systematic review of cost data on AR and AA in selected European countries demonstrated that the majority of the economic burden was indirectly caused by high levels of absenteeism and presenteeism; there was little or no evidence of increasing or decreasing cost trends. Increased awareness of the detrimental effects of AR and/or AA on patients' HRQL and its considerable cost burden might encourage early diagnosis and treatment, in order to minimize the disease burden and ensure beneficial and cost-effective outcomes.

Keywords: Allergic rhinitis, Allergic asthma, Economic burden, Meta-analysis, Systematic review, Quality of life

Background

In Europe, approximately 23 % of the population is affected by allergic rhinitis (AR) [1]. The most common symptoms are sneezing, itchy nose, rhinorrhea, and/or nasal congestion [2], with many patients experiencing symptoms of at least moderate severity; one study estimated that 93 % of patients with AR who consulted general practitioners had symptoms that were moderate-to-severe [3]. Studies of patients consulting general practitioners for AR reported that 18–48 % had symptoms that were not controlled by pharmacotherapy [4, 5]. Despite the bothersome nature of symptoms, AR is often trivialized by the patient; less than half (45 %) seek medical advice or treatment for their condition [4], which results in under-treatment and poor control of symptoms. A UK study found that only 18 % of patients with AR had consulted their doctor about the condition in the preceding 2 years [6]. In a sample of 230 French patients with typical symptoms of AR, 19 % had never consulted their doctor about the problem, despite 90 % reporting that their nasal symptoms affected their daily lives, over half complaining of sleepiness and headaches, and 8 % reporting that they had taken time off work because of their rhinitis [7]. Allergic rhinitis is frequently accompanied by allergic asthma (AA), the prevalence of which increases from less than 2 % in individuals without AR to 10–40 % in those with AR; this combination of upper and lower respiratory symptoms increases the overall impact on the patient [8–10].

There is now considerable evidence that the symptoms of AR and AA negatively affect patients' health-related quality of life (HRQL) [11–20]. This is supported by evidence that successful treatment of symptoms with allergy immunotherapy (AIT) [21–23] or symptomatic treatments [24–31] improves the HRQL of patients with AR. These improvements generally mirror those of conventional clinical outcome measures, such as symptom and medication scores, and lung function tests [32]. Although clinical measures provide information on the affected organ systems, they do not capture the patient's overall perception of the disease burden caused by the

*Correspondence: allan.linneberg@regionh.dk
[1] Research Centre for Prevention and Health, The Capital Region of Denmark, Copenhagen, Denmark
Full list of author information is available at the end of the article

physical, emotional, and social impairments in everyday life [33]. The wider impact of AR on patients' lives is now acknowledged in the allergic rhinitis and its impact on asthma (ARIA) guidelines, which recognize the impact of HRQL on AR, and classify its severity based both on symptoms and its effect on HRQL [32].

There is evidence that AR represents a considerable economic burden [34, 35], with annual costs in the US in 2003 estimated at \$2–\$5 billion USD [34]. Indirect costs resulting from symptoms causing under-performance or loss of productivity in the workplace were particularly high [36–39]. Data published after the present study was completed show that patients with mild AR have less impact on the health economy, with costs of around a quarter of those with moderate-to-severe disease [39].

To date, there has been no systematic review of HRQL data in patients with perennial or seasonal allergies. The objective of this systematic review and meta-analysis was, therefore, to compare HRQL in individuals with AR and/or AA with perennial house dust mite (HDM) or seasonal AR caused by exposure to pollen, or both. As HRQL instruments/questionnaires are included in many clinical studies as a matter of course, HRQL measurements enable comparisons with data from individual studies. In addition, data on the economic burden of AR and AA in selected European countries were systematically reviewed in order to compare direct and indirect costs in patients with perennial HDM and seasonal AR.

Methods

Search and identification of studies

To identify published articles on HRQL in individuals with AR and/or AA, and the economic burden of AR and AA, the following online databases were searched: MEDLINE and MEDLINE In-Process (1946–31 January 2014); EMBASE (1988–2014 week 04); EconLit (1886–January 2014); The Cochrane Library (Cochrane Central Register of Controlled Trials and Cochrane Database of Systematic Reviews); Database of Abstracts of Reviews of Effects; National Institute For Health Research Health Technology Assessment Programme databases; Health Economics Evaluation Database; National Guidelines Clearing House; NHS Evidence; EUROScan; and Clinicaltrials.gov.

The search strategies and keywords used are presented in the Additional file 1. The MEDLINE, EMBASE, EconLit, Cochrane Library, Database of Abstracts of Reviews of Effects, and NIH HTA databases were searched simultaneously using OVID. Unless otherwise stated, the search covered the period from 1 January 2000–31 January 2014 (date of publication).

Study selection

Articles considered for inclusion included randomized, controlled trials, observational and ecological studies, and health economic analyses with HRQL and/or cost as a primary or secondary outcome from one or more of the eight countries of interest: Denmark, France, Germany, Italy, the Netherlands, Spain, Sweden and the United Kingdom. Eligible studies enrolled adults or children diagnosed with (based on positive skin prick tests and/or specific IgE results), and/or treated for, HDM (*Dermatophagoides pteronyssinus* or *Dermatophagoides farinae*) allergy; allergy to grass pollen (orchard, meadow, ryegrass, sweet vernal, and timothy grasses), *Artemisia* pollen, ragweed pollen, or birch pollen; or AA (as defined in the individual studies). Studies of AIT and symptomatic treatments were eligible for inclusion.

Titles and abstracts identified by the literature search were reviewed by NB; a second senior epidemiologist assessed 10 % of the titles and abstracts, and any disagreements were resolved through discussion. Full text versions of potentially eligible studies were obtained and reviewed. Additional relevant articles were identified from the bibliography of some articles, and a report from a clinical trial containing unpublished data was provided by the sponsor. Titles and abstracts of the 20 highest ranked Google Scholar search results were also reviewed and compared with the results of the database search to ensure that no articles had been missed.

Data extraction and meta-analysis

As the aim of this study was to gather information on the HRQL of patients before any intervention, baseline measurements of HRQL (prior to any intervention) in patients with AR and/or AA were extracted from the selected studies. Means and standard deviations (SD) were collected, or where this was not possible, were imputed from available statistics, according to the methods described in [40]. Where data were presented as $p < 0.05$ or $p < 0.01$, values used for imputations were $p = 0.049$ and $p = 0.009$, respectively. Six studies presented data graphically, and values were obtained using a ruler.

Meta-analyses were performed in Microsoft Excel, and heterogeneity was assessed using Q-tables [41]. Differences between subgroups were assessed by ANOVA [42]. Due to the expected differences in study design, random effects models were used to estimate the overall measure of HRQL and the error of the estimate. Pooled mean estimates were presented with standard errors and 95 % Confidence Intervals (CI).

Where possible, HRQL data were grouped by allergen (perennial or seasonal); if the allergen was not stated, data were included in a 'Mixed' group. Some older articles did not specify the sensitizing allergen but categorized patients as suffering from seasonal AR (SAR) or perennial AR (PAR); in these cases PAR was grouped with HDM allergy, and SAR with pollen allergy.

Cost data

Cost data were divided into direct costs (including physician visit, medication costs, hospital stays, comorbidity medication costs, comorbidity physician visits, emergency room visits, acute ward visits, and outpatient care) and indirect costs related to loss of productivity (including absenteeism, presenteeism, production loss, inability to perform usual daily activities, restricted usual daily activities). All costs were converted to 2013 international dollars ($), and expressed as purchasing power parities (PPP).

Results

Search results and selected studies

The electronic search retrieved 2963 abstracts and titles; 2905 were retained for screening, and 2502 of these did not meet the inclusion criteria. Full text copies of 544 articles were screened and 50 were retained for data extraction. One additional reference was identified from the reference section of an article [43] and data were included from an unpublished study report provided by the sponsor [44]. Flow of articles through the selection process and reasons for rejection are shown in Fig. 1. Among the studies reporting HRQL data, 3 included patients with AA; two with PAR+AA, and one with SAR+AA.

Baseline HRQL measurements: RQLQ and mini-RQLQ

The disease-specific rhinitis quality of life questionnaire (RQLQ) is a validated HRQL instrument for adults that measures functional impairments due to seasonal or perennial rhinoconjunctivitis of allergic or non-allergic origin. It comprises seven domains scored on a 7-point scale (from 0 = not impaired at all, to 6 = severely impaired), with higher scores reflecting poorer HRQL [45, 46].

Seventeen studies reported data obtained using RQLQ or mini-RQLQ measured at 'baseline', 'the season before' or on 'a day without symptoms' [5, 24, 43, 47–60]. One study included patients with SAR/pollen allergy only (n = 83) and SAR/pollen allergy with associated AA (n = 52) [49]. Two studies [59, 60] contained data that did not correspond to the recognized RQLQ scale and were excluded from the analysis.

Pooling all the data gave a moderate degree of heterogeneity ($I^2 = 62$ %) with an estimated summary RQLQ of 2.61 ± 0.10 (95 % CI 2.43–2.80). Grouping studies by allergy phenotype [SAR/pollen only, PAR/HDM only, or SAR/pollen and/or PAR ('Mixed' group)] gave I^2 values of 63 % (moderate) for SAR/pollen, 33 % (low) for 'Mixed' group, and −17 % (none) for the PAR/HDM groups. Summary RQLQ estimates for the respective groups were 2.04 ± 0.18 (95 % CI 1.68–2.41) for the SAR/pollen patient group (673 patients in 10 groups from 5 studies); 3.06 ± 0.16 (95 % CI 2.75–3.37) for the Mixed group; and 2.73 ± 0.12 (95 % CI 2.49–2.98) for the PAR/HDM only group (1520 patients in 10 groups from 6 studies) Fig. 2.

Baseline HRQL measurements: SF-36 and SF-12

The 36-Item Short Form Health Survey (SF-36) is a validated, non-disease-specific indicator of overall health status. It comprises 36 items in eight domains that reflect physical and mental functioning, which are scored from 0 to 100, with a lower score indicating poorer HRQL [61]. The SF-12 instrument is a short form of the SF-36 questionnaire, comprising 12 items.

Seven studies reported data using SF-36 or SF-12 [13, 14, 49, 52, 62–64]. One study included patients with SAR/pollen allergy only (n = 83) and SAR/pollen allergy with associated AA (n = 52) [49], and one included PAR/HDM patients with AR (n = 85), AR + AA (n = 62) or rhinitis, asthma and atopic eczema/dermatitis syndrome (n = 31) [63]. Data from one study [64] were insufficient to calculate SDs and this study was excluded from the analysis.

Data for the two main SF-36 composite domains were analyzed, to investigate whether the effects of allergic respiratory disease on physical and mental HRQL differed. Heterogeneity was high when all SF-36 physical component score (PCS) data were pooled ($I^2 = 84$ %). When data were grouped by phenotype, there was no heterogeneity for SAR/pollen ($I^2 = 13$ %) or the PAR/HDM group, ($I^2 = -61$ %), and heterogeneity was low for the Mixed group ($I^2 = 57$ %). Summary estimates of HRQL using the SF-36 PCS for respective phenotypic groups were: SAR/pollen group 64.19 ± 7.89 (95 % CI 48.7–78.6; 201 patients in 4 groups from 2 studies); PAR/HDM group 49.06 ± 1.26 (95 % CI 46.6–51.5; 2255 patients in 6 groups from 2 studies); and 'Mixed' group 50.12 ± 0.52 (95 % CI 49.1–51.1; 4899 patients in 7 groups from 3 studies) Fig. 3.

Heterogeneity between SF-36 Mental Component Scores (MCS) was moderate/high when all studies were pooled ($I^2 = 73$ %). When presented by phenotypic subgroups, there was no heterogeneity for the SAR/pollen group ($I^2 = -8$ %), and heterogeneity was low both in the, 'Mixed' ($I^2 = 46$ %) and PAR/HDM ($I^2 = 32$ %) groups. Summary estimates for the MCS were: SAR/pollen group 50.38 ± 6.46 (95 % CI 37.7–63.0; 201 patients in 4 groups from 2 studies); PAR/HDM group 47.58 ± 1.28 (95 % CI 45.1–50.1; 2255 patients in 6 groups from 2 studies); and 'Mixed' group 44.62 ± 0.39 (95 % CI 43.9–45.4; 4899 patients in 7 groups from 3 studies) Fig. 4.

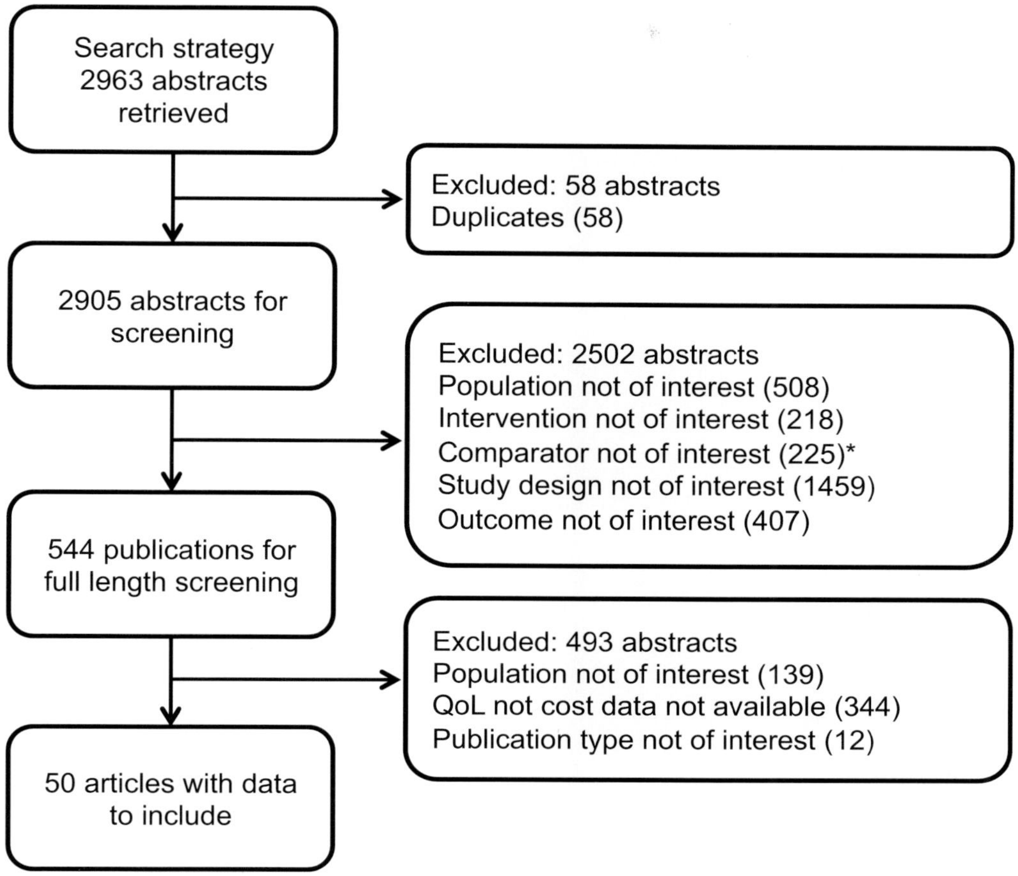

Fig. 1 Schematic diagram of the selection process. *Asterisk* comparator not of interest = environmental control mechanisms, such as mattress protector or humidifier

Comparison of RQLQ total scores between SAR/pollen and PAR/HDM phenotypes

ANOVA indicated that the RQLQ summary estimates of all three groups were different ($F = 3.53$; $p = 0.024$), but that the Mixed and PAR/HDM groups were not different ($F = 0.134$; $p = 0.134$). RQLQ summary scores for the SAR/pollen and PAR/HDM groups were different ($F = 35.9$; $p \leq 0.001$), with the overall HRQL of PAR/HDM patients worse than that of SAR/pollen patients (2.73 ± 0.12 vs. 2.04 ± 0.18; $p \leq 0.001$) Fig. 5a.

Comparison of SF-36 physical and mental component scores between SAR/pollen and PAR/HDM phenotypes

SF-36 PCS summary estimates were different between the three groups ($F = 5.75$; $p = 0.017$), with no difference between the Mixed and PAR/HDM group ($F = 0.857$; $p = 0.355$). The SF-36 PCS summary of the PAR/HDM and SAR/pollen groups was different ($F = 9.867$; $p = 0.002$), with lower HRQL in the patients with PAR/HDM allergy vs. SAR/pollen allergy. Figure 5b shows that the SF-36 PCS of patients in the PAR/HDM group was significantly worse than that of those in the SAR/pollen group (49.06 ± 1.26 vs. 64.19 ± 7.89; $p = 0.002$).

SF-36 MCS summary scores for the three groups were also different ($F = 4.95$; $p = 0.007$), with differences between the Mixed and the PAR/HDM groups ($F = 8.169$; $p = 0.004$), but not between the SAR/pollen and PAR/HDM groups ($F = 0.357$; $p = 0.550$), indicating that HRQL in both groups was equally affected (47.58 ± 1.28 vs. 50.38 ± 6.46, $p = 0.550$). Figure 5b.

Baseline RQLQ and SF-36 domain scores

Eight studies [5, 47, 51–53, 55, 56, 58] reported RQLQ domain scores, or variants thereof. The 'activities' domain showed the highest heterogeneity ($I^2 = 76$ %), with little or no heterogeneity ($I^2 = 9$ %) in 'non-hayfever symptoms', or 'emotional problems' ($I^2 = 18$ %), and medium heterogeneity ($I^2 = 31–35$ %) in the remaining domains

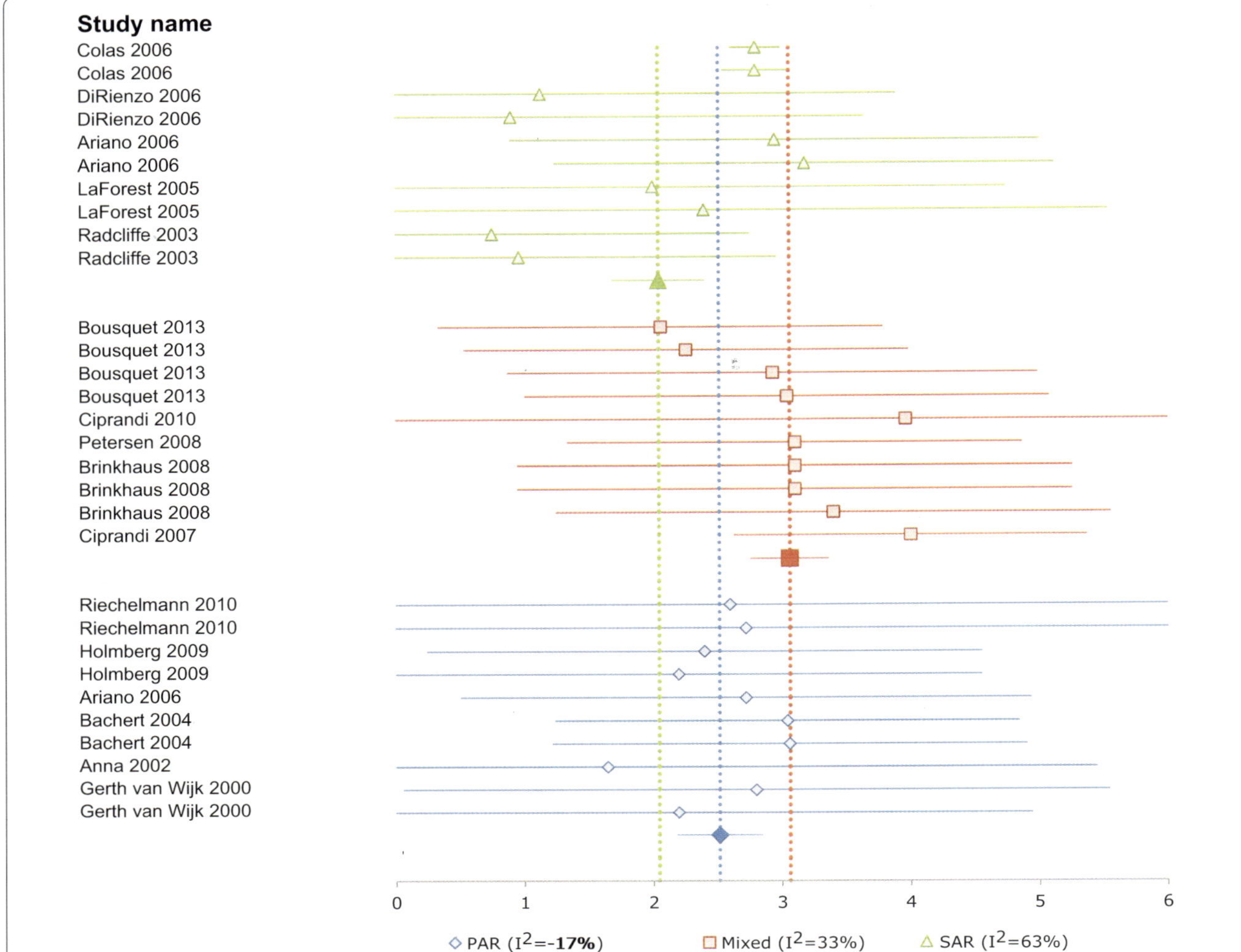

Fig. 2 Forest plot of overall RQLQ baseline scores by phenotype, from 30 groups in 15 studies. Higher scores indicate poorer HRQL

(Additional file 1: Figure S1). 'Practical problems' and 'activities' were the most affected domains, with the 'emotional' domain being the least affected (Fig. 6a).

Four studies [13, 14, 62, 63] reported SF-36 data by domain. The 'role-emotional' domain showed the highest heterogeneity ($I^2 = 43$ %), with little or no heterogeneity in 'physical activity', 'bodily pain', 'general health perception', 'vitality' or 'mental health'. ($I^2 = 0$ % for all; Additional file 1: Figure S2). 'Vitality' was the most affected domain, with 'physical activity' being the least affected domain Fig. 6b. There were insufficient data to compare domain scores by allergy phenotype.

Financial burden of AR and AA

Eleven studies were included in the analysis of direct and indirect costs; nine studies reported data for countries of interest [24, 62, 65–71] and two studies [72, 73] reported information for multiple countries using France and the United Kingdom as reference countries for calculating PPP costs (see Tables 1, 2). No studies that reported AR costs by severity were identified. One of the 17 studies included in the cost analysis was a randomized, controlled trial [72], and may not reflect costs in a real clinical practice setting.

Direct comparison of total direct and indirect costs was complicated by differences in cost assessment in each study. Within countries, specific categories of costs (e.g. GP/specialist/visits, hospitalizations, medications) varied across studies, but we found very limited or no evidence for a trend of increasing or decreasing direct and indirect costs. The majority of the direct costs for AR were borne by the GP services; for patients with AR + AA, the AA

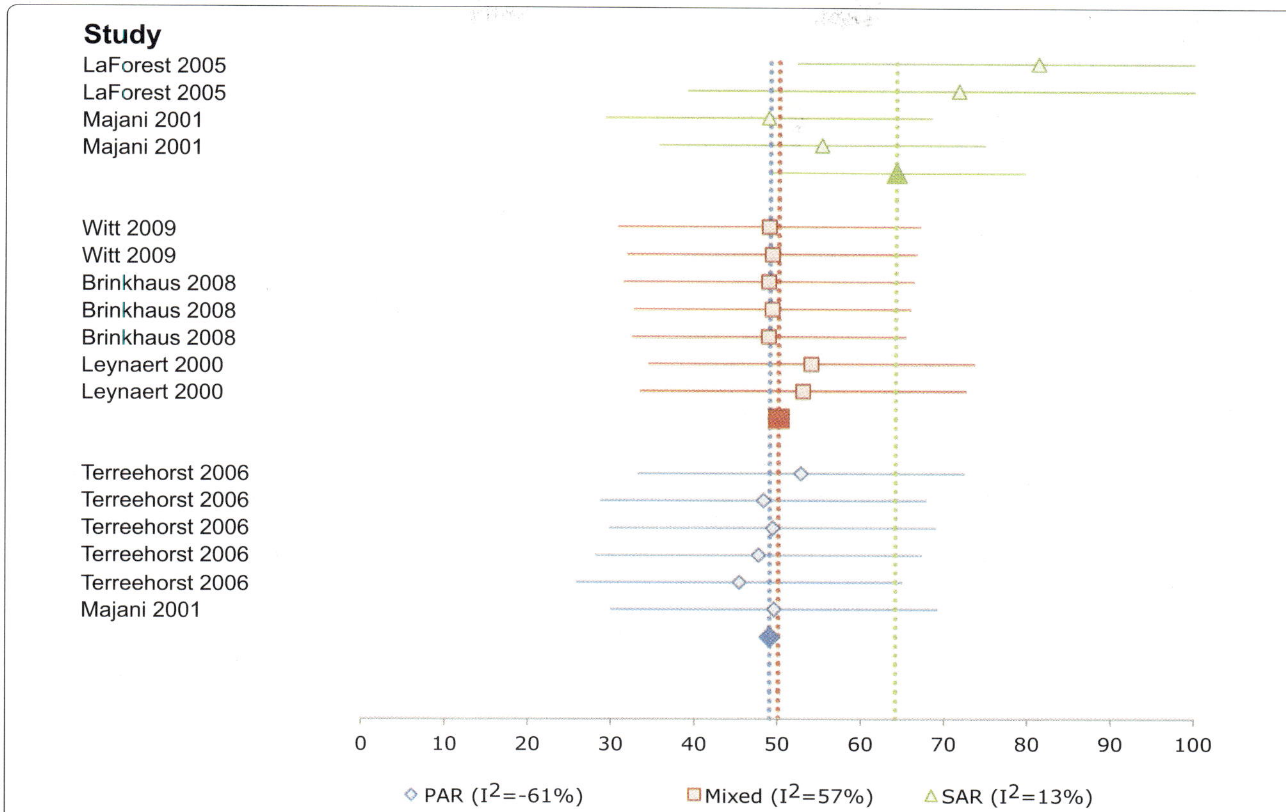

Fig. 3 Forest plot of baseline SF-36/SF-12 physical component scores from 17 groups in six studies by phenotype. 95 % confidence intervals for the Mixed and PAR summary measures are hidden by the *symbols*. Lower scores indicate poorer HRQL

part of the costs concerned medication and hospitalization costs. Medication costs, excluding over-the-counter medications, remained low Table 1.

The majority of the cost burden was indirect (Tables 1, 2) and caused by high absenteeism and presenteeism. Due to the lack of data, it was not possible to determine which had the higher cost; however, based on categories within each country, both were generally greater than the direct costs.

Discussion

Grouping studies by seasonal or perennial symptoms gave an acceptable level of heterogeneity ($I^2 \leq 63$ %) that allowed summary estimates of HRQL from RQLQ and SF-36 instruments to be determined. Heterogeneity was generally higher for the SAR/pollen phenotype than for PAR/HDM, which could reflect the different types of baseline measurements in the selected studies, or the large heterogeneity of SAR. Patients with PAR/HDM allergy had poorer HRQL than those with SAR/pollen allergy when measured by RQLQ, SF-36 total score, and SF-36 PCS. The underlying reason for this difference is unclear, and could be due to differences in symptom frequency, duration, or severity. In Northern Europe, the pollen season is largely confined to the summer months, with the season for grass pollen, which is by far the most frequent cause of pollinosis, usually lasting from mid-May to July [74]; at the height of the pollen season, patients with SAR suffer symptoms approximately 50 % of the time and report an impact on their HRQL [75]. It can be hypothesized that the year-round nature of symptoms might be responsible for the observed poorer HRQL in PAR/HDM allergy; however, published studies report varying results. Bousquet found that the severity of AR was more important in determining HRQL, sleep, daily activities, and work performance than symptom duration [3]. Similar findings were reported by Delgado and colleagues, who observed that HRQL was lower in Spanish patients with olive or grass pollen allergy vs. HDM allergy. This was attributed to the greater severity of symptoms caused by the explosive nature of olive pollination, resulting in sudden and elevated pollen concentrations, in contrast to the more constant concentrations of perennial allergens that were more tolerable for

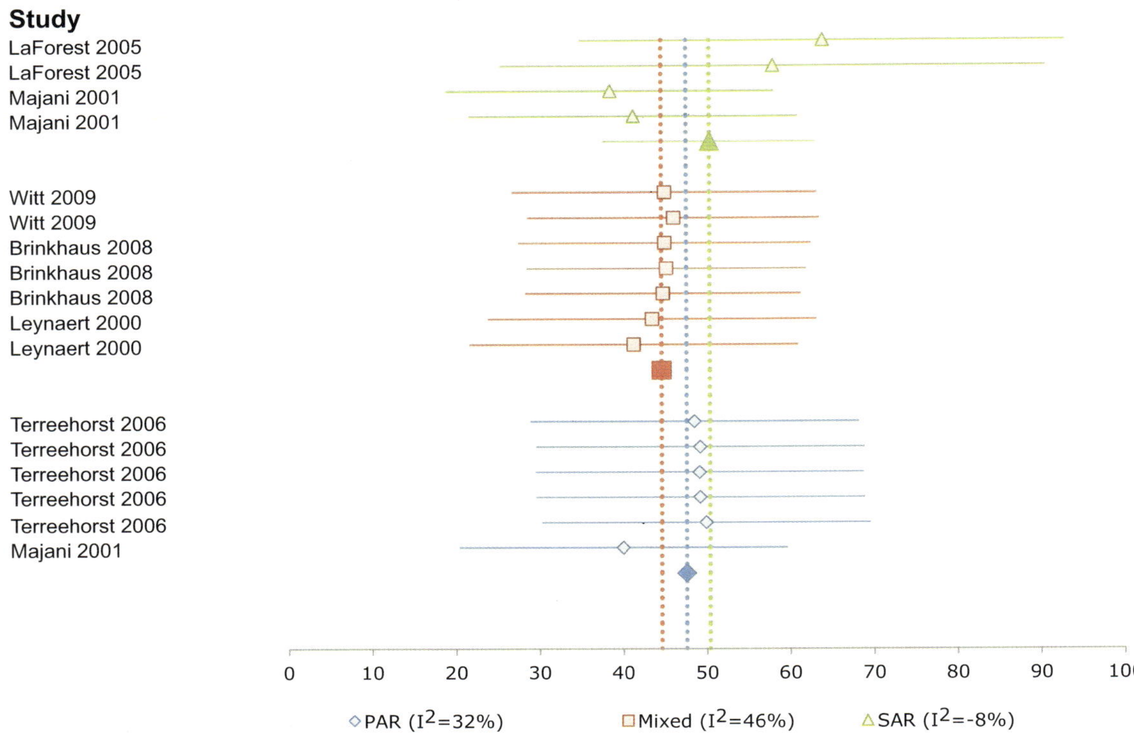

Fig. 4 Forest plot of baseline SF-36/SF-12 mental component scores by phenotype, from 17 groups in six studies. 95 % confidence intervals for the Mixed and PAR summary measures are hidden by the *symbols*. Lower scores indicate poorer HRQL

patients [76]. Another study reported no significant differences in baseline RQLQ scores between patients with HDM, grass pollen, and *Parietaria* pollen allergy [48].

Analysis of SF-36 component scores showed that mental and physical component scores were affected in seasonal and perennial allergy, with HDM/PAR having a greater impact on physical vs. mental component scores. This supports the findings of other studies that report significant emotional problems and poor mental wellbeing in patients with AR, in addition to physical symptoms [13, 33, 77].

Meta-analyses were performed using HRQL measures from generic and disease-specific instruments. Generic questionnaires, like the SF-36, measure a wide range of physical, mental and psychosocial functions; they can be used in different health conditions and in the general population, and have the advantage of allowing comparisons of burden of illness across different disorders. Disease-specific instruments like the RQLQ more accurately reflect the patient's inherent disease-associated problems, but scores cannot be directly compared with other populations. Both the generic and RQLQ instruments show improvements in HRQL in patients treated for AR; disease-specific questionnaires tend to show more important improvements, as they focus on the areas that are impacted by the disease [32]. Nowadays, HRQL questionnaires are used almost routinely in clinical studies of allergy treatments. Observed changes in HRQL generally reflect clinical outcomes; however, some studies report changes in HRQL that are not captured by symptom scores. Therefore, monitoring patients' HRQL in clinical practice has been suggested as a possible strategy to improve the management of AR [78].

Our analysis does not permit comparison of the HRQL of AR patients with that of the general population; however, a Spanish cross-sectional study that investigated the overall HRQL of patients with AR using SF-12 reported that HRQL was 25 % lower than in the general population [79]. Poor HRQL in patients with AR is also supported by evidence that successful treatment of AR symptoms with AIT [21–23] or symptomatic treatment [24–31] improves patient's HRQL scores. A comparison of published EQ-5D utility baseline scores indicated that perennial allergy and/or AA (13 patients with AR and 12 with AR+AA), on a typical day with allergy symptoms, had a score of 0.60 [23], indicating comparable HRQL to diabetes (0.83) [80], cardiovascular disorders (0.73), musculoskeletal disorders (0.63), and psychosomatic disorders (0.57), when measured with the same EQ-5D instrument [81]. Ranges of published EQ-5D scores for AR and/

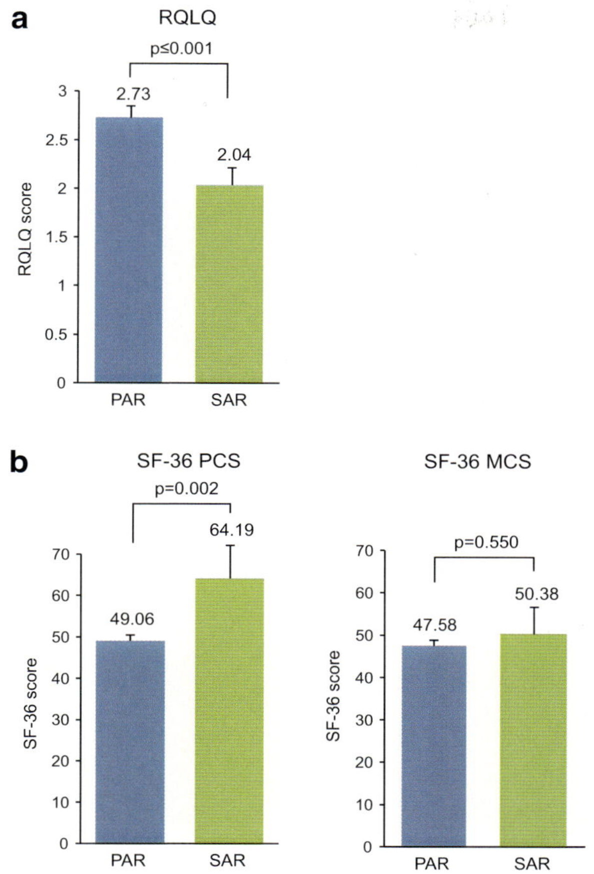

Fig. 5 Overall RQLQ and SF-36 physical and mental component scores for the PAR and SAR phenotypes. **a** RQLQ scores of the PAR and SAR phenotypes; **b** *left* quality of life (QoL) measured by PCS of PAR and SAR patients. *Right* QoL measured by MCS of PAR and SAR patients. *Error bars* represent 95 % CI. Higher RQLQ scores and lower SF-36 scores indicate lower HRQL

or AA and other diseases are summarized in Fig. 7, and indicate that the impact of AR and/or AA on generic HRQL on a day with allergen exposure is not trivial, with an effect that is comparable to chronic conditions, such as liver disease, epilepsy, migraine, and visual disorders [23, 82–86].

There were insufficient data in the present analysis to compare HRQL in patients with AR vs. those with both AR and AA. Delgado and colleagues reported that HRQL associated with AR was worse in patients diagnosed with both AR and asthma than in those with only AR [76]. Using the SF-36 instrument, Leynaert reported that patients with asthma experienced greater impairments in physical functioning that those with AR alone, but asthma did not further impair mental wellbeing of patients with AR [13].

The cost analysis shows variations in direct and indirect AR costs between countries, which may result from true differences in AR costs or from differences in the health systems, diagnostic behavior, or reporting between countries. Indirect costs make up the majority of the cost burden of AR, in line with the outcomes of the most recent European [39] and US studies [34]. A few studies have reported higher direct vs. indirect costs [35, 87]; however, many studies estimate indirect costs by multiplying patients' salaries by the amount of time they are absent from work due to AR. Health impairments associated with AR are often not severe enough to cause absence from work, although they can interfere with cognitive functioning, resulting in fatigue and an impaired ability to learn, concentrate, and make decisions [88], all of which can affect performance in the workplace. In one study, more than a third of patients with AR (36 %) reported reduced workplace performance, or 'presenteeism', which was higher than among patients with asthma (19 %) [89]. In the US, where up to 60 million people are affected by AR [90], annual productivity loss associated with a diagnosis of AR was estimated at $601 million in 1995. When the use of sedating allergy medications and workers' self-assessments of their reduction work productivity due to AR were taken into account, the estimated annual at-work productivity losses increased to $2.4–$4.6 billion [37]. In 2006, the cost of lost productivity in the workplace due to AR was $593 per employee per year, and exceeded that of stress ($518), migraine ($277), depression ($273), and arthritis/rheumatism ($269) [36]. Comorbid AA resulted in higher costs than AR alone [91], or AR with non-allergic asthma [92], indicating its importance in driving costs. The cost of productivity loss is greater than the cost of treating AR symptoms; however, many cost analysis studies do not consider the cost to the patient of over-the-counter AR medications, which could lead to an underestimation of direct costs [34].

Some limitations of the study design should be acknowledged. Search terms were chosen from the RQLQ and SF-36 questionnaires, or were based on the suspected impact of AA and AR on patients' HRQL. The articles identified by the search were mainly safety or efficacy studies that included HRQL as a secondary endpoint. Consequently, abstracts that did not include secondary outcomes would not be identified by the search. This could introduce a bias, such that only studies reporting a change in HRQL were identified. Inclusion of patients with comorbid AA in some groups could also affect HRQL scores, although we estimate any effect to be small. Moreover, the study only included HDM, and not pet allergens, as perennial allergens for perennial allergic rhinitis/asthma. Many of the studies from which data are collated were randomized controlled interventional

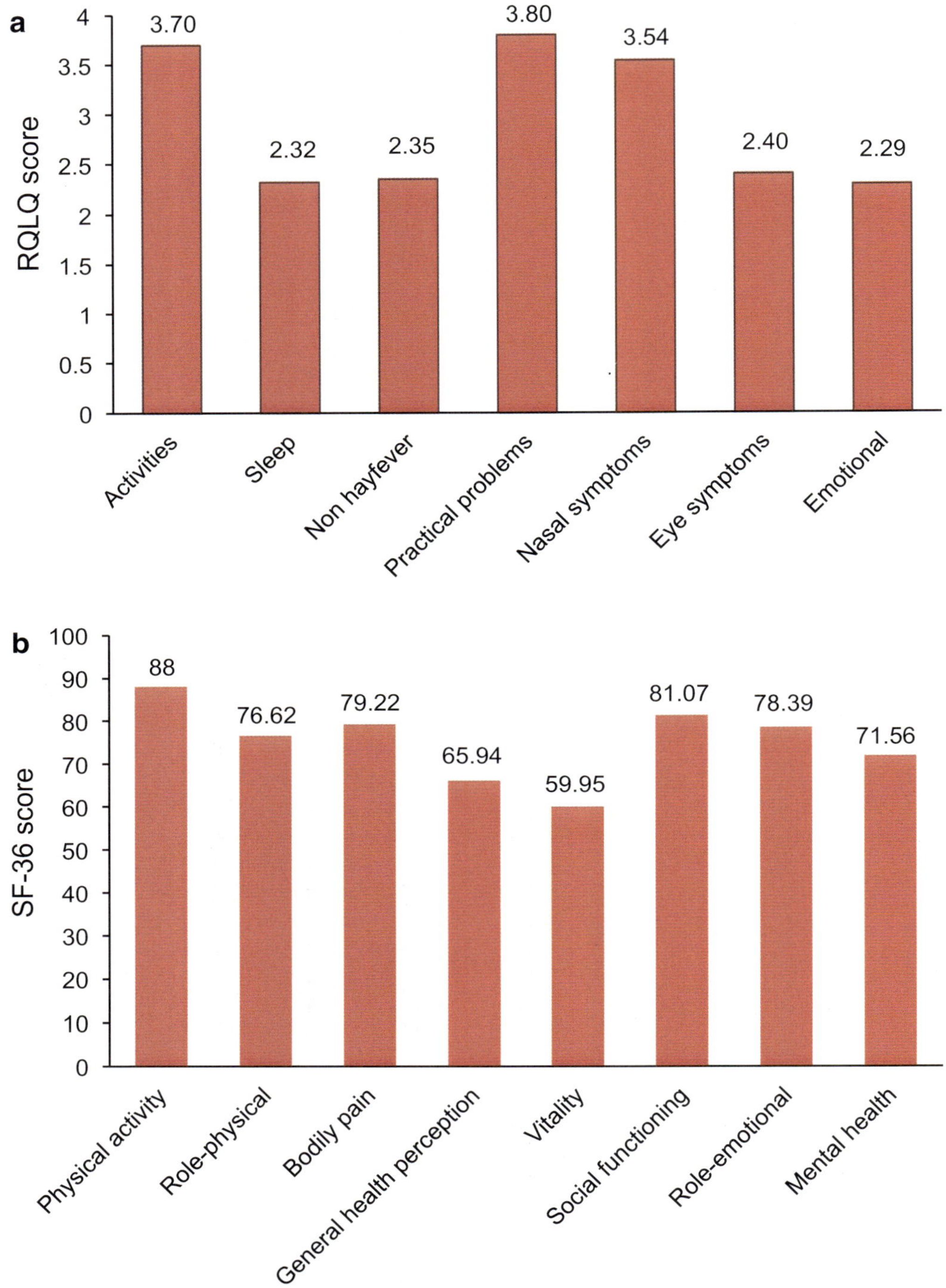

Fig. 6 RQLQ and SF-36 domain scores. **a** RQLQ domain scores in the combined PAR/SAR population; **b** SF-36 domain scores in the PAR/SAR population

Table 1 Direct costs

Country	Ref.	Age group	Direct costs			Values		
			Disease	Allergen	Definition	Country currency	Year of currency	PPP (2013 Int$)
Denmark	[65]	Adult	AR	SAR/grass	GP visit/extra GP visit/acute ward visit/loratadine/budesonide/fluticasone/salbutamol	307.49	2005 (€)	47.19
	[66]	Adult	AR	Mixed	Healthcare	1964.00	2002 (DKK)	300.96
France	[67]	Adult	AR	PAR/HDM	Desloratidine/medication (comorbidity)/medication (additional PAR)/GP visit/comorbidity GP visit	373.32	2007 (€)	492.39
	[68]	Adult	AR	SAR/grass	Direct costs	694.95	2003 (€)	261.64
				PAR/HDM	Direct costs	183.57	2003 (€)	130.71
		Children		SAR/grass	Direct costs	140.33	2003 (€)	200.01
				PAR/HDM	Direct costs	279.33	2003 (€)	398.12
Germany	[62]	Adult	AR	Mixed	GP visit/medication (unspecified)/hospitalization	771.12	2009 (€)	993.71
	[65]	Adult	AR	SAR/grass	GP visit/Extra GP Visit/Acute ward visit/loratadine/budesonide/fluticasone/salbutamol	383.85	2005 (€)	493.88
	[69]	Adult	AR	SAR/grass	Direct costs	356.37	1991 (DEM)	351.56
			AR	PAR/HDM	Direct costs	517.94	1991 (DEM)	884.64
			AR+AA	Mixed	Direct costs	544.02	1991 (DEM)	887.16
Italy	[70]	Adult	AR+AA	Mixed	Medication (unspecified)/outpatient care/emergency department/hospitalization	1589.30	2004 (€)	2568.52
	[71]	Children and adolescent	AR	SAR/grass	Direct costs	500.00	2003 (€)	826.75
				PAR/HDM	Direct costs	518.00	2003 (€)	856.51
				Mixed	Direct costs	506.00	2003 (€)	836.67
Multiple (1)	[72]	Adult	AR	PAR/HDM	GP visit/medication (unspecified)	100.44	2002 (€)	149.07
Multiple (2)	[73]	Adult	AR+AA	SAR/grass	Acute ward visit/asthma medication/budesonide/DESLORATIDINE/Extra GP or specialist visit/fluticasone/GP visit/medication (unspecified)/salbutamol	289.88	2005 (£)	527.27
Sweden	[65]	Adult	AR	SAR/grass	GP visit/extra GP visit/acute ward visit/loratadine/budesonide/fluticasone/salbutamol	595.80	2005 (€)	838.42

DKK Danish Krone, *DEM* Deutsche Mark, *Multiple (1)* Belgium, France, Germany, Italy, Spain, *Multiple (2)* United Kingdom, Germany, the Netherlands, Denmark, Sweden, Spain and Austria

studies, which may tend to include patients with more severe symptoms.

Conclusions

This review presents summary data on HRQL levels in patients with allergic respiratory disease that may be used for comparison with assessments from individual studies. HRQL in PAR/HDM patients was significantly worse than that of SAR/pollen patients, when measured by both disease-specific and generic HRQL instruments, and was reflected by an impact on both physical and mental health. SAR/pollen and PAR/HDM affected MCS to a similar degree, despite a greater impact of PAR/HDM on PCS. A comparison of published EQ-5D utility index scores showed that the impact of PAR, with or without AA, on patients' HRQL was comparable to other chronic diseases. The economic burden of AR is considerable, with indirect costs due to absenteeism and presenteeism making up the majority of costs. Greater awareness of the detrimental effects of AR on HRQL and its cost burden might encourage early diagnosis and treatment in order to minimize the disease burden and ensure beneficial and cost-effective outcomes.

Table 2 Indirect costs

Country	Ref.	Age group	Disease		Indirect costs		Values	
			Disease	Allergen	Definition	Country currency	Year of currency	PPP (2013 Int$)
Denmark	[65]	Adult	AR	SAR/grass	Absenteeism	667.36	2005 (€)	102.26
	[66]	Adult	AR	Mixed	Patient/societal	30606.00	2002 (DKK)	4689.98
France	[67]	Adult	AR	PAR/HDM	Absenteeism/presenteeism/ Wage per work day	1480.68	2007 (€)	1952.95
	[68]	Adult	AR	SAR/grass	Indirect costs	210.86	2003 (€)	229.67
			AR	PAR/HDM	Indirect costs	161.14	2003 (€)	300.52
Germany	[62]	Adult	AR	Mixed	Indirect costs	765.84	2009 (€)	1073.38
	[65]	Adult	AR	SAR/grass	Absenteeism	352.04	2005 (€)	523.04
Italy	[71]	Children and adolescent	AR	SAR/grass	Indirect costs	2222.00	2003 (€)	3674.08
				PAR/HDM	Indirect costs	2057.00	2003 (€)	3401.25
				Mixed	Indirect costs	2166.00	2003 (€)	3581.48
Multiple (1)	[72]	Adult	AR	PAR/HDM	Absenteeism/presenteeism/ Inability to perform usual daily activities/restriction over usual daily activities	4160.40	2002 (€)	6174.94
	[24]	Adult	AR	PAR/HDM	Absenteeism/presenteeism	1826.88	2001 (€)	2711.49
Multiple (2)	[73]	Adult	AR+AA	SAR/grass	Absenteeism/presenteeism/production loss	983.17	2005 (£)	1788.29
Sweden	[65]	Adult	AR	SAR/grass	Absenteeism	384.62	2005 (€)	50.68
Netherlands	[65]	Adult	AR	SAR/grass	Absenteeism	810.12	2005 (€)	1140.01
UK	[65]	Adult	AR	SAR/grass	Absenteeism	408.41	2005 (€)	742.85

DKK Danish Krone, *Multiple (1)* Belgium, France, Germany, Italy, Spain, *Multiple (2)* United Kingdom, Germany, the Netherlands, Denmark, Sweden, Spain and Austria

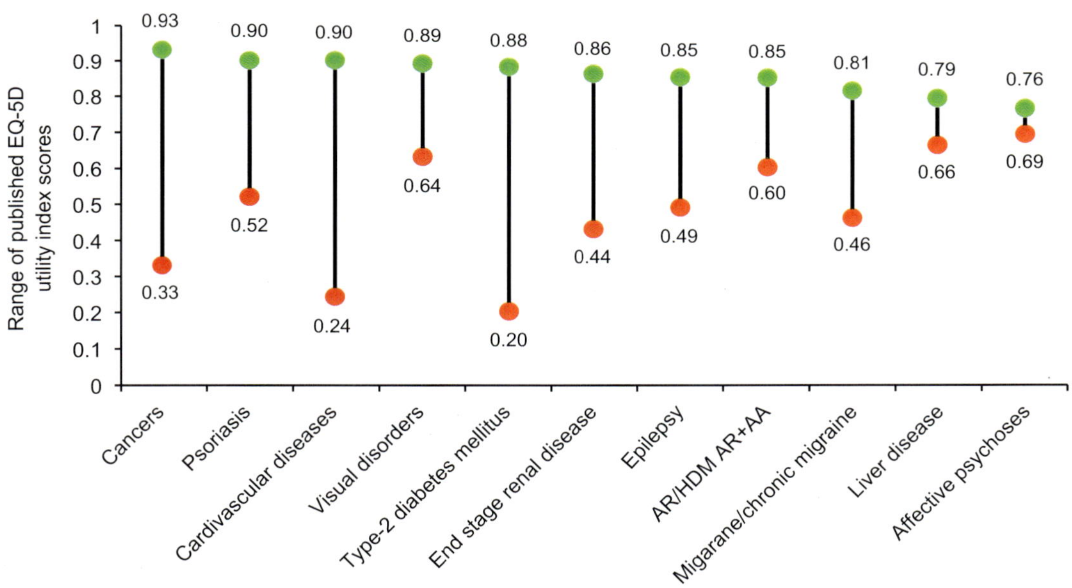

Fig. 7 Range of EQ-5D utility index scores for selected chronic conditions. *Green* and *red circles* represent the upper and lower values, respectively. Values were obtained from published studies in populations with cancer [82], psoriasis [82], cardiovascular diseases [82], visual disorders [82], type-2 diabetes mellitus [82], end stage renal disease [82], epilepsy [83], AR/HDM or AR and AA [23, 84], migraine [84] or chronic migraine [85], liver disease [82], and active psychoses [84, 86]. Lower EQ-5D values indicate lower HRQL

Abbreviations

AA: allergic asthma; AIT: allergy immunotherapy; AR: allergic rhinitis; ARIA: allergic rhinitis and its impact on asthma; GP: general practitioner; HDM: house dust mite; HRQL: health-related quality of life; MCS: mental component score; PAR: perennial allergic rhinitis; PCS: physical component score; PPP: purchasing power parities; RQLQ: rhinitis quality of life questionnaire; SAR: seasonal allergic rhinitis; USD: United States Dollars.

Authors' contributions

AL, NSH and NB designed the study; NB performed the analysis; AL, NSH, JHP, and NB analyzed the data; all authors contributed to the writing of the manuscript. All authors read and approved the final manuscript.

Author details

[1] Research Centre for Prevention and Health, The Capital Region of Denmark, Copenhagen, Denmark. [2] Department of Clinical Experimental Research, Rigshospitalet, Copenhagen, Denmark. [3] Department of Clinical Medicine, Faculty of Health and Medical Sciences, University of Copenhagen, Copenhagen, Denmark. [4] Department of Business and Management, Faculty of Social Sciences, Aalborg University, Aalborg, Denmark. [5] ALK, Hørsholm, Denmark. [6] MAPI, London, UK.

Acknowledgements

The authors thank Dr. Ron Hogg of Copentown UK for medical writing support.

Funding

The study was funded by ALK, Hørsholm, Denmark.

References

1. Bauchau V, Durham SR. Prevalence and rate of diagnosis of allergic rhinitis in Europe. Eur Respir J. 2004;24:758–64.
2. Bousquet J, Van Cauwenberge P, Khaltaev N, Aria Workshop G, World Health O. Allergic rhinitis and its impact on asthma. J Allergy Clin Immunol. 2001;108:S147–334.
3. Bousquet J, Neukirch F, Bousquet PJ, Gehano P, Klossek JM, Le Gal M, Allaf B. Severity and impairment of allergic rhinitis in patients consulting in primary care. J Allergy Clin Immunol. 2006;117:158–62.
4. Canonica GW, Bousquet J, Mullol J, Scadding GK, Virchow JC. A survey of the burden of allergic rhinitis in Europe. Allergy. 2007;62(Suppl 85):17–25.
5. Bousquet PJ, Demoly P, Devillier P, Mesbah K, Bousquet J. Impact of allergic rhinitis symptoms on quality of life in primary care. Int Arch Allergy Immunol. 2013;160:393–400.
6. Jones NS, Smith PA, Carney AS, Davis A. The prevalence of allergic rhinitis and nasal symptoms in Nottingham. Clin Otolaryngol Allied Sci. 1998;23:547–54.
7. Didier A, Chanal I, Klossek JM, Mathieu J, Bousquet J. La rhinite allergique: le point de vue du patient. Revue francaise d'allergologie et d'immunologie clinique. 1999;39:171–85.
8. Spector SL. Overview of comorbid associations of allergic rhinitis. J Allergy Clin Immunol. 1997;99:S773–80.
9. Ozdoganoglu T, Songu M. The burden of allergic rhinitis and asthma. Ther Adv Respir Dis. 2012;6:11–23.
10. Linneberg A, Henrik Nielsen N, Frolund L, Madsen F, Dirksen A, Jorgensen T, Copenhagen Allergy S. The link between allergic rhinitis and allergic asthma: a prospective population-based study. The Copenhagen Allergy Study. Allergy. 2002;57:1048–52.
11. Jaruvongvanich V, Mongkolpathumrat P, Chantaphakul H, Klaewsongkram J. Extranasal symptoms of allergic rhinitis are difficult to treat and affect quality of life. Allergol Int. 2016;65:199–203.
12. Meltzer EO. Quality of life in adults and children with allergic rhinitis. J Allergy Clin Immunol. 2001;108:S45–53.
13. Leynaert B, Neukirch C, Liard R, Bousquet J, Neukirch F. Quality of life in allergic rhinitis and asthma. Am J Respir Crit Care Med. 2000;162:1391–6.
14. Majani G, Biardini I, Giardini A, Senna GE, Minale P, D'Ulisse S, Ciprandi G, Canonica W. Health-related quality of life assessment in young adults with seasonal allergic rhinitis. Allergy. 2001;56:313–7.
15. Stuck BA, Czajkowski J, Hagner AE, Klimek L, Verse T, Hormann K, Maurer JT. Changes in daytime sleepiness, quality of life, and objective sleep patterns in seasonal allergic rhinitis: a controlled clinical trial. J Allergy Clin Immunol. 2004;113:663–8.
16. Song Y, Wang M, Xie J, Li W, Zhang X, Wang T, Tan G. Prevalence of allergic rhinitis among elementary and middle school students in Changsha city and its impact on quality of life. J Laryngol Otol. 2015;129:1108–14.
17. Sritipsukho P, Satdhabudha A, Nanthapisal S. Effect of allergic rhinitis and asthma on the quality of life in young Thai adolescents. Asian Pac J Allergy Immunol. 2015;33:222–6.
18. Adebola SO, Abidoye B, Ologe FE, Adebola OE, Oyejola BA. Health-related quality of life and its contributory factors in allergic rhinitis patients in Nigeria. Auris Nasus Larynx. 2015;43:171–5.
19. Price D, Scadding G, Ryan D, Bachert C, Canonica GW, Mullol J, Klimek L, Pitman R, Acaster S, Murray R, Bousquet J. The hidden burden of adult allergic rhinitis: UK healthcare resource utilisation survey. Clin Transl Allergy. 2015;5:39.
20. Canonica GW, Mullol J, Pradalier A, Didier A. Patient perceptions of allergic rhinitis and quality of life: findings from a survey conducted in europe and the United States. World Allergy Organ J. 2008;1:138–44.
21. Katotomichelakis M, Riga M, Tripsianis G, Balatsouras D, Kourousis C, Danielides G, Giotakis E, Danielides V. Predictors of quality of life improvement in allergic rhinitis patients after sublingual immunotherapy. Ann Otol Rhinol Laryngol. 2015;124:430–6.
22. Durham SR, Yang WH, Pedersen MR, Johansen N, Rak S. Sublingual immunotherapy with once-daily grass allergen tablets: a randomized controlled trial in seasonal allergic rhinoconjunctivitis. J Allergy Clin Immunol. 2006;117:802–9.
23. Petersen KD, Kronborg C, Larsen JN, Dahl R, Gyrd-Hansen D. Patient related outcomes in a real life prospective follow up study: allergen immunotherapy increase quality of life and reduce sick days. World Allergy Organ J. 2013;6:15.
24. Bachert C, Bousquet J, Canonica GW, Durham SR, Klimek L, Mullol J, Van Cauwenberge PB, Van Hammee G. Levocetirizine improves quality of life and reduces costs in long-term management of persistent allergic rhinitis. J Allergy Clin Immunol. 2004;114:838–44.
25. Walter Canonica G, Bousquet J, Van Hammee G, Bachert C, Durham SR, Klimek L, Mullol J, Van Cauwenberge PB. Levocetirizine improves health-related quality of life and health status in persistent allergic rhinitis. Respir Med. 2006;100:1706–15.
26. El Hennawi DE, Ahmed MR, Farid AM. Psychological stress and its relationship with persistent allergic rhinitis. Eur Arch Otorhinolaryngol. 2015;273:899–904.
27. Erdogan BA, Sanli A, Paksoy M, Altin G, Aydin S. Quality of life in patients with persistent allergic rhinitis treated with desloratadine monotherapy or desloratadine plus montelucast combination. Kulak Burun Bogaz Ihtis Derg. 2014;24:217–24.
28. Ciebiada M, Ciebiada MG, Kmiecik T, DuBuske LM, Gorski P. Quality of life in patients with persistent allergic rhinitis treated with montelukast alone

or in combination with levocetirizine or desloratadine. J Investig Allergol Clin Immunol. 2008;18:343–9.
29. Skoner DP, LaForce CF, Nathan RA, Urdaneta ER, Zielinski MA, Sacavage SD, Franklin KB, Wu MM. Effect of cetirizine on symptom severity and quality of life in perennial allergic rhinitis. Allergy Asthma Proc. 2014;35:338–45.
30. Goh BS, Ismail MI, Husain S. Quality of life assessment in patients with moderate to severe allergic rhinitis treated with montelukast and/or intranasal steroids: a randomised, double-blind, placebo-controlled study. J Laryngol Otol. 2014;128:242–8.
31. Amizadeh M, Safizadeh H, Bazargan N, Farrokhdoost Z. Survey on the prevalence of allergic rhinitis and its effect on the quality of high school students' life. Iran J Otorhinolaryngol. 2013;25:79–84.
32. Bousquet J, Khaltaev N, Cruz AA, Denburg J, Fokkens WJ, Togias A, Zuberbier T, Baena-Cagnani CE, Canonica GW, van Weel C, et al. Allergic Rhinitis and its Impact on Asthma (ARIA) 2008 update (in collaboration with the World Health Organization, GA(2)LEN and AllerGen). Allergy. 2008;63(Suppl 86):8–160.
33. Juniper EF. Quality of life in adults and children with asthma and rhinitis. Allergy. 1997;52:971–7.
34. Reed SD, Lee TA, McCrory DC. The economic burden of allergic rhinitis: a critical evaluation of the literature. Pharmacoeconomics. 2004;22:345–61.
35. Schoenwetter WF, Dupclay L Jr, Appajosyula S, Botteman MF, Pashos CL. Economic impact and quality-of-life burden of allergic rhinitis. Curr Med Res Opin. 2004;20:305–17.
36. Lamb CE, Ratner PH, Johnson CE, Ambegaonkar AJ, Joshi AV, Day D, Sampson N, Eng B. Economic impact of workplace productivity losses due to allergic rhinitis compared with select medical conditions in the United States from an employer perspective. Curr Med Res Opin. 2006;22:1203–10.
37. Crystal-Peters J, Crown WH, Goetzel RZ, Schutt DC. The cost of productivity losses associated with allergic rhinitis. Am J Manag Care. 2000;6:373–8.
38. Walker S, Khan-Wasti S, Fletcher M, Cullinan P, Harris J, Sheikh A. Seasonal allergic rhinitis is associated with a detrimental effect on examination performance in United Kingdom teenagers: case-control study. J Allergy Clin Immunol. 2007;120:381–7.
39. Cardell LO, Olsson P, Andersson M, Welin KO, Svensson J, Tennvall GR, Hellgren J. TOTALL: high cost of allergic rhinitis-a national Swedish population-based questionnaire study. NPJ Prim Care Respir Med. 2016;26:15082.
40. Higgins JP, Green S. Cochrane handbook for systematic reviews of interventions. New York: Wiley Online Library; 2008.
41. Neyeloff JL, Fuchs SC, Moreira LB. Meta-analyses and Forest plots using a microsoft excel spreadsheet: step-by-step guide focusing on descriptive data analysis. BMC Res Notes. 2012;5:52.
42. Analysis of Variance Calculator. http://www.danielsoper.com/statcalc3/calc.aspx?id=43. Accessed 1 Feb 2016.
43. Di Rienzo V, Pucci S, D'Alo S, Di Cara G, Incorvaia C, Frati F, Romano A. Effects of high-dose sublingual immunotherapy on quality of life in patients with cypress-induced rhinitis: a placebo-controlled study. Clin Exp All Rev. 2006;6:67–70.
44. Mosbech H. A phase II–III trial assessing the efficacy and safety of three doses of the ALK house dust mite tablet in house dust mite-allergic subjects 81 centres in DE, DK, ES, FR, GB, IT, PL, SE. Copenhagen: National University Hospital; 2009. p. 199.
45. Juniper EF, Thompson AK, Ferrie PJ, Roberts JN. Validation of the standardized version of the rhinoconjunctivitis quality of life questionnaire. J Allergy Clin Immunol. 1999;104:364–9.
46. Juniper EF, Guyatt GH. Development and testing of a new measure of health status for clinical trials in rhinoconjunctivitis. Clin Exp Allergy. 1991;21:77–83.
47. Colas C, Monzon S, Venturini M, Lezaun A. Double-blind, placebo-controlled study with a modified therapeutic vaccine of Salsola kali (Russian thistle) administered through use of a cluster schedule. J Allergy Clin Immunol. 2006;117:810–6.
48. Ariano R, Amoroso S, Astarita C, Bassi M, Bonadonna P, Campi P, Di Gioacchino M, Musarra A, Quercia O, Russello M, et al. Quality of life in allergic rhinitis and impact of high-dose sublingual immunotherapy: a real-life study. Clin Exp All Rev. 2006;6:71–3.
49. Laforest L, Bousquet J, Neukirch F, Aubier M, Pietri G, Devouassoux G, Pacheco Y, Van Ganse E. Influence of sociodemographic factors on quality of life during pollen season in seasonal allergic rhinitis patients. Ann Allergy Asthma Immunol. 2005;95:26–32.
50. Radcliffe MJ. Enzyme potentiated desensitisation in treatment of seasonal allergic rhinitis: double blind randomised controlled study. BMJ. 2003;327:251–4.
51. Petersen KD, Kronborg C, Gyrd-Hansen D, Dahl R, Larsen JN, Lowenstein H. Quality of life in rhinoconjunctivitis assessed with generic and disease-specific questionnaires. Allergy. 2008;63:284–91.
52. Brinkhaus B, Witt CM, Jena S, Liecker B, Wegscheider K, Willich SN. Acupuncture in patients with allergic rhinitis: a pragmatic randomized trial. Ann Allergy Asthma Immunol. 2008;101:535–43.
53. Ciprandi G, Klersy C, Cirillo I, Marseglia GL. Quality of life in allergic rhinitis: relationship with clinical, immunological, and functional aspects. Clin Exp Allergy. 2007;37:1528–35.
54. Riechelmann H, Schmutzhard J, van der Werf JF, Distler A, Kleinjans HAJ. Efficacy and safety of a glutaraldehyde-modified house dust mite extract in allergic rhinitis. Am J Rhinol Allergy. 2010;24:104–9.
55. Holmberg K, Tonnel AB, Dreyfus I, Olsson P, Cougnard J, Mesbah K, Devillier P. Desloratadine relieves nasal congestion and improves quality-of-life in persistent allergic rhinitis. Allergy. 2009;64:1663–70.
56. Anna C-B, Alfonso M, Ernesto E, Pau A, Rosario A, Joan B, Gloria PM. Quality of life after use of environmental control measures together with the application of the acaricide frontac in the environment of patients suffering from allergic respiratory pathology. J Allergy Clin Immunol. 2002;109:S122.
57. Gerth Van Wijk R, Terreehorst IT, Mulder PGH, Garrelds IM, Blom HM, Popering S. Intranasal capsaicin is lacking therapeutic effect in perennial allergic rhinitis to house dust mite. A placebo-controlled study. Clin Exp Allergy. 2000;30:1792–8.
58. Ciprandi G, Cadario G, Valle C, Ridolo E, Verini M, Di Gioacchino M, Minelli M, Gangemi S, Sillano V, Colangelo C, et al. Sublingual immunotherapy in polysensitized patients: effect on quality of life. J Investig Allergol Clin Immunol. 2010;20:274–9.
59. Höiby AS, Strand V, Robinson DS, Sager A, Rak S. Efficacy, safety, and immunological effects of a 2-year immunotherapy with Depigoid® birch pollen extract: a randomized, double-blind, placebo-controlled study. Clin Exp Allergy. 2010;40:1062–70.
60. Cadario G, Ciprandi G, Di Cara G, Fadel R, Incorvaia C, Marcucci F, Marengo F, Puccinelli P, Sensi L, Strazzeri L. Comparison between continuous or intermittent schedules of sublingual immunotherapy for house dust mites: effects on compliance, patients' satisfaction, quality of life and safety. Int J Immunopathol Pharmacol. 2008;21:471–3.
61. McHorney CA, Ware JE Jr, Lu JF, Sherbourne CD. The MOS 36-item short-form health survey (SF-36): III. Tests of data quality, scaling assumptions, and reliability across diverse patient groups. Med Care. 1994;32:40–66.
62. Witt CM, Reinhold T, Jena S, Brinkhaus B, Willich SN. Cost-effectiveness of acupuncture in women and men with allergic rhinitis: a randomized controlled study in usual care. Am J Epidemiol. 2008;169:562–71.
63. Terreehorst I, Duivenvoorden HJ, Tempels-Pavlica Z, Oosting AJ, Monchy JGR, Bruijnzeel-Koomen CAFM, Wijk RG. The effect of encasings on quality of life in adult house dust mite allergic patients with rhinitis, asthma and/or atopic dermatitis. Allergy. 2005;60:888–93.
64. Passalacqua G, Pasquali M, Ariano R, Lombardi C, Giardini A, Baiardini I, Majani G, Falagiani P, Bruno M, Canonica GW. Randomized double-blind controlled study with sublingual carbamylated allergoid immunotherapy in mild rhinitis due to mites. Allergy. 2006;61:849–54.
65. Bachert C, Vestenbæk U, Christensen J, Griffiths UK, Poulsen PB. Cost-effectiveness of grass allergen tablet (GRAZAX®) for the prevention of seasonal grass pollen induced rhinoconjunctivitis ? a Northern European perspective. Clin Exp Allergy. 2007;37:772–9.
66. Petersen KD, Gyrd-Hansen D, Dahl R. Health-Economic Analyses of subcutaneous Specific Immunotherapy for grass pollen and mite allergy. Allergol Immunopathol (Madr). 2005;33:296–302.
67. Sullivan PW, Navaratnam P, Lorber R, Shekar T. The cost-effectiveness of treatment with desloratadine in patients with persistent allergic rhinitis. Curr Med Res Opin. 2010;26:1389–97.
68. Omnes L, Bousquet J, Scheinmann P, Neukirch F, Jasso-Mosqueda G, Chicoye A, Champion L, Fadel R. Pharmacoeconomic assessment of specific immunotherapy versus current symptomatic treatment for allergic rhinitis and asthma in France. Eur Ann Allergy Clin Immunol. 2007;39:148–56.

69. Schädlich PK, Brecht JG. Economic evaluation of specific immunotherapy versus symptomatic treatment of allergic rhinitis in Germany. Pharmacoeconomics. 2000;17:37–52.
70. Dal Negro R, Piskorz P, Vives R, Guilera M, Sazonov Kocevar V, Badia X. Healthcare utilisation and costs associated with adding Montelukast to current therapy in patients with mild to moderate asthma and co-morbid allergic rhinitis. Pharmacoeconomics. 2007;25:665–76.
71. Berto P, Bassi M, Incorvaia C, Frati F, Puccinelli P, Giaquinto C, Cantarutti L, Ortolani C. Cost effectiveness of sublingual immunotherapy in children with allergic rhinitis and asthma. Eur Ann Allergy Clin Immunol. 2005;37:303–8.
72. Bousquet J, Demarteau N, Mullol J, Akker-van Marle ME, Van Ganse E, Bachert C. Costs associated with persistent allergic rhinitis are reduced by levocetirizine. Allergy. 2005;60:788–94.
73. Nasser S, Vestenbaek U, Beriot-Mathiot A, Poulsen PB. Cost-effectiveness of specific immunotherapy with Grazax in allergic rhinitis co-existing with asthma. Allergy. 2008;63:1624–9.
74. D'Amato G, Spieksma FT, Liccardi G, Jager S, Russo M, Kontou-Fili K, Nikkels H, Wuthrich B, Bonini S. Pollen-related allergy in Europe. Allergy. 1998;53:567–78.
75. Small M, Piercy J, Demoly P, Marsden H. Burden of illness and quality of life in patients being treated for seasonal allergic rhinitis: a cohort survey. Clin Transl Allergy. 2013;3:33.
76. Delgado J, Davila ID, Dominguez-Ortega J, Quirce S, Marti-Guadano E, Valero A. Quality of life in patients with respiratory allergy is influenced by the causative allergen. J Investig Allergol Clin Immunol. 2013;23:309–14.
77. Valovirta E, Myrseth SE, Palkonen S. The voice of the patients: allergic rhinitis is not a trivial disease. Curr Opin Allergy Clin Immunol. 2008;8:1–9.
78. Gerth van Wijk R. R. Quality of life, should we bother? Allergy. 2003;58:284–6.
79. Navarro A, Colas C, Anton E, Conde J, Dávila I, Dordal M, Fernández-Parre B, Ibáñez M, Lluch-Bernal M, Matheu V. Epidemiology of allergic rhinitis in allergy consultations in Spain: alergologica-2005. J Investig Allergol Clin Immunol. 2009;19:7–13.
80. Chancellor J, Aballea S, Lawrence A, Sheldon R, Cure S, Plun-Favreau J, Marchant N. Preferences of patients with diabetes mellitus for inhaled versus injectable insulin regimens. Pharmacoeconomics. 2008;26:217–34.
81. Moock J, Kohlmann T. Comparing preference-based quality-of-life measures: results from rehabilitation patients with musculoskeletal, cardiovascular, or psychosomatic disorders. Qual Life Res. 2008;17:485–95.
82. Moller AH, Erntoft S, Vinding GR, Jemec GB. A systematic literature review to compare quality of life in psoriasis with other chronic diseases using EQ-5D-derived utility values. Patient Relat Outcome Meas. 2015;6:167–77.
83. Rogers G, O'Flynn N. NICE guideline: transient loss of consciousness (blackouts) in adults and young people. Br J Gen Pract. 2011;61:40–2.
84. Sullivan PW, Ghushchyan V. Preference-Based EQ-5D index scores for chronic conditions in the United States. Med Decis Making. 2006;26:410–20.
85. Gillard PJ, Devine B, Varon SF, Liu L, Sullivan SD. Mapping from disease-specific measures to health-state utility values in individuals with migraine. Value Health. 2012;15:485–94.
86. Saarni SI, Viertio S, Perala J, Koskinen S, Lonnqvist J, Suvisaari J. Quality of life of people with schizophrenia, bipolar disorder and other psychotic disorders. Br J Psychiatry. 2010;197:386–94.
87. Malone DC, Lawson KA, Smith DH, Arrighi HM, Battista C. A cost of illness study of allergic rhinitis in the United States. J Allergy Clin Immunol. 1997;99:22–7.
88. Fineman SM. The burden of allergic rhinitis: beyond dollars and cents. Ann Allergy Asthma Immunol. 2002;88:2–7.
89. Blanc PD, Trupin L, Eisner M, Earnest G, Katz PP, Israel L, Yelin EH. The work impact of asthma and rhinitis: findings from a population-based survey. J Clin Epidemiol. 2001;54:610–8.
90. Settipane RA, Schwindt C. Chapter 15: allergic rhinitis. Am J Rhinol Allergy. 2013;27(Suppl 1):S52–5.
91. Halpern MT, Schmier JK, Richner R, Guo C, Togias A. Allergic rhinitis: a potential cause of increased asthma medication use, costs, and morbidity. J Asthma. 2004;41:117–26.
92. Lafeuille MH, Gravel J, Figliomeni M, Zhang J, Lefebvre P. Burden of illness of patients with allergic asthma versus non-allergic asthma. J Asthma. 2013;50:900–7.

4

Different clinical allergological features of *Taenia solium* infestation

Paola Lucia Minciullo[1*], Antonio Cascio[2], Stefania Isola[1] and Sebastiano Gangemi[1,3]

Abstract

The tapeworm *Taenia* (*T.*) *solium* can be responsible for two different conditions: taeniasis and cysticercosis. Helminth infections in human host cause an immune response associated with elevated levels of IgE, tissue eosinophilia and mastocytosis, and with the presence of CD4+ T cells that preferentially produce IL-4, IL-5, and IL-13. Individuals exposed to helminth infections may have allergic inflammatory responses to parasites and parasite antigens. PubMed search of human cases of allergic reactions occurring during *T. solium* infestation was performed combining the terms (allergy, urticaria, angioedema, asthma, anaphylaxis) with *T. solium*. A study was considered eligible for inclusion in the review if it reported data on patients with *T. solium* infestation who had signs or symptoms of allergy. In literature we found six articles reporting the association between an allergic reaction and *T. solium* infestation: two cases of urticaria, two cases of relapsing angioedema, one case of asthma and two cases of anaphylaxis. Despite the large diffusion of *T. solium* infestation, we found only a few cases of concomitant allergic reaction and the presence of Taenia in the host. The association between *T. solium* infestation and allergic manifestations has never been clearly demonstrated, and in absence of a well-documented causality the hypotheses are merely speculative. Therefore, the association between Taenia infection and allergy needs to be thoroughly studied to better clarify if this association may really exist and which is the pathogenetic mechanism supported.

Keywords: Allergy, Anaphylaxis, Angioedema, Asthma, Cysticercosis, Urticaria, *Taenia solium*

Background

The tapeworm *Taenia* (*T.*) *solium* can be responsible for two different conditions: taeniasis and cysticercosis. Taeniasis is infection with an adult tapeworm, while cysticercosis is infection with larval stages (of *T. solium*) in body tissues. Taeniasis occurs only in the human host, after ingestion of undercooked pork infected with cysticerci. In taeniasis an adult worm is present in the intestine, and the infestation is usually asymptomatic and generally recognized when segments of proglottids are found in stool specimens. Cysticercosis is caused by ingestion of food contaminated with feces, or by autoinfection. In the latter case, a human infected with adult *T. solium* can ingest eggs produced by that tapeworm, either through fecal contamination or, possibly, from proglottids carried into the stomach by reverse peristalsis. Once eggs are ingested, oncospheres hatch in the intestine invade the intestinal wall, and migrate to striated muscles, as well as the brain, liver, and other tissues, where they develop into cysticerci. Cysticercus consists of a fluid-filled bladder elongate and oval, measuring 5–15 mm with a single protoscolex [1–3]. Cysticercosis of the human nervous system, called neurocysticercosis, may cause different clinical manifestations based on the characteristics of the parasites and the inflammatory response of the host. The intraparenchymal neurocysticercosis mainly causes seizures, whereas the subarachnoid infection with parasite infiltration cause hydrocephalus that may be fatal [4].

Diagnosis of cysticercosis is based on a combination of clinical presentation, imaging findings, history of exposure, and serologic testing as the detection of IgG antibodies to *T. solium* using an ELISA technique. In neurocysticercosis the neuroimaging techniques are considered the gold standard for the diagnosis. However, the detection of specific antibodies against *T. solium*

*Correspondence: pminciullo@unime.it
[1] School and Division of Allergy and Clinical Immunology, Department of Clinical and Experimental Medicine, University Hospital "G. Martino", Messina, Italy
Full list of author information is available at the end of the article

cysticercal antigens in cerebrospinal fluid may be a useful adjunctive diagnostic test. A high rate of patients with neurocysticercosis presents specific IgE and IgG (especially IgG4) that is indicative of intrathecal antibody production [5].

The human immune response to helminth infections is associated with several immunomodulatory mechanisms that can have different and sometime opposite consequences. Asymptomatic carriers often present immunologic hyporesponsiveness and altered cytokine profiles favoring Interleukin (IL)-4 over inflammatory mediators such as IFN-γ and with a prominent role played by IL-10 and TGF-β. On the contrary, patients who develop a symptomatic disease, present loss of the immune tolerance with predominance of Th1 and Th17 responses.

Dendritic cell antigen presentation, B cell antibody production, and epithelial cell alarmin release are other pathways of immune activation suppressed during helminth infection. On the contrary, T regulatory (Treg) and Breg cell differentiation is induced.

Thus, the immunomodulation caused by helminth infection can be useful for the host in protecting from allergic, autoimmune and inflammatory diseases, but, at the same time could be dangerous in reducing tumor immunosurveillance, depending on the characteristics of the parasite, the clinical course of the subject and the chronicity of infection [6].

The inverse association between helminth infection and allergy, first postulated by Bell in 1996 [7] is, today, largely assumed. The global increase in allergy especially in urban areas has led researchers to propose a modified hygiene hypothesis in which the decline in helminth infections is associated with an increase in allergic diseases [8].

However, very little data are available to explain how helminth infection might protect against allergy.

Allergy and helminths induce strongly Th2-skewed responses associated with cytokines such as IL-4, IL-5, and IL-13, with mastocytosis, eosinophilia, and antibody class-switching to produce IgE. However, the two conditions are completely different. Allergy occurs in predisposed people and is due to a polygenic disorder associated with Th2 responses and IgE expression, whereas the Th2 activation during helminth infection is a normal physiological reaction. Moreover, this response is moderated by helminths with the induction of Treg and Breg cells and the production of immunoregulatory cytokines and IgG4 that contrast IgE [9].

However, some helminth infections, especially by *Ascaris lumbricoides* and *Anisakis simplex* are associated with an increased incidence of allergic diseases, such as asthma, allergic rhinoconjunctivitis, atopic dermatitis, chronic urticaria, until to anaphylaxis [10–14]. This is probably due to a cross-reactivity between helminth proteins, as tropomyosin, and specific allergens, especially in *A. lumbricoides* infection [9, 15].

The aim of our study was to depict the different clinical allergological features of *T. solium* infestation.

Literature review

PubMed search of human cases of allergic reactions occurring during *T. solium* infestation was performed combining the terms (allergy, urticaria, angioedema, asthma, anaphylaxis) with *T. solium*. A study was considered eligible for inclusion in the review if it reported data on patients with *T. solium* infestation who had signs or symptoms of allergy.

Results

In literature we found six articles reporting the association between an allergic reaction and *T. solium* infestation: two cases of urticaria, two cases of relapsing angioedema, one case of asthma and two cases of anaphylaxis (Table 1).

Urticaria

Gupta et al. [16] described a case of a 44-year-old woman with a history of urticaria of 1 month duration. No relevant causes of urticaria were established. The patient was treated with antihistamines with a partial response. Subsequently, she presented a painful swelling over right cheek treated with antibiotics without resolution. The patient presented also mild eosinophilia. Ultrasonography on the swelling region revealed the presence of intramuscular cysticercosis with surrounding phlegmon. The woman was treated with albendazole 15 mg/kg for 1 month, initially associated to steroids to reduce inflammatory response. After treatment the Authors observed a reduction in the size of the swelling with no more

Table 1 Different allergic manifestation associated to *Taenia solium* infestation

Allergic manifestation	Sex	Age (years)	Nationality	Reference
Urticaria	Female	44	Indian	Gupta et al. [16]
Urticarial vasculitis	Male	36	Ecuadorian	Shaigany et al. [17]
Angioedema	Female	2	Italian	Accomando et al. [18]
	Male	4	Italian	
Asthma	Female	35	Mexican	Rodríguez Orozco [19]
Anaphylaxis	Male	20	Indian	Singh et al. [20]
	Male	26	Italian	Minciullo et al. [1]

evidence of active cysticercosis in the muscle and also the resolution of urticaria.

A case of urticarial vasculitis associated to neurocysticercosis has been reported [17]. A 36-year-old man presented afebrile seizure and a 3- to 4-month history of intermittent pruritic widespread rash associated with a burning sensation. He had edematous plaques and scattered erythematous papules on both posterior thighs. Skin biopsy showed leukocytoclastic vasculitis, leading to a diagnosis of urticarial vasculitis. The patient presented a cystic lesion in his brain with degenerating cysticercus. Despite the serum antibody testing for cysticercosis was negative and cysticercosis immunoglobulin (Ig)G antibodies had undetectable levels in cerebrospinal fluid, the clinical feature, the exam of the cystic lesion and the MRI images fulfilled the criteria of neurocysticercosis. The patient was treated with albendazole 400 mg twice daily and his urticarial vasculitis resolved within a few days.

Angioedema

Two cases of angioedema related to cysticercosis have been reported by the same Authors [18]. The patients, a 2-year-old female and a 4-year-old male, presented a history of relapsing and migrant angioedema in the upper and lower limbs and in the body trunk and the female patient in the genital region also. The angioedema was associated to prurigo and rash. Blood and stool parasitological exams were normal except for hypereosinophilia; skin prick test for the most common inhalant and food allergens was negative. Test for cysticercosis showed high positivity, however, no presence of *T. solium* cyst was found. Treatment with albendazole 5 mg/kg every 8 h for 4 months led to normal levels of eosinophils and to the disappearance of angioedema.

Asthma

A case of asthma exacerbation related to neurocysticercosis has been reported by Rodriguez Orozco [19]. A 35-year-old female with a 2 years history of mild asthma presented headache, nausea, vomiting and an episode of convulsion in the last 3 months. The electroencephalogram and the neurological evaluation were normal. During the last 2 months the patient presented nocturnal dyspnea, wheezing and a worsening of headache and nausea and she needed hospitalization. She was treated with inhalant corticosteroids and beta-agonists, antileukotrienes and oral corticosteroids. Because of headache and nausea persisted, the patient underwent cerebral tomography that showed the presence of two parenchymal cysts. One was a colloidal cyst interpreted as cyst with a dying parasite, the other one as a dead cyst. The Author concluded that the neurological manifestations were linked to the parasite death. Since asthma exacerbation and neurological symptoms appearance were concomitant, the Author hypothesized that the two entities were related, however, it is difficult to establish in this case if neurocysticercosis is a concomitant event or a trigger factor for asthma exacerbation.

Anaphylaxis

Two case of anaphylaxis related to *T. solium* infestation have been reported [1, 20]. The first was a 20-year-old man who presented with sudden onset of transient generalized urticarial rashes, hypogastric pain that spread to the whole of the abdomen, vomiting, watery diarrhoea and fever of 6 h duration. He also exhibited tachycardia, hypotension, diffuse abdominal tenderness, and rigidity. A diagnosis of appendicular perforation with pelvic collection was made and exploratory laparotomy was normal except for the presence of colourless, odourless gelatinous material in the pelvis. The appendix was histopathologically normal and the histopathological examination of this fluid showed cysticercosis presence. The patient was treated with albendazole 15 mg/kg for 28 days and no other signs of Taenia infestation were present in the follow-up.

The Authors hypothesized a rupture of a cyst in the peritoneal cavity that led to the anaphylactic reaction and the gelatinous content of the cyst caused a peritoneal inflammation mimicking the secondary peritonitis of appendicular perforation [20].

A case of fatal anaphylaxis has been reported by our group [1]. A 26-year-old male died during sleep and death did not seem linked to any previous known diseases. The cadaveric and histologic examinations and the necroscopy concluded that the cause of death was anaphylactic reaction. Specifically, swelling of the larynx, mucous plugging in the airways, pulmonary emphysema, visceral congestion, and splenic eosinophilia supported an allergic reaction. Moreover, in the intestinal loops several meters of a tapeworm with a long series of proglottids were found the worm was identified as *T. solium*.

The most common causes of anaphylaxis (drugs, foods, insect sting) were excluded by interviews with the man's relatives, external examination of the body, and cadaveric examination.

The Authors hypothesized an autoinfection of larval forms by ingestion of eggs present on the man's dirty hands or by reverse peristalsis had occurred and the larval forms developed into cysticercosal cysts. The rupture of a unknown cyst may have triggered the anaphylaxis. At the time of necroscopy, cysticercosal cysts were not searched in the examined tissues, but the presence of *T. solium* in the intestine, the pathologic findings at autopsy, and the absence of other possible causes of anaphylaxis make the association between anaphylaxis and cysticercosis plausible.

Discussion

The association between allergic diseases, especially urticaria, and infectious diseases has been discussed for >100 years [11]. Several chronic persistent bacterial [21], viral [22], parasitic [10, 14] infections have been suspected to trigger allergic symptoms, ranging from urticaria to anaphylaxis.

Taenia solium infestation is endemic in countries in Sub-Saharan Africa, Latin America and Asia where conditions such as inadequate hygiene, poor sanitary conditions, open defecation, free roaming pigs and poverty permit the transmission of the disease [23]. However, three recent reviews indicate that autochthonous human *T. solium* taeniasis/cysticercosis may be possible in Europe [24–26], but current peer reviewed literature is biased towards Western Europe [27].

In this review we reported allergic manifestations related to Taenia infestation. Despite the large diffusion of *T. solium* infestation, we found only seven cases of concomitant allergic reaction and the presence of Taenia in the host. The clinical allergological manifestations reported in these cases are various, including urticaria, angioedema, asthma and anaphylaxis. Moreover, it is interesting to highlight that two cases are reported from India [16, 20], one from Mexico [19], one from USA but the patient was from Ecuador [17], and three from Italy [1, 18].

The association between *T. solium* infestation and allergic manifestations has never been clearly demonstrated, therefore, in absence of a well-documented causality the hypotheses are merely speculative. In some cases the connection between the infection and the allergic reaction is supported by the resolution of the allergic symptoms after surgery and albendazole treatment [16–18]; in other cases it is uncertain if there was just a coexistence of Taenia infection and allergy or if parasite infection was a trigger factor for allergic manifestations.

In any case, the rarity of the co-occurrence of the two entities remains unclear, since helminth infections are usually associated with low rate of allergies. However, in some infections (especially *A. lumbricoides* and *A. simplex*), allergic diseases are increased; this is sometime linked to a cross-reactivity between worm proteins and specific allergens, especially in *A. lumbricoides* infection [9, 15]. Nevertheless, this mechanism has not been observed in Taenia infection.

Therefore, the association between Taenia infection and allergy needs to be thoroughly studied to better clarify if this association may really exist and which is the pathogenetic mechanism supported.

Abbreviations

T.: *Taenia*; Ig: immunoglobulin; IL: interleukin; IFN-γ: interferon-γ; Th: T helper; Treg: T regulatory cells; Breg: B regulatory cells.

Authors' contributions

PLM and SG made substantial contributions to conception and design of this review and participated in critical revision and drafting of final version of the manuscript. AC and SI participated in literature search, acquisition of data and manuscript writing. All authors read and approved the final manuscript.

Author details

[1] School and Division of Allergy and Clinical Immunology, Department of Clinical and Experimental Medicine, University Hospital "G. Martino", Messina, Italy. [2] Department of Health Promotion Sciences and Mother and Child Care "G. D'Alessandro", University of Palermo, Palermo, Italy. [3] Institute of Applied Sciences and Intelligent Systems (ISASI), Messina Unit, Messina, Italy.

References

1. Minciullo PL, Ventura Spagnolo E, Cascio A, Cardia G, Gangemi S. Fatal anaphylactic shock and *Taenia solium* infestation: a possible link? Ann Allergy Asthma Immunol. 2009;103:449–50.
2. Markel EK, Voge M, John DT. Medical parasitology. 7th ed. Philadelphia: WB Saunders Co; 1992. p. 226–60.
3. Garcia HH, Gonzales AE, Evans CA, Gilman RH. *Taenia solium* cysticercosis. Lancet. 2003;362:547–56.
4. Garcia HH, Rodriguez S, Friedland JS, Cysticercosis Working Group in Peru. Immunology of *Taenia solium* taeniasis and human cysticercosis. Parasite Immunol. 2014;36:388–96.
5. Suzuki LA, Rossi CL. Evaluation of cysticercus-specific IgG (total and subclasses) and IgE antibody responses in cerebrospinal fluid samples from patients with neurocysticercosis showing intrathecal production of specific IgG antibodies. Arq Neuropsiquiatr. 2013;71:106–9.
6. Maizels RM, McSorley HJ. Regulation of the host immune system by helminth parasites. J Allergy Clin Immunol. 2016;138:666–75.
7. Bell RG. IgE, allergies and helminth parasites: a new perspective on an old conundrum. Immunol Cell Biol. 1996;74:337–45.
8. Rook GAW. Review series on helminths, immunemodulation and the hygiene hypothesis: the broader implications of the hygiene hypothesis. Immunology. 2009;126:3–11.
9. Fitzsimmons CM, Falcone FH, Dunne DW. Helminth allergens, parasite-specific IgE, and its protective role in human immunity. Front Immunol. 2014;5:61.
10. Wördemann M, Diaz RJ, Heredia LM, et al. Association of atopy, asthma, allergic rhinoconjunctivitis, atopic dermatitis and intestinal helminth infections in Cuban children. Trop Med Int Health. 2008;13:180–6.
11. Wedi B, Raap U, Wieczorek D, Kapp A. Urticaria and infections. Allergy Asthma Clin Immunol. 2009;5:10.
12. Oberholzer C, Nüesch R, Häusermann P. Urticaria and parasites: case report and general view over the most common pathogens of chronic urticaria. Praxis. 2007;96:865–70.
13. Ronellenfitsch U, Bircher A, Hatz C, Blum J. Parasites as a cause of urticaria. Helminths and protozoa as triggers of hives? Hautarzt. 2007;58(133–134):136–41.
14. Minciullo PL, Cascio A, David A, Pernice LM, Calapai G, Gangemi S. Anaphylaxis caused by helminths: review of the literature. Eur Rev Med Pharmacol Sci. 2012;16:1513–8.
15. Santiago HC, Bennuru S, Boyd A, Eberhard M, Nutman TB. Structural and immunologic cross-reactivity among filarial and mite tropomyosin: implications for the hygiene hypothesis. J Allergy Clin Immunol. 2011;127:479–86.

16. Gupta S, Gupta S, Mittal A, Mahendra A, Aggarwal A, Batra R, et al. A rare manifestation of cysticercosis infestation. Acta Med Indones. 2004;46:54–7.
17. Shaigany S, Dabela E, Teich AF, Husain S, Grossman ME. Resolution of urticarial vasculitis after treatment of neurocysticercosis. J Am Acad Dermatol. 2015;72:e32–3.
18. Accomando S, Caserta M, Trizzino A, Amato GM. Two strange cases of hypereosinophilia and child's relapsing angio-oedema. Pediatr Med Chir. 2003;25:367–9.
19. Rodríguez Orozco AR. Neurocysticercosis and asthma. Triggering or concomitant situation. Rev Alerg Mex. 2004;51:36–8.
20. Singh RB, Pavithran NM, Bakshi N. Intraperitoneal rupture of cysticercosal cyst mimicking appendicular perforation. Trop Doct. 2006;36:180–1.
21. Minciullo PL, Cascio A, Barberi G, Gangemi S. Urticaria and bacterial infections. In: Allergy and asthma proceedings, vol. 35, no. 4. Cleveland: OceanSide Publications, Inc.; 2014. p. 295–302.
22. Imbalzano E, Casciaro M, Quartuccio S, Minciullo PL, Cascio A, Calapai G, et al. Association between urticaria and virus infections: a systematic review. In: Allergy and asthma proceedings, vol. 37, no. 1. Cleveland: OceanSide Publications, Inc.; 2016. p. 18–22.
23. Coral-Almeida M, Gabriël S, Abatih EN, Praet N, Benitez W, Dorny P. *Taenia solium* human cysticercosis: a systematic review of sero-epidemiological data from endemic zones around the world. PLoS Negl Trop Dis. 2014;9:e0003919.
24. Del Brutto OH. Neurocysticercosis in Western Europe: a re-emerging disease? Acta Neurol Belg. 2012;112:335–43.
25. Zammarchi L, Strohmeyer M, Bartalesi F, Bruno E, Muñoz J, Buonfrate D, et al. Epidemiology and management of cysticercosis and *Taenia solium* taeniasis in Europe, systematic review 1990–2011. PLoS ONE. 2013;8:e69537.
26. Fabiani S, Bruschi F. Neurocysticercosis in Europe: still a public health concern not only for imported cases. Acta Trop. 2013;128:18–26.
27. Devleesschauwer B, Allepuz A, Dermauw V, Johansen MV, Laranjo-González M, Smit GS, et al. *Taenia solium* in Europe: still endemic? Acta Trop. 2015. doi:10.1016/j.actatropica.2015.08.006.

5

Hypersensitivity reactions due to black henna tattoos and their components: are the clinical pictures related to the immune pathomechanism?

Gianfranco Calogiuri[1], Elisabetta Di Leo[2], Lavjay Butani[3], Stefano Pizzimenti[4], Cristoforo Incorvaia[5], Luigi Macchia[6] and Eustachio Nettis[6*]

Abstract

Hypersensitivity to para-phenylenediamine (PPD) and related compounds induced by temporary black henna tattoos has become a serious health problem worldwide. Different patterns of sensitization with various clinical aspects are described in literature due to PPD associated to henna tattoo and these manifestations are likely correlated with the immunological and dermatological pathomechanisms involved. Henna is the Persian name of the plant *Lawsonia inermis,* Fam. *Lythraceae.* It is a woody shrub that grow in regions of North Africa, South Asia, India and Sri Lanka. Nowadays it is rather frequent to see temporary "tattoos" performed with henna. To make tattoos darker and long-lasting PPD has been associated to henna in tattoo drawings mixtures, so obtaining "*black henna*". In these years there has been a rise of contact sensitization to PPD and in medical literature an increased number of cases have been reported on temporary henna tattoo application. Here we review the various clinical patterns related to PPD and henna tattoo, to investigate the possible link between clinic-morphological pictures and the immunological response to PPD and henna. The literature underlines that different clinical manifestations are related to black henna containing PPD, and its derivative products may cause delayed-type as well as immediate-type reactions. Further studies are needed to investigate the relationship between clinical and morphological aspects of PPD contact dermatitis and the T cell subsets predominance.

Keywords: Para-phenylenediamine, Henna tattoo, Black henna, Contact dermatitis, Allergy

Background

The term "tattoo" derives from two Polynesians words, "TA", which means "to draw" and "TOO" or "TAU" which means "spirit". The whole word means "draw the body". The tattooing procedures have been quite variable in different ages, depending on the cultures involved and thus influencing the perception of a positive or a negative significance. The Hebrews follow Torah exhortations ("you won't make any incision on your body", Deuteronomy, 14 but also Leviticus, 19:28) while for the Maoris the tattoo drawings on the face indicate the social class and status, the profession, the clan and the ability in a battle [1].

Nowadays, in a "liquid society" [2], where nothing is forever, it has become rather frequent to see temporary "tattoos" performed with henna. Painless, highly decorative and, above all, temporary, the henna colour lasts for up to 3 weeks, making it is the perfect way of creating a fashionable look while avoiding the consequences or risks connected to a permanent tattoo.

Henna is the Persian name of the plant *Lawsonia inermis,* Fam. *Lythraceae.* It is a woody shrub, reaching heights up to 3 metres, which grows up mainly in the warm, moist regions of North Africa, South Asia, India

*Correspondence: ambulatorio.allergologia@uniba.it
[6] Section of Allergy and Clinical Immunology, Department of Internal Medicine and Infectious Diseases, University of Bari Medical School, Bari, Italy
Full list of author information is available at the end of the article

and Sri Lanka. Henna plant was identified by Linnaeus, who called it with that name to honour the Scottish doctor of his scientific expedition, Isaac Lawson. The active dying ingredient of henna is a naphtoquinone called *lawsone* (2-hydroxy-1,4-naphthoquinone), constituting about 1% by weight of the crushed leaves [3].

Commercially, henna is available as a green powder, obtained from crushing dried leaves mixed with water and oil to create a paste. Natural henna gives a brownish-orange pigment to the skin when applied (*red henna*), but the colour will darken to brown. Various substances, such as lemon oil, vinegar, eucalyptus oil and coffee, may be added to obtain different colouring effects and a thick paste [4]. The henna is left on the skin to dry for at least 2 h and preferably up to 24 h. The longer henna is put in contact with the skin, the darker the resulting colour will be [3]. As far as allergic reactions are concerned [5, 6], the pure henna is a weak sensitizer and it is poorly responsible for allergic contact dermatitis [7–9], but when para-phenylenediamine (PPD), that is a strong sensitizing agent, is added the frequency of allergic reactions increases. PPD is responsible for professional contact hypersensitivity in photographers, hairdressers and workers manipulating rubber components [10]. PPD can induce different types of hypersensitivity reactions, which may be framed from different points of view, according to the time-pattern onset or according to their morphological aspects.

Methods

We reviewed the available literature concerning the clinical presentations, the morphological pictures associated to allergy to black henna and the immunological mechanisms underlying the allergic reactions.

Results

Clinical manifestations related to a time-pattern onset

Generally, the first signs of allergic contact dermatitis caused by black henna tattoos develop within 1–3 days in those already sensitized, and within 4–14 days in patients who become sensitized by the tattoo [5]. In 2002 Chung et al. suggested that patients sensitized to black henna tattoo should be divided into 2 groups according to their clinical course, that may be acute or subacute. This classification was based on the previous studies of Buckley on photographers [11].

Thus, the clinical features define 2 groups: an acute response to temporary tattooing, typically presenting with intense eczematous responses within 1–2 days of tattooing, and a subacute response, that is, developing lichenoid eruptions slowly in 1–2 weeks [11].

Some reactions may appear 45 days later following the henna tattoo application [12], but sometimes cutaneous reactions may appear few hours following henna tattoo [13, 14]. The latter possibility is caused by a pre-existing sensitization to PPD, probably due to a hidden exposure to cross-reactive compounds belonging to the para-amino group substances [15].

For this reason, beyond the 2 groups identified by Chung et al. there is a third group of patients, whose symptoms onset occurs few hours after a clear exposure to PPD. Their clinical history often includes a previous black henna tattoo, performed months or years ago, which behaves like a silent promoter of sensitization to PPD.

In patients with a silent sensitization to PPD, localized cutaneous manifestations are usually represented by a severe inflammatory dermatitis leading to skin ulcerations following a further henna tattoo [14, 15], but even by a contact urticaria [16] or a contact anaphylaxis due to henna tattoo [17] or henna hair dye [18].

Such clinical expressions are based on a IgE-mediated reaction to vegetable components of henna, and particularly specific IgE towards a 25 kDa henna protein have been detected by immunoblotting [19]. However, when applied as a hair dye, PPD alone with no henna components has been responsible for immediate-type contact anaphylaxis [20–22] or for delayed-type anaphylactic reaction [23], rarely even with a fatal outcome [24].

Another kind of hypersensitivity reactions to PPD is represented by a severe facial angioedema, appearing few hours after a dark hair painting in patients who have previously performed a black henna tattoo [25–27]. This is an acute, severe and even life-threatening condition, sometimes requiring an admission in an Intensive Care Unit [25, 28, 29], because of the involvement of the upper airways frequently in young patients [30–32].

Interestingly, people poisoned by PPD ingestion for suicidal purposes [33, 34] or intoxicated by an extensive black henna tattoo application [35, 36] or by a hair dye [36, 37] show clinical signs of rhabdomyolysis, anemia and acute renal failure always associated to a severe angioneurotic oedema of the upper airway accompanied by a swollen, dry, hard, and protruding tongue.

Morphological clinical pictures

As far as morphological clinical pictures are concerned, they appear to be more various and heterogeneous than time-pattern contact allergy manifestations (Table 1). Thus, beyond the aforementioned urticaria and angioedema or contact anaphylaxis related to black henna tattoo painting and the classical eczematous contact dermatitis [38, 39], have been described lichenoid eruptions [11, 40, 41], lymphomatoid reactions [42, 43], vesicular-bullous lesions [44], which may be very painful and invalidating [45, 46], and erythema multiforme like eruptions

Table 1 Reactions to black henna tattoo: main clinical manifestations and time to onset after the application

Clinical manifestation	Time to onset	Ref
Eczematous contact dermatitis	1–2 days	[11, 49, 50]
Lichenoid eruptions	1–2 weeks	[11, 51, 52]
Contact urticaria and angioneurotic oedema	Few hours–2 days	[19, 33, 34]
Contact anaphylaxis	Few hours	[20]
Lymphomatoid reactions	Few hours–few days	[53, 54]
Vesicular-bullous lesions	1–4 days	[55, 56]
Erythema multiforme like eruptions	2–14 days	[58–60]
Sweet syndrome	3 days	[63]
Wells syndrome	3 days	[64, 65]
Prurigo nodularis	3 months	[66]
Connubial contact dermatitis	Few days	[67, 68]

[29, 47]. Sometimes, the localized eruption may become generalized and associated to systemic symptoms as fever and malaise [50, 51]. Exceptionally, a Sweet syndrome [52], Wells syndrome [53, 54], prurigo nodularis [55] and connubial contact dermatitis [56, 57] have been also described.

It appears obvious that PPD is able to induce different clinical and morphological pattern as it happens in T-cell mediated drug hypersensitivity reactions [58], although PPD is a contact allergen only. Wolkenstein et al. suggested that detoxification enzymatic pathway defects are involved in toxic epidermal necrolysis and other severe cutaneous pathogenesis, allowing reactive metabolites accumulation for drugs as sulfonamides and anticonvulsant [59].

Because keratinocytes exert metabolic activity with two N-acetyltransferases (NAT) 1 and 2 (NAT2), isoenzymes for PPD in the skin [60], in a further in vitro investigation it has been observed that genotyping for NAT1 and NAT2 polymorphisms performed in 147 PPD-sensitized patients, the rapid acetylator NAT1*10 allele were under-represented in PPD-sensitive patients compared with 200 control subjects [61]. Such study suggests PPD slow acetylators NAT2 patients are more prone to develop an erythema multiforme-like reaction [47–50], i.e. a more serious contact allergy, as well as drug induced severe cutaneous eruptions are more frequently observed in slow acetylators [59]. However, in patients with severe cutaneous drug reactions, an expansion of drug specific cytotoxic T CD8+ cell subset and infiltration in cutaneous lesions has been observed in the immuno-histopathologic specimens [62]; T cells subsets and different cytokine patterns are involved in the variability of clinical pictures in drug induced hypersensitivity reactions [58].

By comparing the available data, PPD seems to be a hapten with a peculiar aspect, because it may behave like a systemic drug to elicit a hypersensitivity response. Actually, in PPD sensitized patients specific PPD T cell clones CD4+ CD8+ secreting Th2 cytokine pattern, as IL-4, IL-5, IL-6, IL-8, IL-10, and IL-13, have been identified and isolated in vitro [63, 64]. This was reported also in mice, because PPD-HSA causes a transient activation of CD8+ cytotoxic cells only [63]. However, because vesicular bullous reactions have been reported in patients with contact hypersensitivity to PPD after henna tattoo application [44–46] and two other patterns of T cell activation by PPD have been evidenced in vitro [63], future researches should investigate the relationship between clinical morphological aspect of PPD contact dermatitis and T-cell subsets predominance.

Discussion and conclusions

Henna has been used traditionally for medicinal purposes and as a cosmetic. For medicinal purposes, it has been used as a bitter tea for stomach or intestinal problems, for fever and headache, as a paste to cure ringworm or nail fungus, to reduce chafing and prevent blisters and to soothe irritated, dry or chapped skin [3]. As a cosmetic, henna has been used as a hair thickener, as a nail colorant and conditioner and as a decorative stain for the body. Also, henna has been used as a brown dye for wool, cotton, and silk [3]. Moreover, henna has great significance in all Eastern wedding traditions, and no wedding is complete without drawing floral motifs or geometric decorations on the bride's hands and feet. The increasing use of henna in the 2000s to make temporary tattoos raised the issue of allergic reactions.

Actually, as reported above, the pure henna is a weak sensitizer, but the addition of PPD to make tattoos darker and long-lasting, thus obtaining *black henna*, using mixtures that are often extemporaneously prepared with a variety of materials and sources and very variables concentrations of PPD resulted in a recent exploit of contact sensitization to PPD. In fact, an increased number of cases have been reported through temporary henna tattoo application. Therefore, dermatologists, paediatricians and allergists have alerted about the rising frequency of black henna contact allergy [5, 6]. We reviewed the various clinical patterns related to PPD and henna tattoo to investigate the possible link between clinic-morphological pictures and the immunological response to PPD and henna. The main results may be summarized in a clinical expression with different manifestations related to black henna containing PPD, and in a spectrum of allergic responses including both delayed-type and immediate-type reactions.

Fadden et al. had previously demonstrated that the allergenic component of PPD accumulates in the skin. Hence, intermittent exposure to low concentration of PPD may be equivalent to a higher concentration in a one-off exposure [65]. Because different studies, performed in USA and in United Arab Emirates, have shown that the presence of PPD high concentrations in henna dye mixture ranges from 2 to 29.5% measured through high performance liquid chromatography method [5, 66, 67], it is not unusual that a single henna tattoo, performed as a summer caprice, may be sufficient to induce a silent or clear PPD sensitization.

Actually, no specific IgE to PPD or any related oxidative product have been identified in vitro, but it has been demonstrated that a radio-labelled PPD containing oxidative hair dye applied to human volunteers for 30 min is eliminated predominantly (80–90%) by renal excretion, being accumulated in urine [68]. Such study showed that there is a systemic absorption of PPD through the skin. Goldberg et al. had previously reported that the oxidation product of PPD causing the immediate-type reaction is N′N′-bis(4-aminophenyl)-2,5-diamino-1,4-quinone-dimine [69], also known as Brandowski base (BB), although they were unable to produce a suitable RAST assay [69]. A further investigation has recently shown that, once penetrated in human body, PPD oxidative products bind irreversibly to cysteine at 34 position on human serum albumin [63], so turning to a complete antigen, but it is unclear whether IgE are directed towards the chemical component only or towards the chemically modified albumin which has become immunogenic. Actually, such an IgE-mediated mechanism has been described only in ethylene oxide hypersensitivity [70].

In suggestive clinical pictures, like the urticarial-angioedema-like contact dermatitis, although the mechanisms appears as an IgE-mediated reaction, actually it is an early onset cell-mediated mechanism [26, 27]. It has been suggested, from experimental studies on animals, that specific T-cells with a Th2 cytokines pattern profile specific to PPD could be the effectors cells of delayed response [71]. However, in vitro studies have suggested that also in humans there is a recruitments and activation of Th2 clones in response to PPD exposure [63].

Padovan et al., in their studies on hypersensitivity to beta-lactams antibiotics, reported that Th1 profile, very common in contact allergy, may shift to a Th2 profile depending on the hapten concentration [72]. Because high concentrations of PPD are present in henna tattoo paintings [16, 67], it is possible that PPD contact dermatitis is mediated by specific Th2 cell clones, secreting interleukin (IL)-4 and IL-5. Such a pathomechanism has been confirmed in vitro by the study of Jenkinson et all [63]. To determine whether PPD–HSA was antigenic, these authors assayed the activity of PPD and PPD–HSA on T-cell proliferation, using the lymphocyte transformation test (LTT) and the proliferation and cytokine secretion profile of CD4+ , CD8+ , and CD4/8 double-positive T-cell clones isolated by stimulating T cells from the blood of allergic volunteers with PPD or PPD–HSA. The investigators confirmed that PPD was active in the LTT and that it stimulated CD4+ , CD8+ , and CD4/8 double-positive T-cell clones with a Th2 profile [63].

Moreover, Pichler et al. elaborated the "pharmacological-immune interaction concept" (p-i concept) as they found that some drugs like sulfamethoxazole and lidocaine can bind directly to the HLA peptide complex stimulating T lymphocytes through an HLA restricted processing and metabolism independent pathway [73].

Some in vitro studies have confirmed that such immunological model is working not only for drugs, but even for some contact allergen like PPD [74]. For this reason, in case of direct exposure to high concentration of PPD, the immune response may happen through the "p-i concept" pathways, while the presence memory T-cell clones CD4+ CD45RO+, previously demonstrated in vitro [38], may accelerate the Th2 immune response in patients undergoing to hair dye painting [25–32].

However, further studies are needed to investigate the relationship between clinical and morphological aspects of PPD contact dermatitis and the T-cell subsets predominance.

These observations confirm that the pure henna is a weak sensitizer poorly responsible for allergic contact dermatitis, while PPD represents a strong sensitizing agent responsible for contact hypersensitivity. PPD can induce hypersensitivity reactions involving various pathogenetic mechanisms that are responsible for the time-pattern onset and for their morphological aspects.

Abbreviations

PPD: paraphenylenediamine; NAT: N-acetyltransferases.

Authors' contributions

GC had the idea of the manuscript and was a major contributor in writing the manuscript. EDL was the co-contributor in writing the manuscript. BL revised the manuscript. SP analyzed the pubmed resources. CI participated in coordination and helped to draft the manuscript. LM analyzed the PubMed resources. EN was the co-contributor in creating and drafting the manuscript. All authors read and approved the final manuscript.

Author details

[1] Pneumology and Allergy Department, Hospital Sacro Cuore, Gallipoli, Lecce, Italy. [2] Section of Allergy and Clinical Immunology, Unit of Internal Medicine-"F. Miulli" Hospital, Acquaviva delle Fonti, Bari, Italy. [3] Department of Pediatrics, University of California Davis School of Medicine, Sacramento, USA. [4] Allergy Outpatients' Clinic, ASL-TO3, Ospedale Civile "E. Agnelli", Pinerolo, Turin, Italy. [5] ASST Specialistic Center Gaetano Pini/CTO, Milan, Italy. [6] Section of Allergy and Clinical Immunology, Department of Internal Medicine and Infectious Diseases, University of Bari Medical School, Bari, Italy.

References

1. Levy J, Sewell M, Goldstein N. Á short history of tattooing. J Dermatol Surg Oncol. 1979;5:851–6.
2. Bauman Z. Liquid modernity. 1st ed. Cambridge: Polity Press; 2000.
3. Semwal RB, Semwal DK, Combrinck S, Cartwright-Jones C, Viljoen A. *Lawsonia inermis* L. (henna): ethnobotanical, phytochemical and pharmacological aspects. J Ethnopharmacol. 2014;155(1):80–103.
4. Lestringant GG, Bener A, Frossard PM. Cutaneous reactions to henna and associated additives. Br J Dermatol. 1999;141:598–600.
5. de Groot AC. Side-effects of henna and semi-permanent 'black henna' tattoos: a full review. Contact Dermat. 2013;69:1–25.
6. Calogiuri G, Foti C, Bonamonte D, Nettis E, Muratore L, Angelini G. Allergic reactions to henna-based temporary tattoos and their components. Immunopharmacol Immunotoxicol. 2010;32:700–4.
7. Thami GP, Kaur S, Kanwar AJ. Allergic contact dermatitis to henna. Allergy. 2001;56:1013–4.
8. Öztaş MO, Önder M, Öztaş P, Atahan Ç. Contact allergy to henna. J Eur Acad Dermatol Venereol. 2001;15:91–2.
9. Polat M, Dikilitaş M, Oztaş P, Alli N. Allergic contact dermatitis to pure henna. Dermatol Online J. 2009;15:15.
10. DeLeo VA. Contact allergen of the year: paraphenylenediamine. Dermatitis. 2006;17:53–5.
11. Chung WH, Chang YC, Yang LJ, Hung SI, Wong WR, Lin YJ, Chan HL. Clinicopathologic features of skin reactions to temporary tattoos and analysis of possible causes. Arch Dermatol. 2002;138:88–92.
12. Pegas JR, Criado PR, Criado RF, Vasconcellos C, Pires MC. Allergic contact dermatitis to temporary tattoo by p-paraphenylenediamine. J Invest Allergol Clin Immunol. 2002;12:62–4.
13. Tosti A, Pazzaglia M, Corzza M, Virgili A. Allergic contact dermatitis caused by mehindi. Contact Dermat. 2000;42:356.
14. Ballard MS. Contact dermatitis after henna skin tattooing. J R Army Med Corps. 2006;152:242–3.
15. Arroyo MP. Black henna tattoo reaction in a person with sulphonamide and benzocaine drug allergies. J Am Acad Dermatol. 2003;48:301–2.
16. Temesvari E. Contact urticaria from paraphenylenediamine. Contact Dermat. 1984;11:125.
17. Abdullah K, McDavidson N. A woman who collapsed after painting her soles. Lancet. 1996;348:658.
18. Cronin E. Immediate type hypersensitivity to henna. Contact Dermat. 1979;5:198–9.
19. Bolhar ST, Mulder M, van Ginkel CJW. IgE mediated allergy to henna. Allergy. 2001;56:248.
20. Mavrolein G, Begishvili B, Frew AJ. Anaphylaxis to hair dye: a case report. Clin Exp Allergy. 1998;28:121–2.
21. Fukunaga T, Kawagoe R, Hozumi H, Kanzaki T. Contact anaphylaxis due to paraphenylenediamine. Contact Dermat. 1996;35:185–6.
22. Pasche-Koo E, French L, Piletta-Zanin PA, Hauser C. Contact urticarial and shock to hair dye. Allergy. 1998;53:904–5.
23. Sahoo B, Handa S, Penchalla K, Kumab H. Contact anaphylaxis due to hair dye. Contact Dermat. 2000;43:244.
24. Belton AL, Chira T. Fatal anaphylactic reaction to hair dye. Am J Forensic Med Pathol. 1997;18:290–2.
25. Shavit I, Hoffmann Y, Shachor-Meyouhas Y, Knaani-Levinz H. Delayed hypersensitivity reaction from black henna tattoo manifesting as severe facial swelling. Am J Emerg Med. 2008;26:515e3–4.
26. Gulen F, Zeyrek D, Altinoz S, Perer E, Demir E, Tanac R. Urticaria and angioneurotic edema due to the temporary henna tattoo. Minerva Ped. 2006;58:583–5.
27. Tukenmez Demirci G, Kivanc Altunay I, Atis G, Kucukunal A. Allergic contact dermatitis mimicking angioedema due to paraphenylenediamine hypersensitivity: a case report. Cutan Ocul Toxicol. 2011;31:1–3.
28. Jasmin ZF, Darling JR, Handley JM. Severe allergic contact dermatitis to paraphenylenediamine in hair dye following sensitization to black henna tattoos. Contact Dermat. 2005;52:116–7.
29. Broides A, Sofer S, Lazar I. Contact dermatitis with severe scalp swelling and upper airway compromise due to black henna hair dye. Pediatr Emerg Care. 2011;27:745–6.
30. Kind F, Scherer K, Bircher AJ. Contact dermatitis to paraphenylenediamine in hair dye following sensitization to black henna tattoos: an ongoing problem. J Deuscht Dermatol Gesel. 2012;10:572–7.
31. Redlick F, DeKoven J. Allergic contact dermatitis to paraphenylenediamine in hair dye after sensitization from black henna tattoos: a report of 6 cases. Can Med Assoc J. 2007;176:445–6.
32. Sosted H, Johanssen JD, Andersen KE, Menné T. Severe allergic hair dye reaction in 8 children. Contact Dermat. 2008;54:87–91.
33. Suliman SM, Homeida M, Aboud OI. Paraphenylenediamine induced acute tubular necrosis following hair dye ingestion. Hum Toxicol. 1983;2:633–5.
34. D'Arcy PF. Fatalities with the use of henna dye. Pharm Intern. 1982;3:217–8.
35. Hashim M, Hamza YO, Yahia B. Poisoning from henna dye and paraphenylenediamine mixtures in children in Karthoum. Ann Trop Pediatr. 1992;12:3–6.
36. Brown JH, Conway B, Hill CM. Chronic renal faiure associated with topical application of paraphenylenediamine. Br J Med. 1987;294:155.
37. Abdelraheem MB, El-Tigani MA, Hassan EG, Ali MA, Mohamed IA, Nazik AE. Acute renal failure owing to paraphenylene diamine hair dye poisoning in Sudanese children. Ann Trop Paediatr. 2009;29:191–6.
38. Le Coz CJ, Lefebvre C, Keller F, Grosshans E. Allergic contact dermatitis caused by skin painting (pseudotattooing) with black henna, a mixture of henna and p-phenylenediamine and its derivatives. Arch Dermatol. 2000;136:1515–7.
39. Jovanovic DL, Slavkovic-Jovanovic MR. Allergic contact dermatitis from temporary henna tattoo. J Dermatol. 2009;36(1):63–5.
40. Rubegni P, Fimiani M, de Aloe G, Andreassi L. Lichenoid reaction to temporary tattoo. Contact Dermat. 2000;42:117–8.
41. Sharma VK, Mandal SK, Sethuraman G, Bakshi NA. Para-phenylenediamine-induced lichenoid eruptions. Contact Dermat. 1999;41:40–1.
42. Calzavara-Pinton P, Capezzera R, Zane C, Brezzi A, Pasolini G, Ubiali A, et al. Lymphomatoid allergic contact dermatitis from para-phenylenediamine. Contact Dermat. 2002;47:173–4.
43. Paley K, Geskin LJ, Zirwas MJ. Cutaneous B-cell pseudolymphoma due to paraphenylenediamine. Am J Dermatopathol. 2006;28:438.
44. Choovichian V, Chatapat L, Piyaphanee W. A Bubble Turtle: bullous contact dermatitis after a black henna tattoo in a backpacker in Thailand. J Travel Med. 2015;22:287–8.
45. Jung P, Seszttak-Greinecker G, Wantke F, Gotz M, Jarisch R, Hemmer W. A painful experience: black henna tattoo causing severe bullous contact dermatitis. Contact Dermat. 2005;54:219–20.
46. Van den Keybus C, Morren MA, Goossens A. Walking difficulties due to an allergic reaction to a temporary tattoo. Contact Dermat. 2008;53:180–1.
47. Barrientos N, Abajo P, de Vega MM, Dominguez J. Erythema multiforme-like eruption following allergic contact dermatitis in response to para-phenylenediamine in a temporary henna tattoo. Int J Dermatol. 2014;53:348–50.
48. Jappe U, Hausen BM, Petzoldt D. Erythema-multiforme-like eruption and depigmentation following allergic contact dermatitis from a paint-on henna tattoo, due to para-phenylenediamine contact hypersensitivity. Contact Dermat. 2001;45:249–50.
49. Sidwell RU, Francis ND, Path FRC, Basarab T, Morar N. Vescicular erythema multiforme like reaction to paraphenylenediamine in a henna tattoo. Pediat Dermatol. 2008;25:201–4.
50. Neri I, Giacomini F, Raone B, Patrizi A. Generalized erythema multiforme after localized allergic dermatitis from dark henna tattoo. Pediatr Dermatol. 2009;26:496.
51. Mohamed M, Nixon R. Severe allergic contact dermatitis induced by paraphenylenediamine in paint-on temporary tattoos. Australas J Dermatol. 2000;41:168–71.

52. Rosmaninho A, Machado S, Amorim I, Lobo I, Selores M. Henna tattoo and Sweet syndrome: a possible relation. Eur J Dermatol. 2009;19:642–3.
53. Nacaroglu HT, Celegen M, Karkıner CS, Günay I, Diniz G, Can D. Eosinophilic cellulitis (Wells' syndrome) caused by a temporary henna tattoo. Postepy Dermatol Allergol. 2014;31:322–4.
54. Lönngren V, Young E, Simanaitis M, Svedman C. Neutrophilic and eosinophilic dermatitis caused by contact allergic reaction to paraphenylenediamine in hair dye. Arch Dermatol. 2012;148:1299–301.
55. Verma P, Yadav P. Paraphenylenediamine dye allergic contact dermatitis of mustache region manifesting as prurigo nodularis-like lesions. Dermatitis. 2014;25:91–2.
56. Lopez IE, Turrentine JE, Cruz PD. Clues to diagnosis of connubial contact dermatitis to paraphenylenediamine. Dermatitis. 2014;25:32–3.
57. Goldenberg A, Matiz C, Eichenfield LF. Religious allergic contact dermatitis. Pediatr Dermatol. 2015;32:191–2.
58. Pichler WJ, Adam J, Daubner B, Gentinetta T, Keller M, Yerly D. Drug hypersensitivity reactions: pathomechanism and clinical symptoms. Med Clin North Am. 2010;94:645–64.
59. Wolkenstein P, Charue D, Laurent P, Revuz J, Roujeau JC, Bagot M. Metabolic predisposition to cutaneous adverse drug reactions. Role in toxic epidermal necrolysis caused by sulfonamides and anticonvulsants. Arch Dermatol. 1995;131:544–51.
60. Kawakubo Y, Merk HF, Masaoudi TA, Sieben S, Blömeke B. N-Acetylation of paraphenylenediamine in human skin and keratinocytes. J Pharmacol Exp Ther. 2000;292:150–5.
61. Blömeke B, Brans R, Coenraads PJ, Dickel H, Bruckner T, Hein DW, et al. Para-phenylenediamine and allergic sensitization: risk modification by N-acetyltransferase 1 and 2 genotypes. Br J Dermatol. 2009;161:1130–5.
62. Rozieres A, Vocanson M, Saïd BB, Nosbaum A, Nicolas JF. Role of T cells in non-immediate allergic drug reactions. Curr Opin Allergy Clin Immunol. 2009;9:305–10.
63. Jenkinson C, Jenkins R, Aleksic M, Pirmoahamed M, Naisbit D, Park BK. Characterization of para-phenylenediamine-albumin binding sites and T-cell responses to hapten modified protein. J Investig Dermatol. 2010;110:732–42.
64. Coulter EV, Jenkinson C, FarrellJ Lavergne SN, Pease C, White A, et al. Measurement of CD4þ and CD8þ T-lymphocyte cytokine secretion and gene expression changes in para- phenylenediamine allergic patients and tolerant individuals. J Investig Dermatol. 2010;130:161–74.
65. White J, Basketter D, Pease C, Sanders D, McFadden J. Intermittent exposure to low concentration paraphenylenediamine can be equivalent to single higher-dose exposure. Contact Dermat. 2007;56:262–5.
66. Brancaccio RR, Brown LH, Chang YT, Fogelman JP, Mafong EA, Cohen DE. Identification and quantification of para-phenylenediamine in a temporary black henna tattoo. Am J Contact Dermat. 2002;13:15–8.
67. Al Suwaidi A, Ahmed H. Determination of paraphenylenediamine (PPD) in henna in the United Arab Emirates. Int J Environ Res Public Health. 2010;7:1681–93.
68. Hueber-Becker F, Nohyneck G, Meuling W, Beneech-Keffer F, Toutain H. Human systemic exposure to a 14-C-paraphenylenediamine containing oxidative hair dye and correlation with in vitro percutaneous absorption in human or pig skin. Food Chem Toxicol. 2004;42:1227–36.
69. Goldberg JB, Herman FF, Hirata I. Systemic anaphylaxis due to an oxidation product of para-phenylenediamine in hair dye. Ann Allergy. 1987;7:38–40.
70. Grammer LC, Paterson BF, Roxe D, Daugirdas JT, Ing TS, Ivanovich PT, et al. IgE against ethylene oxide-altered human serum albumin in patients with anaphylactic reactions to dialysis. J Allergy Clin Immunol. 1985;7:511–4.
71. Yokozeki H, Wu MH, Sumi K, Igawa Y, Miyazaki Y, Katayama I, et al. Th2 cytokines, IgE and mast cells play a crucial role in the induction of paraphenylenediamine induced contact hypersensitivity in mice. Clin Exp Immunol. 2003;132:385–92.
72. Padovan E, von Greyerz S, Pichler WJ, Weltzien HU. Antigen-dependent and -independent IFN-gamma modulation by penicillins. J Immunol. 1999;162:1171–7.
73. Zanni M, von Greyter S, Schneyder B, Wendland T, Pichler WJ. Allele unrestricted presentation of lidocaine by HLA DR molecules to alpha/beta+ T cells clones. Int Immunol. 1998;10:507–15.
74. Sieben S, Kawakubo Y, Al Masaoudi T, Merk HF, Blomeke B. Delayed type hypersensitivity reaction to para-phenylenediamine is mediated by 2 different pathways of antigen recognition by specific alpha/beta human T cell clones. J Allergy Clin Immunol. 2002;109:1003–11.

6

Different co-sensitizations could determine different risk assessment in peach allergy? Evaluation of an anaphylactic biomarker in Pru p 3 positive patients

Carina Gabriela Uasuf[1], Danilo Villalta[2], Maria Elisabetta Conte[2], Caterina Di Sano[1], Maria Barrale[3], Vincenzo Cantisano[3], Elisabetta Pace[1], Mark Gjomarkaj[1], Sebastiano Gangemi[4*] and Ignazio Brusca[3]

Abstract

Background: In Italy, the nsLTP (Pru p 3) has been identified as the most frequent cause of food allergy and anaphylaxis. In order to estimate the risk assessment in peach allergy, we investigated the presence of correlations between the levels of sIgE to Pru p 3 with the severity of the clinical symptoms in two Pru p 3 positive populations from two different areas of Italy.

Methods: 133 consecutively Pru p 3 positive patients were recruited from South Italy, where the prevalence of PR-10 and profilin sensitization is low, and from North-East Italy, where the sensitization to pathogenesis related protein -10 (PR-10) and profilin is higher. Skin prick test (SPT) to peach extract and sIgE to peach panallergens were performed.

Results: All 133 patients were positive to SPT to peach extract and to sIgE to Pru p 3. The North-East population was simultaneously positive to Pru p 1 (42.8 %) and Pru p 4 (12.7 %), while no Southern patients were positive to PR-10 or to profilin. A significant difference in the levels of sIgE to Pru p 3 was found only in South Italy Pru p 3 + patients vs. asymptomatic patients ($p = 0.01$) and in mild reactions vs. severe reactions ($p = 0.0008$). In South Italy patients, it was also found a significant correlation between the severity of the clinical reaction and the levels of sIgE to Pru p 3 ($p = 0.001$).

Conclusion: Level of sIgE to Pru p 3 indicates the possibility of development a severe food allergic reaction. Pru p 3 positive patients from different geographical areas and with different co-sensitizations to Pru p 1 and/or Pru p 4 could have a different risk assessment in peach allergy.

Keywords: nsLTP, Peach allergy, sIgE to Pru p 3, Anaphylactic biomarker, Risk assessment, Co-sensitization, Molecular allergy based diagnosis

Background

The possibility to predict, by in vitro approaches, the development of symptoms related to food allergy (FA) has been studied by different research groups and several data have been published focusing on this point. Interestingly, some results have demonstrated that the levels of specific IgE (sIgE) for food allergens can be considered a reliable marker of a positive "in vivo" challenge test. [1–3]. Currently, the risk assessment of FA can be predicted in a more accurate way since the development of the molecular allergy based diagnosis, although it's still not possible to distinguish between patients who are asymptomatic from those symptomatic.

In FA, the molecular allergy based diagnosis has the peculiarity of identify different type of sensitizations depending on the geographical area. For example, it has been shown that the sensitization to the panallergen

*Correspondence: gangemis@unime.it
[4] School and Division of Allergy and Clinical Immunology, Department of Clinical and Experimental Medicine, University of Messina, Messina, Italy
Full list of author information is available at the end of the article

non-specific lipid transfer protein (nsLTP) increases from North Europe to the Mediterranean area, while the sensitization to the pathogenesis related protein-10 (PR-10) increases in the opposite direction. By contrast, the frequency of sensitization to profilin is almost invariable.

Several studies showed that Pru p 3, the peach nsLTP, is the more frequent cause of food-induced allergy and anaphylaxis in Italy [4–6]. The clinical manifestations of nsLTP sensitization range from those of minor entity, like contact itch or oral allergic syndrome (OAS), to anaphylactic shock. [7].

The sensitization to this heat and proteolytic digestion resistant protein is potentially very dangerous [8]. Cross reactions between peach nsLTP and nsLTP from other foods, have been described with other members of the Rosaceae family, seed, nuts, cereals, and other foods from plant origin [9–19].

The relationship between the levels of sIgE, the severity of the clinical reactions and the presence of symptoms with foods containing nsLTP different from peach, is presently controversial [20–23].

In consideration of the potential hazard of the sensitization to Pru p 3, it is evident how important is to identify a biomarker able to predict both the severity of an allergic reaction and the potential cross reactions with other nsLTP foods.

The aim of this study was to investigate a possible correlation between an anaphylactic biomarker, such as sIgE to Pru p 3, with the severity of symptoms in two Pru p 3 sensitized populations from different geographical areas of Italy. In addition, we performed the ROC curve analysis of the sIgE to Pru p 3 in order to identify patients at a higher risk of anaphylaxis and compare our results with the data published in literature.

Methods

Patients

133 consecutively allergic patients who attended the observation were recruited. A common selection criteria was used in all participating center: (a) clear history of an allergic reaction after being in contact with/or after the consumption of peach, (b) skin prick test (SPT) positive to peach extract, (c) positive sIgE to Pru p 3, (d) positive oral open food challenge or in case the challenge could not been performed, a well-documented severe allergy had been exhibited, e) patients positive to SPT to peach and to sIgE to Pru p 3 but asymptomatic. None of the patients were under oral corticosteroid or antihistamine.

All 71 patients who attended the outpatient Allergy Unit of C.N.R. and Buccheri La Ferla Hospital were born and live in Palermo (South Italy). All 62 patients who attended the outpatient Allergy Unit of Santa Maria degli Angeli Hospital were born and live in Pordenone (North-East, Italy).

Patients were divided into four groups based on severity of symptoms: asymptomatic, OAS, mild systemic reactions (Mueller classification grade 1–2), and severe systemic reactions (Mueller classification grade 3–4) (Table 1) [24].

Skin prick tests

SPTs to peach extract (ALK-Abello, Milan, Italy) were performed consecutively by the same investigator in the South population and by another investigator in the North-East population, on the volar surface of the forearm by using a standard 1 mm tip lancet, according to the recommendations of the European Academy of Allergy and Clinical Immunology group. Histamine hydrochloride (10 mg/mL) and saline (ALK-Abello, Milan, Italy), respectively, were used as positive and negative controls.

The SPT results were considered positive if the difference between the mean diameter of the wheal and the negative control was at least of 3 mm.

sIgE dosage

sIgE anti-rPru p 1, anti-rPru p 3, and anti-rPru p 4 were consecutively determined using the ImmunoCAP system (Thermofisher/Phadia Diagnostics, Uppsala, Sweden). Results were expressed in kUA/L and a value >0.15 kUA/L was considered positive.

All serum samples were consecutively analysis by both Buccheri La Ferla and Maria degli Angeli laboratories. The calibration test was done when the ImmunoCAP 250 required. Every day, new reagents were used due to the high number of samples analysed by both laboratories. During every single session, two control curves and one quality control (given by Thermofisher/Phadia Diagnostics) were performed. In addition, measurements of sIgE to peach and to Pru p 3 were done using a "house control" (obtained from a serum pool frozen at −80 °C).

Table 1 Demographic and clinical characteristics of sensitized peach patients from North-East and South Italy

	South Italy	North-East Italy
Patients (n)	71	62
Sex (f/m)	41/30	34/28
Age (mean, years)	25.7	38.03
Clinical manifestation (n)		
Asymptomatic	5	13
OAS	7	28
Mild reactions	40	17
Severe reactions	19 (7 anaphylactic shock)	4 (1 anaphylactic shock)

Both laboratories have been participated to external VEQ specific allergy programs: Buccheri La Ferla laboratory has been participated to the Sicilian Region CRQ and the laboratory from Pordenone, to the NEQAS UK.

To be sure the results were reproducible, all 133 serum samples were analysed by Buccheri La Ferla laboratory, during a single session, using the same batch of reagents.

Table 2 Difference in sensitization to peach allergens between the North-East and the South Italian patients

	Pru p 1	Pru p 4	Pru p 3
Palermo n = 71 (%)	0*	0**	100
Pordenone n = 62 (%)	42.8	12.7	100

* $p < 0.0001$

** $p = 0.005$

Oral food challenge

Patients with OAS reintroduced peaches under our supervision and experienced local symptoms of OAS. In view of the observational nature of the study and of the fear of several patients of a possibly severe adverse reaction, patients with systemic reactions were not challenged because of documented severe peach allergy [25].

The study was performed with the approval of the ethics committee of Policlinico—Giaccone Hospital—Palermo Italy (7/2013–12.06.2013) and was in agreement with the Helsinki Declaration. Written consent form was obtained from the patients.

Statistical methods

The association between levels of sIgE to Pru p 3 in asymptomatic vs. symptomatic patients with local and systemic reactions were analyzed by Mann–Whitney test.

The ROC analysis was carried out to determine the optimal cut-off value of sIgE to Pru p 3 to distinguish asymptomatic from symptomatic patients both in South and North-East Italian populations.

Correlations between sIgE levels and symptom severity were assessed using Spearman rank correlation (rho). In addition, the odds ratio of sIgE levels to Pru p 3 was calculated to assess the risk of severe reactions. The latest test was not done in the North-East group due to the low number of patients with severe reactions.

Medcalc 11.4.4.0 was used for the statistical analyses. A *p* value of <0.05 was considered significant.

Results

All South and North-East Italian patients were positive (mean diameter > 3 mm) to SPT to peach extract and to sIgE to Pru p 3. The sensitization to other panallergens differs according to the geographical area: the North-East population was simultaneously positive to Pru p 1 (42.8 %) and Pru p 4 (12.7 %), while no Southern patients were positive to PR-10 or to profilin (Table 2).

The levels of sIgE to Pru p 3 from the two populations are shown in Fig. 1.

In the South population, it was found a significant difference in the levels of sIgE to Pru p 3 between all symptomatic patients (OAS, mild, and severe systemic reactions) vs. asymptomatic patients ($p = 0.01$), and between patients with mild systemic reactions compare with patients with severe systemic reactions ($p = 0.0008$). On the other hand, in the North-East population, not significant differences were found in the levels of sIgE to Pru p 3 between symptomatic (OAS, mild, and severe systemic reactions) vs. asymptomatic patients ($p = 0.08$) and between patients with mild systemic reactions compared with patients with severe systemic reactions ($p = 0.09$).

Interestingly, in the South population was found a correlation between the severity of the clinical reactions and the levels of sIgE to Pru p 3 (Spearman's test = 0.366; $p = 0.001$). Unfortunately, in the North-East population, not correlation test was done due to the low number of patients with severe allergic reactions.

The ROC curve analysis from all South Pru p 3 positive patients identified a value of sIgE to

Pru p 3 of 2.87 kUA/L as the best value discriminating asymptomatic from symptomatic (OAS, mild, and severe systemic reactions) patients [sensitivity 91.04 % (95 % CI 81.5–96.6); specificity 75 % (95 % CI 19.4–99.4); LR + 3.64 (95 % CI 2.1–6.4); Fig. 2].

A value of sIgE to Pru p 3 of 5.87 kUA/L has a sensitivity of 67.16 % (95 % CI 54.6–78.2) and a specificity of 100 % (95 % CI 39.8–100.0).

The ROC curve analysis from all North-East Pru p 3 positive patients identified a value of sIgE to Pru p 3 of 2.68 kUA/L as the best value that discriminated asymptomatic from symptomatic (OAS, mild, and severe systemic reactions) patients [sensitivity 36.0 % (95 % CI 22.9–50.8); specificity 69.2 % (95 % CI 38.6–90.9); LR + 1.17 (95 % CI 0.7–2.0); Fig. 2].

In the South group, the value of sIgE to Pru p 3 of 10.2 kUA/L was the best value that discriminated severe reactions from other clinical reactions [sensitivity 70.0 % (95 % CI 45.7–88.1); specificity 88.9 % (95 % CI 65.3–98.6); LR + 6.30 (95 % CI 4.5–8.8)]. Due to the low number of severe reactions in the North-East population, it was not possible identify a value of sIgE to Pru p 3 able to discriminate severe reactions from other clinical reactions (Fig. 3).

The area under curve (AUC) of symptomatic (OAS, mild, and severe systemic reactions) vs. asymptomatic

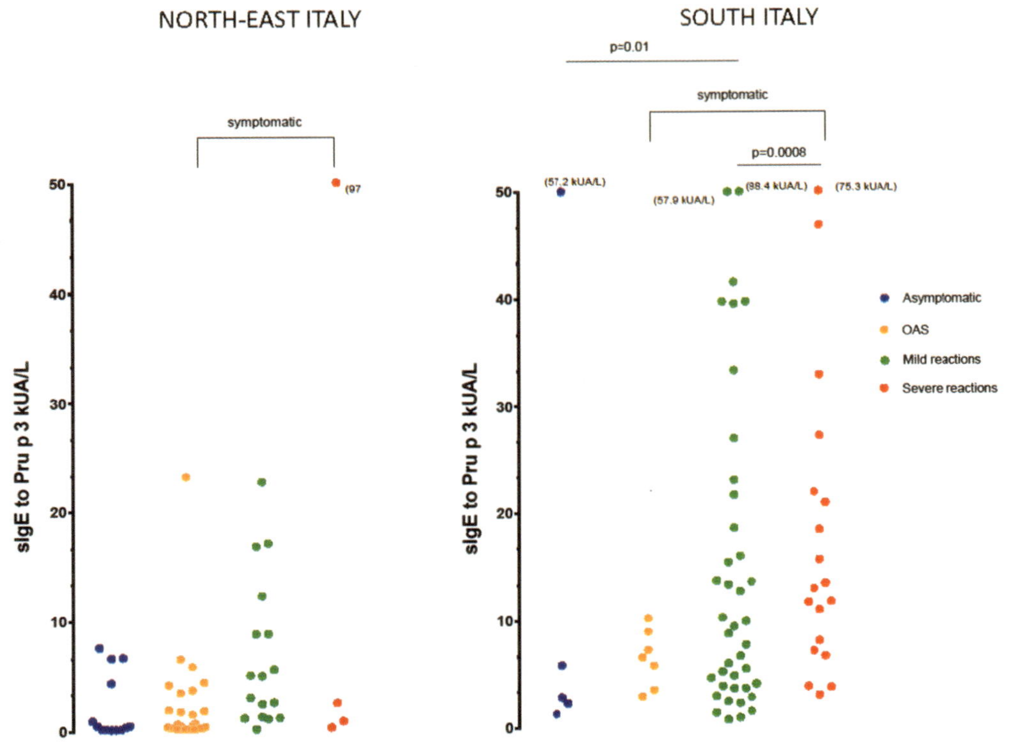

Fig. 1 Levels of sIgE to Pru p 3 in peach allergic patients from South and North-East Italy according to the clinical reactions

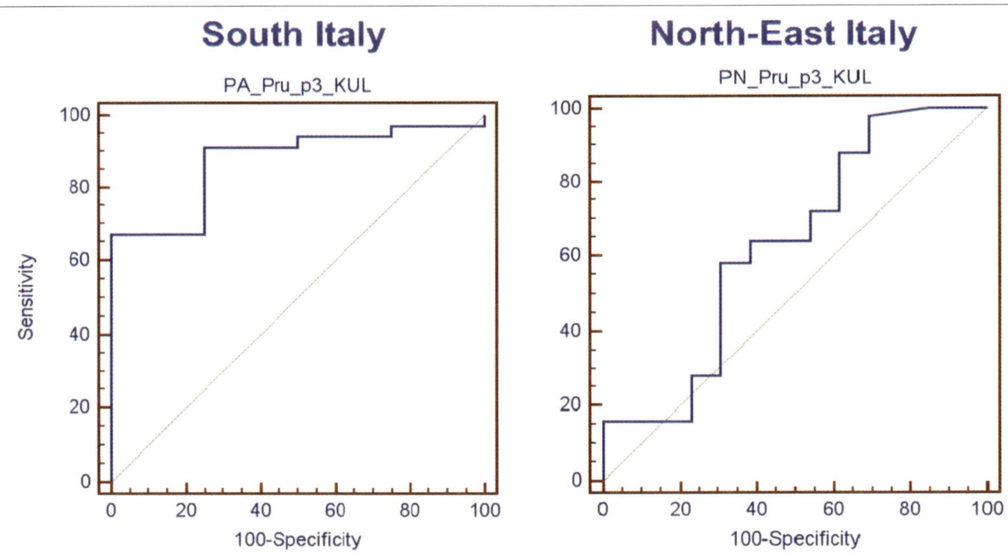

Fig. 2 ROC curves for sIgE to Pru p 3 values in all peach allergic patients from South and North-East Italy

patients living in South Italy and North-East Italy were 0.873 and 0.631 ($p < 0.0001$; $p = 0.1116$), respectively. AUC of patients with clinical severe reaction vs. all other reactions were 0.819 and 0.755 ($p < 0.0001$; $p = 0.12$), respectively.

The risk assessment of severe allergic reactions was the following: for a value of sIgE to Pru p 3 >7.5 kUA/L, the odds ratio 95 % CI was 69 (2.3–2028; $p = 0.01$) and >10 kUA/L, the odds ratio 95 % CI was 225 (3.9–13,114; $p = 0.009$).

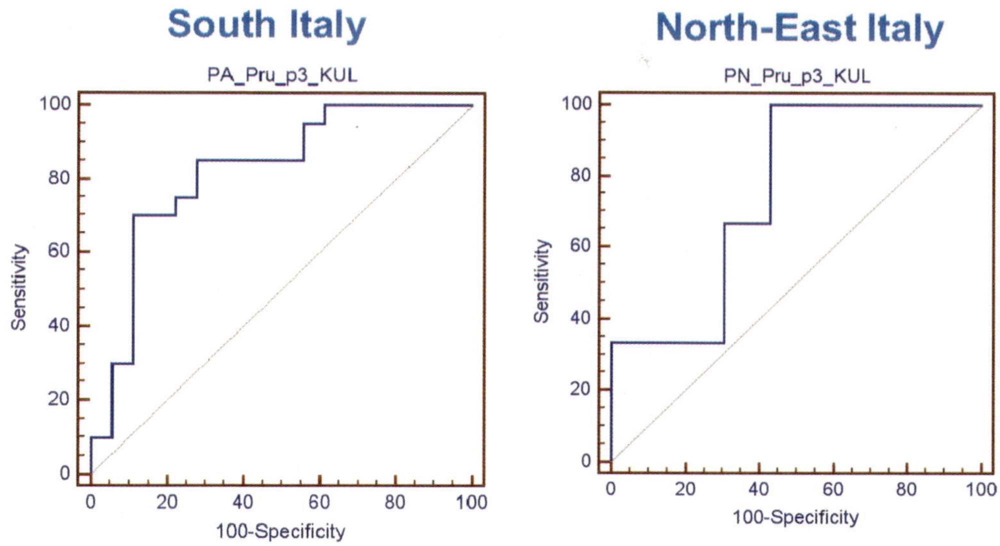

Fig. 3 ROC curve for sIgE to Pru p 3 values in patients with severe allergic reactions from South and North-East Italy

Discussion

For the first time, a study evaluates the usefulness of an anaphylactic biomarker in the risk assessment of Pru p 3 positive patients from different geographical areas of the same country.

In this study, we investigated the presence of correlations between the levels of sIgE to Pru p 3 with the severity of the clinical reactions in a South Italian population and compared them, with the results from a Nord-East Italian population, where the prevalence of sensitization to birch pollen is similar to North Europe.

All patients were assigned to one of the four groups according to their clinical manifestations: asymptomatic, OAS, mild systemic reactions and severe systemic reactions. We found that levels of sIgE to Pru p 3 (Mann–Whitney test) in the South population was significantly different between asymptomatic vs. symptomatic (OAS, mild and severe systemic reactions) Pru p 3 positive patients and between patients with mild systemic reactions in comparison to those with severe systemic reactions. Surprising, we could not found any significant differences in the levels of sIgE to Pru p 3 (Mann–Whitney test) in none of the groups from North-East Italy.

Few studies have assessed the relationship between the levels of sIgE to Pru p 3 and the severity of the clinical reactions, and taken all together provided contradictory results. Gaier et al. [26] have reported that the presence of sIgE to Pru p 3 in peach allergic patients who live in a geographical area with a high sensitization to birch pollen, may be considered a marker of severe reactions. On the other hand, Novembre et al. [21] have not found any relations between the levels of sIgE and the severity of the clinical reaction in a pediatric population; while Pastorello et al. [23] have found sIgE levels to Pru p 3 significantly higher in patients with severe OAS than in patients with mild OAS. In this study, we found a significant correlation between the severity of the clinical reaction and the levels of sIgE to Pru p 3. The differences in the results obtained could be attributed to the different type of population included in the studies.

An important result of this study was the determination of a cut-off level for sIgE to Pru p 3 values that can better discriminate asymptomatic patients from those symptomatic (2.87 kUA/L for the South Italian population and 2.69 kUA/L for the North-East population) and within this group, identify those patients at a higher risk for developing severe allergic reactions.

Pastorello et al. [23] have identified a cut-off value of sIgE to Pru p 3 of 2.69 kUA/L with a lower sensitivity 63.9 % but similar specificity 75 % that better discriminated peach-allergic patients at a higher risk for developing more severe symptoms.

Interestingly, we found a value of sIgE to Pru p 3 higher than 10.2 kUA/L (sensitivity almost of 90 %) that was present in 70 % of the patients with severe systemic reactions from South Italy. In the North-East group, with the same value of sIgE to Pru p 3, we have a higher specificity but a lower sensitivity. However, we cannot exclude that these results are probably affected by a bias due to the low numbers of patients with severe allergic reactions included in this population.

Although it has been shown that panallergens differ according to the geographical areas [4–6], up to now, nobody has studied the prevalence of peach panallergen in Sicily. The high sensitization to nsLTP and the lower prevalence of sensitization to profilin have been previously reported in a study done with Sicilian and Austrian patients allergic to Parietaria judaica [27]. In this regard, a study done in allergic patients (Uasuf et al. 2014 unpublished data) to assess the prevalence of panallergens in South Italy, has found that in 599 positive molecular ImmunoCAP tests performed, the prevalence of profilin was 3.6 % and of PR-10 was only 1 %.

The different clinical manifestations present in the two Italian populations could be attributed not only to the existence of different co-sensitization to the panallergens but also to the levels of sIgE to Pru p 3. Therefore, lower levels of sIgE to Pru p 3 and the co-existence of positivity to Pru p1 and/or Pru p 4 could explain the minor frequency of severe reactions in the North-East patients with respect to the South patients, monosensitized and with higher level of sIgE to Pru p 3. On a speculative level, this fact supports the hypothesis that patients positive to Pru p 3 and simultaneously positive to Pru p 1 and/or Pru p 4, have a sort of 'protective' effect against the development of severe symptoms induced by Pru p 3 [23].

Conclusion

Our results show that the level of an anaphylactic biomarker like sIgE to Pru p 3, indicates the possibility of development a severe food allergic reaction. In addition, Pru p 3 positive patients from different geographical areas and with different co-sensitizations could have a different risk assessment in peach allergy.

This study could be a model to extrapolate to other geographical areas with different co-sensitizations to identify probably high risk group in food allergy.

Further studies, including multicentre studies are necessary to confirm and expand these results.

Abbreviations

nsLTP: non specific lipid transfer protein; sBT: serum basal tryptase; FA: food allergy; sIgE: specific immunoglobulin E; CRD: component resolved diagnosis; PR-10: pathogenesis related protein-10; OAS: oral allergic syndrome; SPT: skin prick test.

Authors' contributions

CU has made substantial contributions to conception and design of the study, acquisition of data and drafting the manuscript. DV, MEC have made substantial contributions to conception and design of the study and acquisition of data. CDS, MB, VC have carried out the in vitro immunoassays. EP, MG have been involved in drafting the manuscript. SG has revised the manuscript critically for important intellectual content. IB has made substantial contributions to conception and design of the study, analysis and interpretation of data. All authors read and approved the final manuscript.

Author details

[1] Allergy Diseases Center "Prof. G. Bonsignore", Institute of Biomedicine and Molecular Immunology "A. Monroy"(IBIM)-National Research Council (CNR), Palermo, Italy. [2] Allergy and Clinical Immunology Unit, A.O "S. Maria degli Angeli di Pordenone", Pordenone, Italy. [3] Clinical Pathology, Allergy Unit, Buccheri La Ferla Hospital, Palermo, Italy. [4] School and Division of Allergy and Clinical Immunology, Department of Clinical and Experimental Medicine, University of Messina, Messina, Italy.

References

1. Sampson HA, Ho DG. Relationship between food-specific IgE concentrations and the risk of positive food challenges in children and adolescents. J Allergy Clin Immunol. 1997;100(4):444–51.
2. Yunginger JW, Ahlstedt S, Eggleston PA, Homburger HA, Nelson HS, Ownby DR, Platts-Mills TA, Sampson HA, Sicherer SH, Weinstein AM, Williams PB, Wood RA, Zeiger RS. Quantitative IgE antibody assays in allergic diseases. J Allergy Clin Immunol. 2000;105:1077–84.
3. Sampson HA. Utility of food-specific IgE concentrations in predicting symptomatic food allergy. J Allergy Clin Immunol. 2001;107(5):891–6.
4. Asero R, Antonicelli L, Arena A, Bommarito L, Caruso B, et al. Causes of food-induced anaphylaxis in Italian adults: a multi-centre study. Int Arch Allergy Immunol. 2009;150:271–7.
5. Fernandez-Rivas M, Bolhaar S, Gonzalez-Mancebo E, Asero R, van Leeuwen A, et al. Apple allergy across Europe: how allergen sensitization profiles determine the clinical expression of allergies to plant foods. J Allergy Clin Immunol. 2006;118:481–8.
6. Zuidmeer L, van Ree R. Lipid transfer protein allergy: primary food allergy or pollen/food syndrome in some cases. Curr Opin Allergy Clin Immunol. 2007;7(3):269–73.
7. Egger M, Hauser M, Mari A, Ferreira F, Gadermaier G. The role of lipid transfer proteins in allergic diseases. Curr Allergy Asthma Rep. 2010;10:326–35.
8. Wijesinha-Bettoni R, Alexeev Y, Johnson P, Marsh J, Sancho AI, et al. The structural characteristics of nonspecific lipid transfer proteins explain their resistance to gastroduodenal proteolysis. Biochemistry. 2010;49:2130–9.
9. Asero R, Mistrello G, Roncarolo D, Amato S, Caldironi G, Barocci F, van Ree R. Immunological cross-reactivity between lipid transfer proteins from botanically unrelated plant-derived foods: a clinical study. Allergy. 2002;57:900–6.
10. Sánchez-Monge R, Lombardero M, García-Selles FJ, Barber D, Salcedo G. Lipid transfer proteins are relevant allergens in fruit allergy. J Allergy Clin Immunol. 1999;103:514–9.
11. Pastorello EA, Vieths S, Pravettoni V, Farioli L, Trambaioli C, Fortunato D, Lüttkopf D, Calamari M, Ansaloni R, Scibilia J, Ballmer-Weber BK, Poulsen LK, Wütrich B, Hansen KS, Robino AM, Ortolani C, Conti A. Identification of hazelnut major allergens in sensitive patients with positive double-blind, placebo-controlled food challenge results. J Allergy Clin Immunol. 2002;109:563–70.
12. Asero R. Lipid transfer protein cross-reactivity assessed in vivo and in vitro in the office: pros and cons. J Investig Allergol Clin Immunol. 2011;21(2):129–36.
13. Pastorello EA, Farioli L, Pravettoni V, Ispano M, Scibola E, Trambaioli C, Giuffrida MG, Ansaloni R, Godovac-Zimmermann J, Conti A, Fortunato D, Ortolani C. The maize major allergen, which is responsible for food-induced allergic reactions, is a lipid transfer protein. J Allergy Clin Immunol. 2000;106:744–51.
14. Pastorello EA, Farioli L, Pravettoni V, Robino AM, Scibilia J, Fortunato D, Conti A, Borgonovo L, Bengtsson A, Ortolani C. Lipid transfer protein and vicilin are important walnut allergens in patients not allergic to pollen. J Allergy Clin Immunol. 2004;114:908–14.
15. Lauer I, Dueringer N, Pokoj S, Rehm S, Zoccatelli G, Reese G, Miguel-Moncin MS, Mistero Bahima A, Enrique E, Lidholm J, Vieths S, Scheurer S. The non-specific lipid transfer protein, Ara h 9, is an important allergen in peanut. Clin Exp Allergy. 2009;39:1427–37.

16. Díaz Perales A, Lombardero M, Sánchez-Monge R, García-Selles FJ, Pernas M, Fernández-Rivas M, Barber D, Salcedo G. Lipid-transfer proteins as potential plant panallergens: cross-reactivity among proteins of Artemisia pollen, Castanea nut and Rosaceae fruits, with different IgE-binding capacities. Clin Exp Allergy. 2000;30:1403–10.
17. Ciardiello MA, Palazzo P, Bernardi ML, Carratore V, Giangrieco I, Longo V, Melis M, Tamburrini M, Zennaro D, Mari A, Colombo P. Biochemical, immunological and clinical characterization of a cross-reactive nonspecific lipid transfer protein 1 from mulberry. Allergy. 2010;65(5):597–605.
18. Pastorello EA, Farioli L, Stafylaraki C, Scibilia J, Giuffrida MG, Mascheri A, Piantanida M, Baro C, Primavesi L, Nichelatti M, Schroeder JW, Pravettoni V. Fennel allergy is a lipid-transfer protein (LTP)-related food hypersensitivity associated with peach allergy. J Agric Food Chem. 2013;61(3):740–6.
19. Pastorello EA, Scibilia J, Farioli L, Primavesi L, Giuffrida MG, Mascheri A, Piantanida M, Mirone C, Stafylaraki C, Violetta MR, Nichelatti M, Preziosi D, Losappio L, Pravettoni V. Rice allergy demonstrated by double-blind placebo-controlled food challenge in peach-allergic patients is related to lipid transfer protein reactivity. Int Arch Allergy Immunol. 2013;161(3):265–73.
20. Asero R, Mistrello G, Roncarolo D, Amato S. Relationship between peach lipid transfer protein specific IgE levels and hypersensitivity to non-Rosaceae vegetable foods in patients allergic to lipid transfer protein. Ann Allergy Asthma Immunol. 2004;92:268–72.
21. Novembre E, Mori F, Contestabile S, Rossi ME, Pucci N. Correlation of anti-Pru p 3 IgE levels with severity of peach allergy reactions in children. Ann Allergy Asthma Immunol. 2012;108(4):271–4.
22. Pastorello EA, Farioli L, Stafylaraki C, Mascheri A, Scibilia J, Pravettoni V, Primavesi L, Piantanida M, Nichelatti M, Asero R. Anti-rPru p 3 IgE levels are inversely related to the age at onset of peach-induced severe symptoms reported by peach-allergic adults. Int Arch Allergy Immunol. 2013;162(1):45–9.
23. Pastorello EA, Farioli L, Pravettoni V, Scibilia J, Mascheri A, Borgonovo L, Piantanida M, Primavesi L, Stafylaraki C, Pasqualetti S, Schroeder J, Nichelatti M, Marocchi A. Pru p 3-sensitised Italian peach-allergic patients are less likely to develop severe symptoms when also presenting IgE antibodies to Pru p 1 and Pru p 4. Int Arch Allergy Immunol. 2011;156(4):362–72.
24. Mueller HL. Diagnosis and treatment of insect sensitivity. J Asthma Res. 1966;3:331–3.
25. Bindslev-Jensen C, Ballmer-Weber BK, Bengtsson U, Blanco C, Ebner C, Hourihane J, Knulst AC, Moneret-Vautrin DA, Nekam K, Niggemann B, Osterballe M, Ortolani C, Ring J, Schnopp C, Werfel T. Standardization of food challenges in patients with immediate reactions to foods—position paper from the European Academy of Allergology and Clinical Immunology. Allergy. 2004;59:690–7.
26. Gaier S, Oberhuber C, Hemmer W, Radauer C, Rigby NM, Marsh JT, Mills CEN, Shewry PR, Hoffmann-Sommergruber K. Pru p 3 as a marker for symptom severity for patients with peach allergy in a birch pollen environment. J Allergy Clin Immunol. 2009;124(1):166–7.
27. Stumvoll S, Westritschnig K, Lidholm J, Spitzauer S, Colombo P, Duro G, Kraft D, Geraci D, Valenta R. Identification of cross-reactive and genuine *Parietaria judaica* pollen allergens. J Allergy Clin Immunol. 2003;111(5):974–9.

A survey on the perception of allergy specialists about the reimbursed grass pollen tablets for seasonal allergic rhinitis in Italy

Ilaria Massaro[1*], Oliviero Rossi[2], Cristoforo Incorvaia[3] and Carlo Lombardi[4]

Abstract

Background: Sublingual immunotherapy (SLIT) is a feasible option to classical subcutaneous immunotherapy to treat respiratory allergy and is increasingly prescribed in Europe. However, the lack of reimbursement may limit its prescription. In 2015, the 5-grass pollen tablets was authorized by the European Medicine Agency to treat grass-pollen induced rhinitis and was approved in Italy for full reimbursement. We evaluated the opinions of allergy specialists after the availability of the reimbursed 5-grass pollen tablets.

Methods: A multiple choice questionnaire composed by six questions was used to assess the specialists opinion. The questionnaire was uploaded on the free access online platform SurveyMonkey. The link to access the platform was sent to all members of the Società Italiana di Asma, Allergologia e Immunologia Clinica (SIAAIC). The access to the questionnaire was anonymous. At survey ending, the access was closed and data were downloaded directly from SurveyMonkey website.

Results: The questionnaire was filled by 70 allergists. The majority of allergists felt as most important the concept of SLIT as a drug, the content of allergen extract mirroring the natural exposure, the pre-coseasonal schedule as the most patient's oriented, the very good profile of tolerability and safety, the importance of the build-up phase, and the importance of checking the patient after starting immunotherapy.

Conclusions: The opinions of the Italian allergy specialists about the reimbursed 5-grass-pollen tablets are very positive and make likely an appropriate prescription of SLIT for grass-pollen induced rhinitis in the next years.

Background

Allergen immunotherapy (AIT) is an efficacious, evidence-based treatment for allergic rhinitis [1]. Sublingual immunotherapy (SLIT) is a feasible option to classical subcutaneous immunotherapy (SCIT), that has its main advantages over SCIT in a better safety and in a lower cost [2, 3]. Actually, SLIT is increasingly prescribed also in countries where SCIT has been dominant, such as Germany [4] and is the most used form of AIT in Italy [5]. The allowance of allergen extracts for AIT by the different regional health systems in Italy is uneven, and in a study that evaluated the factors influencing the AIT prescription by a questionnaire submitted to about 450 specialists, the cost of treatment and the reimbursement were listed among the factors possibly influencing the prescription [6]. In 2015, the 5-grass pollen tablets, based on the fulfillment of all the requirements by the European Medicine Agency (EMA), that resulted in the authorization of the product to treat grass-pollen induced rhinitis, was approved by the Agenzia Italiana per il Farmaco (AIFA) for full reimbursement, i.e. class A, as for drugs [7].

We aimed this study at evaluating the opinions of allergy specialists after the availability of the reimbursed 5-grass pollen tablets.

*Correspondence: massaroilaria81@gmail.com
[1] Cell Therapy and Transfusion Medicine, Azienda Ospedaliero Universitaria Careggi, Florence, Largo Brambilla 1, 50134 Florence, Italy
Full list of author information is available at the end of the article

Methods

A multiple choice questionnaire developed by a group of allergists of the Società Italiana di Asma, Allergologia e Immunologia Clinica (SIAAIC) and composed by six questions (reported in Table 1) was used to assess the specialists opinion. The questionnaire was uploaded on the free access online platform SurveyMonkey (http://www.surveymonkey.com) on March 1 2016. The link to access the platform and the optional answers to the questionnaire was sent to all SIAAIC members by the SIAAIC scientific secretary. The access to the questionnaire was anonymous. On April 7 2016 the access was closed and data were downloaded directly from SurveyMonkey website.

Results

Seventy allergists anonymously filled in the questionnaire. Figures 1 2, 3, 4, 5 and 6 depict the data obtained. The majority of allergists chose as most important the concept of AIT as a drug for question 1, the content of allergen extract mirroring the natural exposure for question 2, the pre-coseasonal schedule as the most patient's oriented for question 3, a very good profile of tolerability and safety for question 4, the importance of the build-up

Table 1 Questions and answers choices

Questions	Choices
According to your experience, what was changed by the reimbursement of the grass-pollen tablets for seasonal rhinitis?	a. Accessibility to sublingual immunotherapy b. Possibility to adequately treat patients with moderate to severe seasonal rhinitis c. Possibility to treat all ARIA stages of rhinitis d. The concept of AIT as a drug
According to your opinion, how important is that the content of the allergen extract mirror the patient's natural exposure?	a. Very important b. Not important c. I do not know
Which is the treatment schedule for grass pollen-induced rhinitis more oriented toward patient's preference?	a. Perennial b. Pre-coseasonal c. Indifferent
According to your experience, the registered sublingual immunotherapy has a tolerability and safety profile	a. Very good b. Good c. Quite low
In performing sublingual immunotherapy, is the build-up phase important?	a. Yes b. No c. I do not know
After starting registered sublingual immunotherapy, do you check the patient after some weeks/months?	a. Always b. Sometimes c. Never

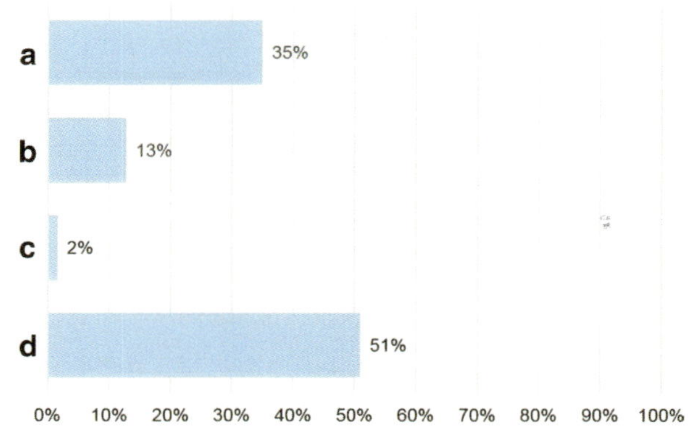

Fig. 1 Answers to the question "According to your experience, what was changed by the reimbursement of the grass-pollen tablets for seasonal rhinitis?"

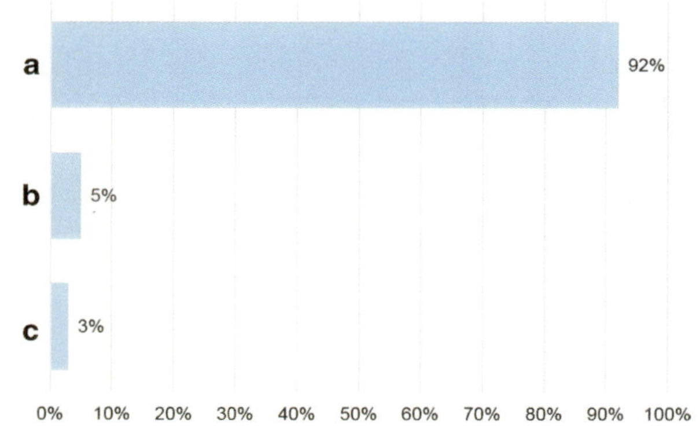

Fig. 2 Answers to the question "According to your opinion, how important is that the content of the allergen extract mirror the patient's natural exposure?"

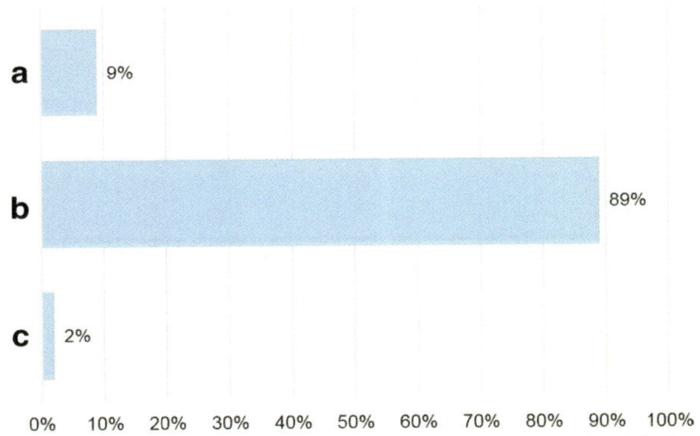

Fig. 3 Answers to the question "Which is the treatment schedule for grass pollen-induced rhinitis more oriented toward patient's preference?"

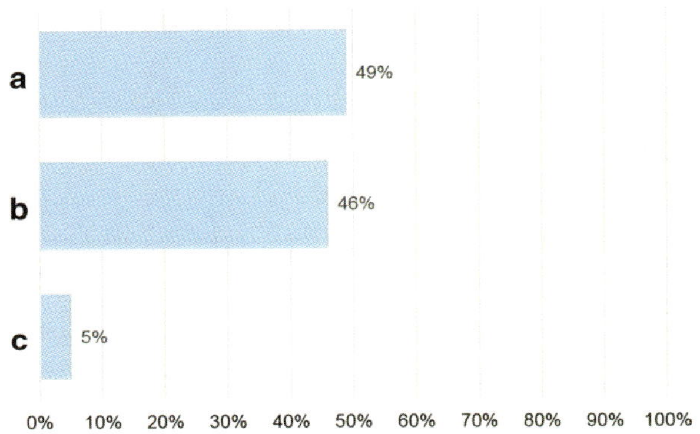

Fig. 4 Answers to the question "According to your experience, the registered sublingual immunotherapy has a tolerability and safety profile"

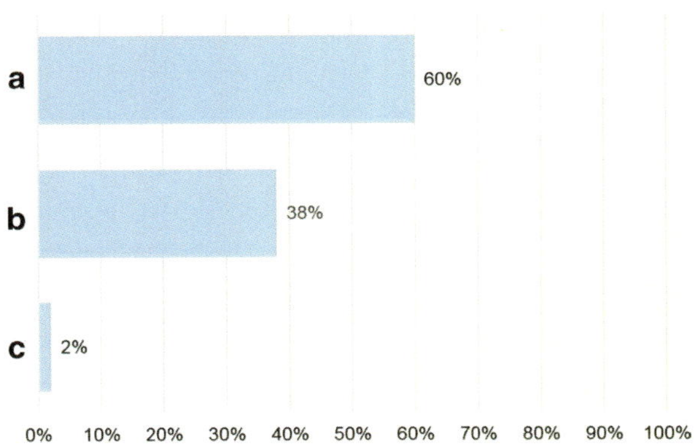

Fig. 5 Answers to the question "In performing sublingual immunotherapy, is the build-up phase important?"

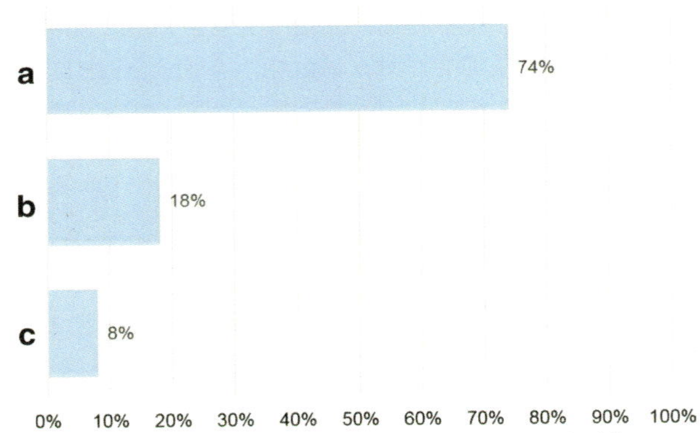

Fig. 6 Answers to the question "After starting registered sublingual immunotherapy, do you check the patient after some weeks/months?"

phase for question 5, and the importance of checking the patient after starting immunotherapy for question 6.

Discussion

The registration of grass pollen tablets as pharmaceutical quality products for grass pollen-induced rhinitis was a breakthrough in the history of AIT [7]. In fact, the commonly used AIT products were defined as Named Patient Products (NPP), because they were individual preparations that were not considered by the regulatory agencies as registered products [8]. The large placebo-controlled trials with grass pollen tablets performed to obtain the authorization by EMA as registered products clearly demonstrated the efficacy and safety of SLIT and paved the way to the modern AIT [9, 10]. In particular, the registration of the 5-grass-pollen tablets, as well as the data obtained from post marketing studies dealing with pharmacoeconomic impact [11] and patients' phenotyping [12] has led to the approval for full reimbursement by AIFA as a treatment for seasonal allergic rhinitis. Soon after, the one-grass (*Phleum pratense*) pollen tablet was also approved. In this survey we evaluated the opinions of the Italian allergy specialists about the reimbursed grass-pollen tablets, including the differences between the 5 grass-pollen and the 1-grass pollen tablets. The number of allergy specialists participating to the survey was not large, but the decision to fill in the questionnaire was spontaneous and no repeated invitation was sent. The overall opinion on the grass-pollen tablets identified as key factors the concept of AIT products as drugs (indicated by 51% of the allergists) and the utility of patient's monitoring after starting the treatment (indicated by 74% of the allergists). The other four issues allowed to highlight the perceived differences between the two products. Concerning the question assessing the value of an allergen content mirroring the natural exposure of patients to grass pollen, 92% of the allergists attributed to such factor a pivotal importance. Indeed, the superior adequacy of SLIT by a mix of five grasses over only *P. pratense* in Italian patients was indicated by both botanical and immunological studies. From the botanical point of view, phenologic analyses were performed on a number of grasses, by sampling every 10 days, starting in April, in 50 stations distributed across Italy. The flowering phase was assessed using a stereomicroscopy-based method for the detection of spreading stamens, and the data were compared to those from the official pollen calendar. Relevant differences were found between grass pollen count and effective flowering of the grass species as assessed by phenology. In fact, only some species contributed to the pollen peak, while important *Pooideae*, such as *P. pratense*, were not present during the pollen peak in northern and central Italy [13]. Immunological data supported the botanical observation, based on the results obtained with RAST-inhibition using sera of grass allergic patients from central Italy, that showed a significantly higher binding by the 5-grass extract compared with the *P. pratense* extract when grass pollens other than *P. pratense* were tested [14]. The questions concerning the pre-coseasonal schedule as the most patient's oriented, the profile of tolerability and safety and the importance of the build-up phase pertain to the same issue. In fact, a pre-coseasonal protocol, as indicated for the 5-grass pollen tablets, is defined as optimal for pollen allergy [15], while the protocol indicated for *P. pratense* tablet is perennial. In addition, the build-up phase and the safety are apparently related, as shown by the fact that the majority of severe adverse reactions occurred with the administration of the first dose of the *P. pratense* tablet, that has no build-up phase [16, 17]. On the other hand, in the position paper endorsed by the World Health Organization allergen immunotherapy is defined as "the practice of administering gradually increasing quantities of an allergen extract to an allergic subject to ameliorate the symptoms associated with subsequent exposure to the causative allergen" [18]. Thus, an AIT schedule with no build-up phase is not adherent to such definition.

In conclusion, the opinions of the Italian allergy specialists about the reimbursed 5-grass-pollen tablets are very positive and make likely an appropriate prescription of SLIT for grass-pollen induced rhinitis in the next years. Expanding this kind of survey to other specialists and including in the questionnaires also a comparison between AIT registered tablets and the common NPP is likely to further improve our knowledge on physicians opinion on AIT.

Authors' contributions

All authors were equally involved in the conception and design, analysis and interpretation of the data, and drafting of the paper; all authors agree to be accountable for all aspects of the work. All authors read and approved the final manuscript.

Author details

[1] Cell Therapy and Transfusion Medicine, Azienda Ospedaliero Universitaria Careggi, Florence, Largo Brambilla 1, 50134 Florence, Italy. [2] Allergy Unit, Azienda Ospedaliero Universitaria Careggi, Florence, Florence, Italy. [3] Cardiac/Pulmonary Rehabilitation, Centro Specialistico Gaetano Pini/CTO, Milan, Italy. [4] Allergy and Pneumology Departmental Unit, Fondazione Poliambulanza Hospital, Brescia, Italy.

Competing interests

Cristoforo Incorvaia is a scientific consultant for Stallergenes, Milan, Italy. Ilaria Massaro, Oliviero Rossi and Carlo Lombardi declare that they have no competing interests.

References

1. Jutel M, Agache I, Bonini S, Burks AW, Calderon MA, Canonica GW. International consensus on allergy immunotherapy. J Allergy Clin Immunol. 2015;136(3):556–68.
2. Bauer CS, Rank MA. Comparative efficacy and safety of subcutaneous versus sublingual immunotherapy. J Allergy Clin Immunol. 2014;134(3):765–75.
3. Dranitsaris G, Ellis AK. Sublingual or subcutaneous immunotherapy for seasonal allergic rhinitis: an indirect analysis of efficacy, safety and cost. J Eval Clin Pract. 2014;20(3):225–38.
4. McDonell AL, Wahn U, Demuth D, Richards C, Hawes C, Andreasen JN. Allergy immunotherapy prescribing trends for grass pollen-induced allergic rhinitis in Germany: a retrospective cohort analysis. Allergy Asthma Clin Immunol. 2015;11(1):19.
5. Musarra A, Bilò MB, Bonini S, Canonica GW, Senna GE. Consensus on allergen specific immunotherapy. Eur Ann Allergy Clin Immunol. 2013;45(suppl 3):1–49.
6. Frati F, Incorvaia C, Cadario G, Fiocchi A, Senna GE, Rossi O, et al. Factors influencing the prescription of allergen immunotherapy: the allergen immunotherapy decision analysis (AIDA) study. Eur Ann Allergy Clin Immunol. 2013;45(suppl 2):11–6.
7. Ciprandi G. A major step forward for sublingual immunotherapy: the quality of 5-grass pollen tablet is recognized also in Italy. J Asthma Allergy. 2015;8:25–7.
8. Kaul S, May S, Lüttkopf D, Vieths S. Regulatory environment for allergen-specific immunotherapy. Allergy. 2011;66(6):753–64.
9. Dahl R, Kapp A, Colombo G, de Monchy JG, Rak S, Emminger W, et al. Efficacy and safety of sublingual immunotherapy with grass allergen tablets for seasonal allergic rhinoconjunctivitis. J Allergy Clin Immunol. 2006;118(2):434–40.
10. Didier A, Malling HJ, Worm M, Horak F, Jäger S, Montagut A, et al. Optimal dose, efficacy, and safety of once-daily sublingual immunotherapy with a 5-grass pollen table for seasonal allergic rhinitis. J Allergy Clin Immunol. 2007;120(6):1338–45.

11. Ruggeri M, Oradei M, Frati F, Puccinelli P, Romao C, Dell'Albani I, et al. Economic evaluation of 5-grass pollen tablets versus placebo in the treatment of allergic rhinitis in adults. Clin Drug Invest. 2013;33(5):343–9.
12. Frati F, Dell'Albani I, Passalacqua G, Bonini S, Rossi O, Senna G, et al. A survey of clinical features of allergic rhinitis in adults. Med Sci Monit. 2014;20:2151–6.
13. Frenguelli G, Passalacqua G, Bonini S, Fiocchi A, Incorvaia C, Marcucci F, et al. Bridging allergological and botanical knowledge in seasonal allergy: a role for phenology. Ann Allergy Asthma Immunol. 2010;105(3):223–7.
14. Marcucci F, Sensi L, Di Cara G, Incorvaia C, Puccinelli P, Scurati S, et al. Which allergen extract for grass pollen immunotherapy? An in vitro study. Immunol Invest. 2010;39(6):635–44.
15. Lombardi C, Incorvaia C, Braga M, Senna G, Canonica GW, Passalacqua G. Administration regimens for sublingual immunotherapy to pollen allergens: what do we know? Allergy. 2009;64(6):849–54.
16. de Groot H, Bijl A. Anaphylactic reaction after the first dose of sublingual immunotherapy with grass pollen tablet. Allergy. 2009;64(6):963–4.
17. Galip N, Bahceciler N. Rare adverse events due to house dust mite sublingual immunotherapy in pediatric practice: two case reports. Immunotherapy. 2015;7(12):1235–9.
18. Bousquet J, Lockey R, Malling HJ. Allergen immunotherapy: therapeutic vaccines for allergic diseases. A WHO position paper. J Allergy Clin Immunol. 1998;102(4):558–62.

8

Clinical management, expectations, and satisfaction of patients with moderate to severe allergic rhinoconjunctivitis treated with SQ-standardized grass-allergen tablet under routine clinical practice conditions in Spain

Tomás Chivato[1*], Pedro Álvarez-Calderón[2], Carmen Panizo[3], Ricardo Abengozar[4], César Alías[5], Ali Al-Baech[6], José Arias-Irigoyen[6], M. José Caballero[7], Lluis Conill[8], Silvia de Miguel[9], Rafael Laguna[10], Joan Martínez-Benazet[11], Francisco Matoses[12], Jose Camilo Martínez-Alonso[13], Lourdes Mendizábal[14], Celsa Pérez-Carral[15], Carlos Puerto[16], Joan Serra-Batllés[17], Adolfo Vélez[18], Jonathan Vicente[19] and Fernando de la Torre[20]

Abstract

Background: Sublingual immunotherapy has been proven as a well-tolerated and effective treatment for allergic rhinitis. Within this type of treatment, GRAZAX® is the most documented product in terms of safety and efficacy. The objective of this study was to identify the patients' expectations and level of treatment satisfaction, as well as the clinical management of patients with moderate/severe allergic rhinoconjunctivitis treated with GRAZAX®.

Methods: This was a non-interventional, observational, multi-centre, open-label study involving a total of 131 adult patients aged 18–66 years with confirmed diagnosis of grass-allergy and initiated treatment with GRAZAX® between June 2010 and April 2011.

Results: In the pollen season after starting treatment, 56.6% of patients stated that their symptoms were much less/less intense, 86% needed less symptomatic medication for control of their symptoms, and 74.4% manifested to have improved (quite/a lot) as regards their allergic disease since treatment was initiated as compared with previous grass pollen season. The patient satisfaction with GRAZAX® was measured using a visual analogue scale (VAS) between 0 (minimum satisfaction) and 100 (maximum satisfaction) comprising five different items: effectiveness, tolerability, cost, convenience and overall satisfaction. The results obtained for each item were [mean (SD)]: 74.7 (18.1), 70.3 (36.1), 39.3 (25.8), 86.2 (12.6), 78.4 (15.8) respectively. The patient's level of satisfaction is highly influenced, especially in terms of assessment of effectiveness, tolerability and convenience, by the information provided by the specialist.

Conclusions: In summary, it can be concluded that improved communication leads to increased patient knowledge, greater patient compliance, and increased patient satisfaction.

Keywords: Allergic rhinitis, Allergen immunotherapy tablet, Satisfaction, Expectations, Clinical management

*Correspondence: tchivato@ceu.es
[1] Decanato. Facultad de Medicina, Facultad de Medicina Universidad CEU San Pablo. Grupo Hospitales HM, Avda. Montepríncipe s/n, Boadilla del Monte, 28668 Madrid, Spain
Full list of author information is available at the end of the article

Background

Despite not being considered a life-threatening disease, allergic rhinitis or rhinoconjunctivitis cause functional problems (physical, emotional, social, and occupational) that tend to worsen with time. Moreover, this disease represents a high cost burden for healthcare systems, often exceeding those derived from more serious conditions; allergic rhinoconjunctivitis is very common [1], affecting around one in four people of the total population. In a large-scale study that included over 9500 patients from Western European countries, the prevalence of allergic rhinitis was found to be around 23%. Because it is frequently considered not to be a life-threatening disease, it often remains undiagnosed, resulting in inadequate control of the symptoms [1].

From an economic point of view, the consequences of allergic rhinoconjunctivitis are considerable in terms of direct (treatments and visits to the GP/specialist) and indirect (i.e., sick leave from work or school, sleep disorders, and disruption of daily activities) costs.

Grasses are one of the most common causes of allergic rhinitis, having a clear impact on patients' quality of life [2]. There are various options for the management of this condition: symptomatic medication for the relief of the symptoms and avoidance of allergen exposure. On the other hand, the underlying cause of the allergic disease can be targeted through allergen-specific immunotherapy. Although proven effective, subcutaneous administration of the allergen can be uncomfortable and time-consuming. Sublingual allergen immunotherapy has been the subject of clinical development over the last 20 years. A Cochrane review published in 2011 [3] concluded that the use of sublingual immunotherapy for allergic rhinitis and rhinoconjunctivitis is effective and is not associated with significant adverse events.

Regarding sublingual immunotherapy, the grass allergen tablet GRAZAX® (*Phleum pratense* 75,000 SQ-T/2800 BAU, ALK, Denmark) is the most documented product in terms of safety and efficacy in children and adults [4–12].

However, several aspects of this therapeutic alternative, which tend to be closely associated with therapeutic adherence, have not been thoroughly examined, as for example: patients' expectations and their knowledge concerning a certain treatment [13, 14], the administration routes for immunotherapy [15], patient satisfaction with this treatment [16], and certain clinical management and patient education factors that may help reinforce positive patient behaviour regarding the treatment [17, 18].

The purpose of this study is to determine the expectations and level of satisfaction of patients (using the data collected from a questionnaire), as well as to collect information regarding the clinical management of patients with moderate/severe allergic rhinoconjunctivitis treated with GRAZAX®.

Methods

Design, treatment, and patients

Non-interventional, observational, multicenter, open-label study that included one hundred and thirty-one (131) adult patients aged between 18 and 66 years. All study subjects had a confirmed diagnosis of grass pollen allergy, reached through routine clinical practice (positive prick test and/or specific IgE) and had initiated treatment with GRAZAX® between June 2010 and April 2011 (i.e., had started treatment at least 2 months before the beginning of the 2011 grass pollen season). Two patients were excluded from the study because they were under 18 years of age.

Written informed consent was obtained from all patients before their inclusion in the study. The corresponding health authorities and the ethics committee approved the study.

Patients enrolled in the study were provided with a questionnaire comprising 18 questions and a visual analogue scale (VAS). The questionnaire was answered by the study subjects and aimed to assess their state of health and knowledge and expectations regarding the treatment with GRAZAX®; the VAS scoring ranged from *not at all satisfied* (0) to *maximum satisfaction* (100).

Variables

In this exploratory, descriptive study, no primary endpoint was established. Instead, a cluster of three relevant variables were assessed using an ad hoc questionnaire

- *Current patient satisfaction* to our knowledge, there is no standardised validated tool for this patient population. Thus, this variable was assessed through items specifically designed for this study. The ad hoc items in the study included Likert-type response options or visual analogue scorings.
- *Patients' expectations at the start of treatment and at present* a series of ad hoc items were drawn up. Data regarding the information patients received about their illness and treatment were also collected.
- *Clinical management received by patients* certain characteristic aspects of patients' perception regarding their clinical management.

Study data was collected retrospectively the year before the inclusion of the patients in the study. There was no follow-up of the participants as the study consisted of a single visit for data collection. Sociodemographic and clinical data were also collected.

Statistical analysis

Nonparametric tests (bilateral Kolmogorov–Smirnov test with 95% confidence level) were used to assess the normal distribution of the variables. Statistical inference was obtained by bivariate or multivariate analyses. The bivariate analyses were parametric (Chi squared, Student's t distribution, ANOVA) or bilateral nonparametric (Fisher's exact, Mann–Whitney, Kruskal–Wallis), with a 95% confidence level.

Results

Characteristics of patients

Mean age was 33.9 ± 12.9 years (53.5% female and 46.5% male). All study patients suffered from allergic rhinitis (see the characteristics of the disease in Table 1), as diagnosed by the ARIA guidelines [2]. Sixty-seven (67) patients had allergic asthma associated with rhinitis (73.1% intermittent, 14.9% mild persistent, 11.9% moderate, as per the Spanish Guidelines for the Management of Asthma -GEMA-) [19]. Median of time of treatment: 13 months (Q1–Q3: 11–17).

35.7% of study patients were monosensitized to grass, from which 64.3% were sensitized to grass and other allergens (these patients were considered as polysensitized). The most frequent allergens affecting the latter group were pollens (*Olea*: 33.7%; *Cupressus*: 26.5%; *Plantago*: 24.1%), mites (*D. pteronyssinus*: 28.9%), moulds (*Alternaria*: 9.6%), and epithelia (cat: 24.1%; dog: 20.5%).

Patients' expectations at the beginning of the treatment and at present

Patients were asked about their knowledge and expectations regarding their treatment with GRAZAX®. The results are summarized in Table 2.

Table 1 Clinical characteristics of the rhinitis

Characteristics of allergic rhinitis	% of patients
Intermittent	43.7
Persistent	56.3
Mild	20.2
Moderate-severe	79.8
Sleep interference	24.0
Interference with daily activities	43.4
Interference with working activities or studies	42.6
Troublesome symptoms	68.2
Symptomatic medication used for rhinitis	
Topical antihistamines	17.5
Oral antihistamines	73.0
Topical corticosteroids	44.4
Oral corticosteroids	4.8
Antileukotrienes	17.5

Table 2 Knowledge and expectations regarding the allergen immunotherapy tablet

	n	%
In your opinion, which is the aim of an allergen treatment? (n = 126)		
Improve quality-of-life	83	65.9
Reduce the number of attacks	34	27.0
Prevent life-threatening events	5	4.0
Avoid the development of new allergies	4	3.2
What do you expect from your treatment with the allergen immunotherapy tablet? (n = 128)		
Complete cure of the allergy	79	61.7
Some improvement of the symptoms	33	25.8
Avoid the development of new allergies	4	3.1
Prevent the onset of asthma symptoms	12	9.4
When do you think the allergen immunotherapy tablet will start to be effective? (n = 123)		
In a few days or weeks	41	33.3
In a few months	66	53.7
In a few years	16	13.0
Do you think the treatment could be dangerous or cause adverse events? (n = 115)		
The *allergen immunotherapy tablet* is safe	34	29.6
Sometimes	39	33.9
Rarely	42	36.5

When the answers in different subgroups of patients based on age, sex, mono-/polysensitized, years of evolvement of the allergic disease, or type and severity of allergic rhinitis were analysed, statistically significant differences were only found for the expectations regarding treatment. Thus, whereas 41.7% of patients with mild rhinitis expected a complete cure, this percentage increased to 64.9% ($p = 0.042$) in patients with moderate-severe rhinitis.

Clinical management of the patients

All study patients were asked on the type of information received from their allergologist regarding their allergic disease and treatment with GRAZAX®. The main results are included in Table 3.

During the pollen season, 56.6% of patients stated their symptoms were much less/less intense, 86% required less symptomatic medication for the control of their allergic symptoms, and 74.4% stated the allergic disease had improved (quite/a lot) since the initiation of the treatment with GRAZAX® in comparison with the previous grass pollen season.

Level of satisfaction of patients treated with GRAZAX®

Patients´ satisfaction with GRAZAX® was measured using a visual analogue scale (VAS) with a range of scores between 0 (minimum satisfaction) and 100 (maximum

Table 3 Clinical information received by the patients

	n	%
Did you receive information about your disease before starting the treatment with the allergen immunotherapy tablet? (n = 128)		
Yes, in detail	114	89.1
Yes, a little	14	10.9
Did you receive information about the different treatments for your disease? (n = 129)		
Yes, in detail	102	79.1
Yes, a little	25	19.4
I received no information	2	1.6
Did you receive information about the characteristics of the allergen immunotherapy tablet? (n = 128)		
Yes, in detail	107	83.6
Yes, a little	20	15.6
I received no information	1	0.8
Did you receive written information about your disease or its treatment? (n = 128)		
Yes	58	45.3
No	70	54.7

satisfaction) comprising five items: effectiveness, tolerability, cost, convenience, and overall satisfaction. The following results, expressed as means (SD), were obtained for each item: 74.7 (18.1), 70.3 (36.1), 39.3 (25.8), 86.2 (12.6), 78.4 (15.8), respectively. No statistically significant differences were found between these variables regarding the age and sex of the patients.

Considering the duration of the disease (<6 years, 6–12 years, or >12 years), significant differences were found for the variable "effectiveness" (78.2 (16.3) vs. 76.4 (18.3) vs. 69.7 (19.0), respectively; $p = 0.025$). Statistical differences were also found for the degree of severity of the allergic rhinitis (Table 4).

Table 5 shows how patients´ satisfaction level is highly influenced by the information provided by the specialist, particularly in terms of assessment of effectiveness and convenience.

Finally, overall patient satisfaction with GRAZAX® with respect to previous immunotherapy treatments showed that 56.36% of the patients considered GRAZAX® as "much better" and 30.9% as "better".

Discussion

Allergic rhinoconjunctivitis and rhinitis are independent risk factors for asthma. These two conditions increase the social and economic impact of asthma and represent an important burden for the healthcare system [2, 20]. Data on drug intake, healthcare resources, days of work missed, and loss of productivity associated to allergic rhinitis were collected by the Spanish Society of Allergy and Clinical Immunology (SEAIC).

The management of allergic rhinitis involves different strategies, including patient education, allergen avoidance, and symptomatic and etiological treatments. Within this latter option, GRAZAX® is the only product authorized for treating grass pollen allergy with a registered disease-modifying effect [21]. According to the results obtained in the clinical trials performed with GRAZAX®, a significant clinical benefit is achieved after the first 4 months of treatment [9]. For this reason the authors assumed that 1 year of treatment could be an acceptable time for evaluating the satisfaction and expectations of patients.

The healthcare system could benefit from an annual increase in the number of patients treated with specific immunotherapy in terms of additional cost savings and improved health status for the patients [20]. In this study we show that 86% of patients treated with GRAZAX® take less symptomatic medication after starting the treatment, which implies lower costs for the national healthcare system. These findings are in line with a previous study by Donahue et al. [22]. who found immunotherapy to be a less cost-intensive strategy than standard pharmacotherapy over a 10-year period. Treatment with GRAZAX® has been described in the literature to be a cost-effective intervention for the prevention of grass pollen-induced rhinoconjunctivitis [23, 24]. However, factors related to patient satisfaction and expectations have not been thoroughly studied, despite their key role in the therapeutic strategy.

The relevance of quality of life for these patients is reflected in the fact that 65.9% consider an improvement in this aspect to be the main treatment goal. On the other hand, opinions among patients regarding treatment safety are divided and complete information is

Table 4 Degree of satisfaction with the allergen immunotherapy tablet *as per* the severity of the allergic rhinitis (VAS scale: 0 -not at all satisfied-, 100 -maximum satisfaction-)

AR type	n	Effectiveness Mean (SD)	Adverse effects Mean (SD)	Cost Mean (SD)	Convenience Mean (SD)	Overall Mean (SD)
Mild	24	80.42 (16.15)	83.54 (30.16)	55.21 (25.64)	89.17 (13.73)	82.29 (17.00)
Moderate/severe	93	72.42 (18.85)	66.02 (37.18)	36.61 (24.36)	85.86 (12.33)	77.08 (16.17)
p value[1]		0.032	0.041	0.002	0.092	0.058

[1] The p value was calculated using bilateral Student's parametric t test (or the nonparametric Mann–Whitney U test) with a 95% confidence level

Table 5 Relationship between patient satisfaction and disease- and treatment-related information received

	n	Mean (SD)	Effectiveness Mean (SD)	Adverse events Mean (SD)	Cost Mean (SD)	Convenience Mean (SD)
Before starting the treatment, did your doctor speak to you about the disease?						
Yes, at length	112	76.34 (17.6)	69.91 (36.35)	40.0 (25.86)	86.74 (13.10)	79.63 (15.12)
Yes, a little	14	62.50 (17.84)	77.86 (31.85)	33.2 (25.91)	82.50 (8.03)	72.14 (15.65)
p value[1)]		0.002	0.446	0.272	0.050	0.108
Did your doctor speak to you about the different possible treatments for your disease?						
Yes, at length	100	76.70 (17.56)	70.40 (36.57)	40.45 (26.45)	87.70 (12.50)	78.85 (15.73)
Yes, a little	25	69.40 (17.52)	68.80 (36.15)	35.20 (23.07)	80.00 (11.99)	77.72 (16.20)
p value[1]		0.012	0.959	0.577	0.007	0.491
Did your doctor speak to you about the characteristics of GRAZAX®?						
Yes, at length	105	76.33 (18.00)	68.62 (37.65)	39.38 (26.47)	87.57 (12.39)	78.84 (15.95)
Yes, a little	20	69.50 (15.30)	77.75 (28.07)	39.50 (22.59)	78.75 (12.23)	77.50 (15.09)
p value[1]		0.023	0.904	0.460	0.008	0.237

[1] The p value was calculated using the bilateral ANOVA parametric test (or nonparametric Kruskal–Wallis) with a 95% confidence level

crucial to ensure treatment adherence. A recent study with GRAZAX® [25] showed that all but one of the adverse reactions registered with the first dose occurred within the observation period specified in the SmPC for the used dose. The appropriate management of the patient´s reaction to this first dose, along with medical support, can help prevent treatment withdrawal. Physician-patient agreement, physician's ability to deal with all the patient's problems, and taking into consideration his/her expectations, feelings, and ideas are key for the final outcome.

It is generally accepted that better clinical benefits are achieved when treatment is started in early stages of a disease. In this study, patients who have had the disease for a shorter time, asses the effectiveness of the allergen immunotherapy tablet significantly better in comparison with patients who have suffered the condition for a longer time (<6 years: 78.2, 6–12 years: 76.4, >12 years: 69.7, $p = 0.025$).

In the Table 2, 33.9 and 36.5% feel that immunotherapy may be "sometimes" or "rarely" dangerous or may produce adverse events, respectively. With GRAZAX® the adverse reactions are more frequent in the beginning of the treatment and, in many patients, with the administration of the first dose and most of reaction occurred during the observation period after the administration of the first dose. When the doctor explains the type of adverse reactions that can be expected by the treatment, and considering that GRAZAX® is self-administered at patient´s home, the authors considered as relevant the perception of patients about the safety of treatment.

As for treatment adherence, most patients said to have received complete information about the disease and the treatment, although there was no written information (i.e., leaflets, etc.). Patients' expectations are essential for adherence, and in this study a high percentage (between 25 and 40.5%) of the patients expected the treatment to have an effect "in days or weeks". Patients should be encouraged to ask questions and be given clear verbal information by their physician, supplemented, whenever possible, by emotional support and written information packages.

Although it is clear that the intensity of the clinical management (number duration of the visits) affects various aspects of patient´s satisfaction, it is a non-linear effect, implying that other variables may influence this relationship. Determining whether physicians' communication strategies have a direct effect on patient satisfaction ratings is not straightforward [26, 27]. Cohort studies to assess the effect of communication measures have to be designed and developed; however, strategies to promote treatment adherence should be based on the concept of user-friendly information and improved patient-health professional communication.

In summary, the level of satisfaction is closely related to the information given to the patients; satisfaction increases with the amount and type of explanations received from the physician (e.g., time explaining the disease, existing treatments, or specific information about the new tablet-based treatment). A better communication leads to increased patient knowledge, compliance, and satisfaction.

Authors' contributions

All the authors included patients and review the manuscript. Tomás Chivato wrote the manuscript. Fernando De la Torre performed the statistical analysis and contributed to the manuscript writing. All authors read and approved the final manuscript.

Author details

[1] Decanato. Facultad de Medicina, Facultad de Medicina Universidad CEU San Pablo. Grupo Hospitales HM, Avda. Montepríncipe s/n, Boadilla del Monte, 28668 Madrid, Spain. [2] Hospital Clínico Universitario de Santiago, La Coruña, Spain. [3] Hospital Ntra Sra del Prado, Toledo, Spain. [4] Hospital Virgen del Valle, Toledo, Spain. [5] Clínica Corachán, Barcelona, Spain. [6] Private Office, Huelva, Spain. [7] Clínica ASISA, Córdoba, Spain. [8] Hospital Can Misses, Ibiza, Spain. [9] Policlínico Salud 4, Madrid, Spain. [10] Private Office, Madrid, Spain. [11] Hospital Ntra Sra de Meritxell, Escaldes-Engordany, Andorra. [12] Hospital General, Valencia, Spain. [13] Hospital Virgen de la Concha, Zamora, Spain. [14] Clínica Virgen de Fátima, Seville, Spain. [15] Hospital Comarcal da Costa, Lugo, Spain. [16] Private Office, Asturias, Spain. [17] Hospital de Vic, Barcelona, Spain. [18] Hospital San Juan de Dios, León, Spain. [19] Hospital General, Soria, Spain. [20] ALK-Abelló, S.A, Madrid, Spain.

Acknowledgements

We thank Eva Baro (3D-Health) for her technical support.

References

1. Bauchau V, Durham SR. Prevalence and rate of diagnosis of allergic rhinitis in Europe. Eur Respir J. 2004;24:758–64.
2. Bousquet J, van Cauwenberge P, Khaltaev N, ARIA Workshop Group, World Health Organization. Allergic rhinitis and its impact on asthma (ARIA). J Allergy Clin Immunol. 2001;108(5 Suppl):S147–334.
3. Radulovic S, Calderon MA, Wilson D, Durham S. Sublingual immunotherapy for allergic rhinitis (Review) 2011. Cochrane Database Syst Rev. 2010;12:CD002893.
4. Malling HJ, Lund L, Ipsen H, Poulsen L. Safety and immunological changes during sublingual immunotherapy with standardized quality grass allergen tablets. JIACI. 2006;16:162–8.
5. Durham S, Yang WH, Pedersen MR, Johansen N, Rak S. Sublingual immunotherapy with once-daily grass allergen tablets: a randomized controlled trial in seasonal allergic rhinoconjunctivitis. JACI. 2006;117:802–9.
6. Calderon MA, Birk AO, Andersen JS, Durham SR. Prolonged preseasonal treatment phase with SLIT increases clinical efficacy. Allergy. 2007;62:958–61.
7. Bufe A, Eberle P, Franke-Beckmann E, Funck J, Kimming M, Klimek L, Knect R, Stephan V, Tholstrup B, Weißhaar C, Kaiser F. Safety and efficacy in children of an SQ-standardized grass allergen tablet for sublingual immunotherapy. J Allergy Clin Immunol. 2009;123:167–73.
8. Kleine-Tebbe J, Ribel M, Herold DA. Safety of a SQ-standardised grass allergen tablet for sublingual immunotherapy: a randomized, placebo-controlled trial. Allergy. 2006;61:181–4.
9. Dahl R, Kapp A, Colombo G, de Monchy JGR, Rak S, Emminger W, Fernández Rivas M, Ribel M, Durham S. Efficacy and safety of sublingual immunotherapy with grass allergen tablets for seasonal allergic rhinoconjunctivitis. JACI. 2006;118:434–40.
10. Durham S, Emminger W, Kapp A, Colombo G, de Monchy JGR, Rak S, Scadding GK, Andersen JS, Riis B. Long-term clinical efficacy in grass pollen rhinoconjunctivitis after treatment with SQ standardized grass allergy immunotherapy tablet. J Allergy Clin Immunol. 2010;125:131–8.
11. Rak S, Yang WH, Pedersen MR, Durham S. Once-daily sublingual allergen-specific immunotherapy improves quality of life in patients with grass pollen-induced allergic rhinoconjunctivitis: a double-blind, randomised study. Qual Life Res. 2007;16:191–201.
12. Frølund L, Durham SR, Calderon M, Emminger W, Andersen JS, Rask P, Dahl R. Sustained effect of SQ-standardized grass allergy immunotherapy tablet on rhinoconjunctivitis quality of life. Allergy. 2010;65:753–7.
13. Sade K, Berkun Y, Dolev Z, Shalit M, Kivity S. Knowledge and expectations of patients receiving aeroallergen immunotherapy. Ann Allergy Asthma Immunol. 2003;91:444–8.
14. Mahesh PA, Vedanthan PK, Amrutha DH, Giridhar BH, Prabhakar AK. Factors associated with non-adherence to specific allergen immunotherapy in management of respiratory allergy. Indian J Chest Dis Allied Sci. 2010;52:91–5.
15. Pajno GB, Vita D, Caminiti L, Arrigo T, Lombardo F, Incorvaia C, Barberio G. Children's compliance with allergen immunotherapy according to administration routes. J Allergy Clin Immunol. 2005;116:1380–1.
16. Ferrer M, Morais-Almeida M, Guizova M, Khanferyan R. Evaluation of treatment satisfaction in children with allergic disease treated with an antihistamine: an international, non-interventional, retrospective study. Clin Drug Investig. 2010;30:15–34.
17. Vita D, Caminiti L, Ruggeri P, Pajno GB. Sublingual immunotherapy: adherence based on timing and monitoring control visits. Allergy. 2010;65:668–9.
18. Incorvaia C, Rapetti A, Scurati S, Puccinelli P, Capecce M, Frati F. Importance of patient's education in favouring compliance with sublingual immunotherapy. Allergy. 2010;65:1341–2.
19. GEMA (Guía española para el manejo del asma). Arch Bronconeumol. 2009;45(Supl 7):2–35.
20. Nathan RA. The burden of allergic rhinitis. Allergy Asthma Proc. 2007;28:3–9.
21. Grazax® Summary of product characteristics.
22. Donahue JG, Greineder DK, Connor-Lacke L, Canning CF, Platt R. Utilization and cost of immunotherapy for allergic asthma and rhinitis. Ann Allergy Asthma Immunol. 1999;82:339–47.
23. Canonica GW, Poulsen PB, Vestenbæk U. Cost-effectiveness of GRAZAX® for prevention of grass pollen induced rhinoconjunctivitis in Southern Europe. Respir Med. 2007;101:1885–94.
24. Bachert C, Vestenbaek U, Christensen J, Griffiths UK, Poulsen PB. Cost-effectiveness of grass allergen tablet (GRAZAX®) for the prevention of seasonal grass pollen induced rhinoconjunctivitis—a Northern European perspective. Clin Exp Allergy. 2007;37:772–9.
25. Armentia A, Carballada F, Carretero P, de Paz S, Lobera T, Marcos C, Martínez JC, Rodríguez I, Soto T, Venturini M, de la Torre F. Postmarketing study for assessment of tolerability of a grass allergen immunotherapy Tablet (GRAZAX®) in patients with rhinitis or rhinoconjunctivitis. J Investig Allergol Clin Immunol. 2012;22:485–90.
26. Stewart MA. Effective physician-patient communication and health outcomes: a review. Can Med Assoc J. 1995;152:1423–33.
27. Williams S, Weinman J, Dale J. Doctor-patient communication and patient satisfaction: a review. Fam Pract. 1998;15:480–92.

9

Tolerated drugs in subjects with severe cutaneous adverse reactions (SCARs) induced by anticonvulsants and review of the literature

Fabrizio De Luca[1], Laura Michelina Losappio[1], Corrado Mirone[1], Jan Walter Schroeder[1], Antonella Citterio[2], Maria Gloria Aversano[1], Joseph Scibilia[1] and Elide Anna Pastorello[1*]

Abstract

Background: Anticonvulsant hypersensitivity syndrome represents a rare but potentially fatal kind of adverse drug reaction. This clinical picture often hampers the flexibility with which alternative anticonvulsants or even other classes of drugs are prescribed in these patients, negatively affecting the efficacy of treatment and the course of the disease. The aim of this study was to analyse a group of six patients with severe cutaneous drug reactions induced by anticonvulsants and to report which alternative antiepileptic drugs and which drugs of other classes were tolerated.

Case presentation: A total of six patients (2 males and 4 females, age 11–73 years) are described in this study. In all the patients the onset of the severe cutaneous drug reactions was 2–4 weeks after initiating the anticonvulsant therapy: 2 out of 6 patients presented with a drug reaction with eosinophilia and systemic symptoms under therapy with phenytoin; 2 out of 6 presented with Stevens–Johnson syndrome under therapy with lamotrigine; and 2 out of 6 presented with a toxic epidermal necrolysis, one of them under therapy with valproic acid, and the other one under therapy with lamotrigine. Alternative anticonvulsants tolerated after the reaction were: clonazepam, levetiracetam, diazepam, delorazepam and lormetazepam.

Conclusions: In our cases we observed that non aromatic anticonvulsants and benzodiazepines were well tolerated as alternative treatments in six patients with reactions to aromatic anticonvulsivants and that the risk of hypersensitivity reactions to other drug classes was not increased as compared to general population.

Keywords: Anticonvulsants, Drug hypersensitivity, Anticonvulsant hypersensitivity syndrome, Stevens–Johnson syndrome, Toxic epidermal necrolysis, Drug reaction with eosinophilia and systemic symptoms, Severe cutaneous adverse reactions

Background

Anticonvulsant hypersensitivity syndrome (AHS) represents a rare but potentially fatal kind of adverse drug reaction. The antiepileptic drugs (AEDs) most commonly involved are the aromatic anticonvulsants such as phenytoin, phenobarbital, carbamazepine, and lamotrigine; however, in the literature several cases induced by valproic acid are also reported [1–3]. Clinical presentations are highly variable and include either simple pruritic eruptions or severe forms such as Stevens–Johnson syndrome (SJS), toxic epidermal necrolysis (TEN) and drug reaction with eosinophilia and systemic symptoms (DRESS) [4, 5]. SJS and TEN are characterized by detachment of the epidermis and erosions of mucous membranes and are considered to be the same disease, the only difference being the extent of skin detachment, < 10% of total body surface area in SJS, and > 30% in TEN [6]. DRESS is characterized by eosinophilia, skin rash, fever, lymphadenopathy, and visceral organ involvement [7]. The clinical symptoms usually develop from 1 to 8 weeks after starting the antiepileptic therapy; adults older than 64 years are at the highest risk for severe

*Correspondence: elide.pastorello@ospedaleniguarda.it
[1] Department of Allergology and Immunology, Ospedale Metropolitano Niguarda Ca' Granda, Piazza Ospedale Maggiore, 3, 20162 Milan, Italy
Full list of author information is available at the end of the article

cutaneous adverse reactions (SCARs) [8]. The estimated incidence of mucocutaneous severe reactions to AEDs with internal organ involvement ranges from 1 in 1000 to 1 in 10,000 drug exposures [9]. In SJS/TEN necrosis of the skin and mucous membranes characterizes the disease; apoptosis of keratinocytes is mediated by the Fas–FasL interaction or through cytotoxic T-cell release of granulysin [10]. A genetic background confers an increased risk to develop severe forms of AHS in some ethnic groups, as demonstrated by several associations between HLA-A and -B haplotypes and severe anticonvulsant reactions, as reported in Table 1 [11–16].

As it has been demonstrated in the last decade, the T cell activation at the basis of SCARs is explainable by the so called "p-i mechanism" that does not imply any processing or metabolism of the drug, making thus reasonable a definite HLA restriction [17].

Infections play an important role in the pathogenesis of these reactions through an aspecific activation of immunological response, so that, for example the human herpes virus 6 (HHV-6) reactivation in DRESS is considered a relevant diagnostic marker [18]. Moreover, viral infections as well as other cell damaging events such surgery or severe cardiac diseases, represent the so called 'danger' factors able to prepare the pathogenetic background favouring the appearance of SCARs. All these aspects are crucial points to address in order to evaluate the risk of hypersensitivity reactions to alternative anticonvulsants or other types of drug. However, more studies will be necessary to better define the kind of genetic/environmental interaction that are at the basis of these syndromes. As a result, SCARs often restrict the use of alternative anticonvulsants or of other classes of drugs that have to be prescribed in these patients, negatively affecting the efficacy of treatment and the course of the disease.

The aim of this study was to describe a group of six patients with SCARs induced by anticonvulsant drugs and to report which alternative antiepileptic drugs and drugs of other classes were tolerated.

Case reports

A total of 6 caucasian patients (2 males and 4 females, age 11–73 years), admitted to Niguarda Ca' Granda Metropolitan Hospital for SCARs, are described in this study. In all of the patients the onset of the SCARs was 2–4 weeks after initiating the anticonvulsant therapy. For each patient we collected data regarding medical and pharmacological history. They were evaluated according to the diagnostic criteria based on RegiSCAR (Registry for Serious Cutaneous Reactions) classification (i.e. both clinical and histological features). In order to identify the inducing drug, we obtained a detailed and thorough medication history. Furthermore, a standard set of laboratory tests was performed including blood count, renal function, liver function, inflammatory markers, lactate dehydrogenase (LDH). Moreover, samples for antinuclear antibodies (ANA), and immunoglobulins against HHV-6, hepatitis virus B (HBV) and C (HCV), herpes simplex virus (HSV) type 1 and 2, human immunodeficiency virus (HIV), Epstein–Barr virus (EBV), and cytomegalovirus (CMV), blood cultures and urine cultures, were collected in order to exclude other diseases. Among the six cases, we found two cases of DRESS, two cases of SJS, and two cases of TEN. Tables 2 and 3 summarize the clinical characteristics of the study patients. Table 4 shows treatment, culprit and tolerated drugs after and during SCARs.

Cases of DRESS

Two patients, an 11-year old male (P1) and a 32-year old female (P2) presented SCARs and relevant eosinophilia after 3 weeks of therapy with phenytoin, prescribed as prophylactic anticonvulsant for surgical removal of glioblastoma in P1 and neurosurgery due to the rupture of a middle cerebral artery aneurysm in P2. Both patients developed generalized papular rash, fever, asthenia, lymphadenopathy, leukocytosis, eosinophilia, and signs

Table 2 Demographics and risk factors

Patient	Sex/age	Risk factors
P1	M/11	Surgery treatment of cerebral cancer
P2	F/32	Surgery for rupture of middle cerebral artery aneurysm
P3	M/73	Severe cachexia
P4	F/53	Acute disseminated encephalomyelitis
P5	F/41	Head trauma
P6	F/21	None

Table 1 Associations between HLA-A and -B haplotypes and severe anticonvulsant reactions

Disease	Culprit drug	HLA haplotype	Population	Authors (ref. number)
SJS /TEN	Carbamazepine	HLA-B*15:02	Asians	[11–13]
SJS/TEN and DRESS	Carbamazepine	HLA-A*31:01	Europeans	[14, 15]
SJS/TEN and DRESS	Phenytoin	HLA-B*15:13 and -B*15:02	Malaysians	[16]

SJS: Stevens Johnson syndrome, TEN: toxic epidermal necrolysis, DRESS: drug reaction with eosinophilia and systemic symptoms

Table 3 Clinical and laboratory data at the diagnosis

	P1	P2	P3	P4	P5	P6
Eosinophils (%)	12	39	5.1	4.6	2.3	2.2
Leukocytes (10^9/L)	34.67	40.23	15.0	16.0	5.6	4.7
Atypical lymphocytes	+	+	–	–	–	–
GOT/GPT (IU/L)	1034/906	1068/960	56/50	89/63	510/702	503/731
CRP (mg/dL)	9.2	9.6	13.6	11.3	1.1	1.0
LDH (IU/L)	1780	1890	1230	1360	1450	423
HHV-6 infection	+	+	–	–	–	–
HCV, HBV, CMV, HSV-1 and -2, EBV, HIV infection	–	–	HSV-2	–	–	
Blood cultures	–	–	Candida albicans	MRSA	Staphylococcus capitis	MRSA
Urine cultures	–	–	–	–	Enterococcus faecalis	–
ANA	–	–	–	–	–	–
Skin biopsy	Acantholytic cells, skin detachment, mild lymphocytic infiltration	ND	ND	Apoptotic keratinocytes, spongiosis, subepidermal blister and dermal inflammatory infiltrate	Dermal infiltrate of lymphocytes and monocytes	Apoptotic keratinocytes, epidermal necrosis and dermal infiltrate of lymphocytes

CRP: C-reactive protein, GOT: glutamate oxaloacètique transaminase, GPT: glutamane pyruvate transaminase, LDH: lactate dehydrogenase, ANA: antinuclear antibodies, MRSA: methicillin-resistant *Staphylococcus aureus*, *ND*: not done, +: positive, –: negative

Table 4 Treatment, culprit and tolerated drugs after and during SCARs

Patient	SCARs	Culprit drug	Latency (weeks)	Treatment	Tolerated anticonvulsants	Other tolerated drugs
P1	DRESS	Phenytoin	3	Methylprednisolone for 3 months	Clonazepam	Ibuprofen, clarithromycin
P2	DRESS	Phenytoin	3	Prednisone for 1 year	Levetiracetam	Metamizole, tramadol, amoxicillin, clarithromycin, ketoprofen, metoclopramide, rituximab, lercanidipine
P3	SJS	Lamotrigine	4	Hydrocortisone bolus, prednisone for 1 month and immunoglobulin intravenously	Delorazepam and lormetazepam	Echinocandin
P4	SJS	Phenytoin	4	Hydrocortisone bolus, prednisone for 1 month and immunoglobulin intravenously	Diazepam	Teicoplanin, haloperidol
P5	TEN	Valproic acid	2	Prednisone for 1 month and immunoglobulin intravenously	Diazepam and levetiracetam	Meropenem
P6	TEN	Lamotrigine	2	Prednisone for 1 month and immunoglobulin intravenously	Diazepam and levetiracetam	Teicoplanin

SCARs: severe cutaneous adverse reactions, SJS: Stevens–Johnson syndrome, DRESS: drug reaction with eosinophilia and systemic symptoms, TEN: toxic epidermal necrolysis

of liver damage, as reported in Table 3. Eosinophilia, lymphadenopathy, skin biopsy in P1, and HHV-6 DNA positivity confirmed the diagnosis of DRESS. Other diagnostic tests were carried out to better characterize the extent of the organ involvement and possible complications. Abdominal ultrasound showed splenomegaly in P1 and was normal in P2. Positron emission tomography-computed tomography and cervical lymph node biopsy performed to investigate the relevant lymphoadenomegaly in P2 demonstrated only reactive lymphadenopathy, thus excluding a lymphoproliferative disorder. Anticonvulsants were discontinued in both the patients after the diagnosis and a treatment with methylprednisolone 40 mg daily for 40 days was given to P1; a complete and stable remission of symptoms was observed after a slow tapering of methylprednisolone over a period of 2 months. P2 underwent therapy with prednisone 70 mg daily for 10 days; glucocorticoid was then interrupted for a few days in order to perform lymph nodal biopsy that confirmed the reactive lymphadenopathy: a severe clinical relapse was observed characterized by macular papular rash, systemic lymphadenopathy, itching and asthenia. Prednisone was readministered at a dosage of 50 mg daily for 15 days, reduced to 25 mg and slowly tapered off 5 mg every 2 weeks under strict medical control. Normalization of inflammatory and necrosis markers was observed in P2 after 4 months from the beginning of glucocorticoid therapy; subsequently P2 showed relevant adverse effects: hypertension, headache, acne, hair loss and osteoporosis. In both cases a new anticonvulsant drug was necessary for a relapse of seizures. In P1 clonazepam was introduced after few days of glucocorticoid premedication treatment and was well tolerated in the following months. P2 underwent treatment with levetiracetam for seizure relapse and the drug was well tolerated in the following months. Other drugs were well tolerated after the reaction despite the fear of clinical relapse, such as ibuprofen and clarithromycin in P1; metamizole, tramadol, amoxicillin, clarithromycin, ketoprofen, lercanidipine, and metoclopramide in P2. One month after definitive suspension of glucocorticoids P2 manifested an abrupt increase in blood pressure, dysarthria, confusional state and headache not responsive to treatment. The patient was again hospitalized and the following blood values were observed: Hb 7.8 g/dL, platelets count 11,000 × 10^9/L, LDH 1560 IU/L, haptoglobin 10 mg/dL, the presence of schistocytes in peripheral blood, total bilirubin 2.2 mg/dL, and ADAMTS13 activity at 7%. After hospital admission the patient manifested purpuric lesions. Brain magnetic resonance imaging was carried out and showed micro hemorrhages. The diagnosis of thrombotic thrombocytopenic purpura (Moskowitz syndrome) was made so treatment with rituximab at dose of 375 mg/m^2, i.e. once weekly for 4 weeks plus prednisone at 50 mg daily for 2 weeks with tapering after 1 month was instituted. The complete resolution of the clinical picture required a total of 14 months.

Cases of SJS

Two patients, a 73-year old male (P3) and a 53-year old female (P4) presented SCARs after 4 weeks of therapy with lamotrigine, prescribed to P3 for bipolar disorder with prevailing depressive symptoms in severe cachexia, and phenytoin prescribed to P4 as prophylaxis after acute disseminated encephalomyelitis. Both had developed diffuse maculopapular rash, fever, and 24 h later ulcerations of the oral mucosa, blistering skin lesions, epithelial detachment, conjunctivitis, and diffuse pain. HSV-2 IgM positivity was observed in P3. The clinical pictures and skin biopsy performed in P4 confirmed the diagnosis of SJS (Table 3). Abdominal ultrasound, echocardiogram and chest CT excluded organ involvement. After suspected SJS diagnosis, anticonvulsants were immediately discontinued; both P3 and P4 were treated with hydrocortisone 1 g bolus, followed by prednisone 50 mg/daily for 10 days tapered in the subsequent month. During the hospitalization the patients were treated with intravenous immunoglobulins (IV Ig) 0.4 g/kg daily for 5 days, and with topical agents. Enteral feeding and crystalloid were also required. New anticonvulsants were given: lormetazepam and diazepam in P3 and diazepam in P4. Moreover, P4 developed psychosis as an adverse effect of glucocorticoid therapy and was treated with haloperidol. Echinocandin and teicoplanin were administered for 2 weeks because of prolonged fever and positive blood cultures for *Candida albicans* and methicillin-resistant *Staphylococcus aureus* (MRSA) in P3 and P4, respectively. Both antibiotics were well tolerated by the patients and they were discharged after 3 weeks in good clinical conditions.

Cases of TEN

Two females, 41 year old (P5), and 21 year old (P6), presented SCARs after 2 weeks of therapy with valproic acid, given to P5 consequently to head trauma, and with lamotrigine, used in P6 for epilepsy. Both patients developed diffuse maculopapular rash and in addition P6 showed severe asthenia and conjunctivitis. Their clinical pictures progressed rapidly to TEN, showing epidermal detachment, mucosal involvement with severe bleeding requiring blood transfusions. In particular, epidermal detachment involved 45 and 95% of the body surface in P5 and P6, respectively. During the hospitalization, P6 developed respiratory distress requiring mechanical ventilation. Diagnostic routine work up on the diagnosis showed leukocytosis and sign of liver damage in both the patients. Infections were detected by urine cultures that showed *Enterococcus faecalis* in P5 and by blood cultures that were positive for *Staphylococcus capitis* and MRSA in P5 and in P6, respectively. Clinical pictures and skin biopsy confirmed the TEN diagnosis (Table 3). Ultrasound abdomen showed hepatomegaly in both patients, and echocardiograms were normal. Based on the diagnosis of TEN, anticonvulsants were stopped and the patients were treated with topical medications, IV Ig at 0.4/kg daily for 5 days and with prednisone 50 mg daily during 2 weeks of the hospitalization with slow tapering with complete remission after 1 month from the discharge. Meropenem and teicoplanin were administered for 2 weeks to treat secondary infections in P5 and P6 respectively and enteral feeding and crystalloid were also required. Antibiotics were perfectly tolerated also after glucocorticoid tapering. In both cases, new anticonvulsant were considered necessary and levetiracetam and diazepam were introduced in P5 and P6 respectively, a few days after the start of cortisone treatment, and were well tolerated in the following months.

Conclusions

The principal aim of this study was to describe the course of six patients affected by SCARs to anticonvulsants. These drugs, as well as allopurinol, have been already regarded as one of the most common causes of SCARs [19, 20]. The analysis of our clinical data allowed us to determine the tolerance to alternative anticonvulsants and to different drug classes that in the routine practice are often not administered for the fear of a relapse. According to a prospective RegiSCAR study, aromatic AEDs, in particular carbamazepine, phenytoin, and lamotrigine, were considered responsible for the reaction in the 35% of cases. Additional culprit drugs were allopurinol, sulfonamides and other antibiotics involved in another 41% of cases [19]. Two out of 6 SCARs from our study were induced by lamotrigine, three by phenytoin and one by valproic acid. In a recent review 172 cases of DRESS associated with 44 drugs were analyzed: the most frequently implicated was carbamazepine, followed by lamotrigine and phenytoin [21]. In SJS/TEN, an association with 12 "highly suspect" medication was reported that included anticonvulsants, mostly carbamazepine, oxcarbazepine, phenytoin and lamotrigine [20]. These observations confirmed previous clinical data [22, 23]. The reactions in our patients occurred on the first exposure to the drug, with a latency time from 2 to 4 weeks after the beginning of therapy, as already observed [1, 9]. Several potential risk factors for AED hypersensitivity were reported: previous history of AED-induced eruption [24], autoimmune diseases, treatment with corticosteroids, family history of SCARs [25], age below 12 years or above 64 associated with altered drug metabolism [8], head injury, surgery, genetic markers such as HLA-B*15:02 and HLA-A*31:01, and reactivation of HHV-6 and -7, EBV and CMV virus [26, 27].

In our patients we identified several of the above quoted risk factors, in particular: surgery (P1, P2), head trauma (P5), and herpes viral infections in P1, P2 (i.e. HHV-6), and in P3 (i.e. HSV 2); of note, this last patient also suffered from recurrent airway infections due to a cachectic state. All these situations have been reported to potentially determine severe distress and injury to cells that in turn can release internal molecules able to act as damage or danger signals stimulating toll-like receptors on antigen presenting cells activating thus the immune response.

The culprit drugs were identified only by clinical data as up to now no standardized diagnostic test has been adopted in delayed T-cell mediated drug allergy reactions except in contact dermatitis IVa type [28]. Although different skin tests (SPT, ID, patch tests) have been suggested as useful tools for the diagnosis of SCARs [29], more recently drug patch test was reported as the only convenient and safe tool for identifying culprit drugs in DRESS; on the contrary, this procedure was not recommended in SJS/TEN [30, 31]. We did not perform in vivo tests because our patients assumed only AEDs at the onset of SCARs. The clinical course worsened after discontinuation of the culprit drug, as already reported in DRESS [32]. Liver was the extracutaneous organ more frequently affected in our patients, as usually observed in DRESS (70–95%), and in SJS/TEN [33]. In DRESS, hepatic damage was more severe after phenytoin [34], as observed also in our two DRESS patients (P1 and P2). We observed no heart or kidney damage. Signs of renal damage were reported just in the 11% of DRESS patients, mainly, after allopurinol administration [19]. In P1 and P2, a diffuse lymphadenopathy was observed, as already reported in DRESS in nearly 75% of the cases [35]. In particular, in P2 lymph node biopsy showed a benign lymphoid hyperplasia, one of the two histological patterns reported in this syndrome, besides pseudolymphoma [7]. The most common complications we observed were secondary infections i.e. septicemia (4 out of 6 patients; 66%). A transient respiratory failure appeared in one case (P6). P2 developed an autoimmune disease, a sequelae already reported in DRESS especially if not treated with steroids [36]. However, in our patient a thrombotic thrombocytopenic purpura (Moskowitz syndrome) was developed nevertheless a previous high dose steroid therapy followed for several months. The time for complete resolution of the hypersensitivity reaction ranged from 2 to 12 months, compared to a period of 14–345 days reported by others [19, 36].

In respect to the culprit drugs, 5 out of 6 SCARs cases were induced by aromatic anticonvulsant drugs to confirm an increased risk of severe reactions to these molecules in comparison with other AEDs. In two cases (P3 and P6) the culprit drug was lamotrigine, a molecule already associated with a high risk of SJS and TEN [23], through a dose dependent effect [37]. Both lamotrigine and phenytoin, culprit drugs in P3, P4 and P6, were regarded as "highly suspect" compounds associated with SJS/TEN in a pharmacovigilance study [20]. Cross-reactivity between aromatic anticonvulsants ranged from 30 to 58% [38, 39], for this reason in our cases we selected non aromatic drugs, i.e. benzodiazepines and levetiracetam, as an alternative treatment. This choice relied on previous reports suggesting non aromatic AEDs, like gabapentin, as agents with low allergenic potential [39], in particular levetiracetam, was a drug associated with lower rash rates (0–6%) [24].

Some authors advised against treatment with antibiotics or NSAIDs in the DRESS acute period, for unexplained cross-reactivity able to worsen the clinical picture [27]. However, alternative antimicrobials were administered without adverse effects in 16 out of 17 patients affected with antibiotic-related DRESS [40]. Our experience showed that in AED-induced SCARs the risk of hypersensitivity reactions to other drug classes was not increased in comparison with general population. Recently, a strict relationship between SCARs induced by allopurinol and carbamazepine and definite HLA-aplotypes has been identified. This observation might implicate a tight HLA restriction also in adverse reactions to different drugs and consequently a low risk of additional events [41]. In fact, other drugs tolerated were: ibuprofen, clarithromycin, amoxicillin, metamizole, tramadol, ketoprofen, metoclopramide, rituximab, lercanidipine, echinocandin, teicoplanin, haloperidoland meropenem. In our patients, we discontinued the culprit drug and administered steroid therapy at high dosage, a treatment suggested in other studies [42, 43]. High doses of steroid might have an immunosuppressive effect preventing a relapse due to other compounds [41]. The management of our patients differed according to the Unit in which they were admitted: DRESS subjects were treated in our Centre with high doses of steroids, while SJS/TEN subjects were treated in Burn Unit with IVIG, steroids and topic therapy. High doses of IVIG was effective in our SJS/TEN patients, as already reported in some studies [44], although this treatment was considered useless by other Authors [45]. The prognosis was good also as a consequence of careful supportive treatment conducted in specialized Burn Units.

In conclusion, on the basis of our case reports, we can suggest that non aromatic drugs, i.e. benzodiazepines and levetiracetam, are the most safe alternative treatment in SCARs due to the anticonvulsants. Moreover, we observed that drugs belonging to other classes were well tolerated in these patients confirming thus indirectly an

HLA restriction for hypersensitivity reactions to other anticonvulsant drugs as well as to carbamazepine and phenytoin.

Abbreviations

AHS: anticonvulsant hypersensitivity syndrome; AEDs: antiepileptic drugs; SJS: Stevens–Johnson syndrome; TEN: toxic epidermal necrolysis; DRESS: drug reaction with eosinophilia and systemic symptoms; SCARs: severe cutaneous adverse reactions; RegiSCAR: Registry for Serious Cutaneous Reactions; LDH: lactate dehydrogenase; ANA: antinuclear antibodies; HBV: hepatitis virus B; HCV: hepatitis virus C; HSV: herpes simplex virus; HIV: human immunodeficiency virus; EBV: Epstein–Barr virus; CMV: cytomegalovirus.

Authors' contributions

FDL collected data. LML wrote the draft paper and analyzed the data. CM, MGA wrote the draft paper. JWS followed clinical course of the patients. AC and JS revised the draft paper. EAP designed the study, wrote and revised the draft paper. All authors read and approved the final manuscript.

Author details

[1] Department of Allergology and Immunology, Ospedale Metropolitano Niguarda Ca' Granda, Piazza Ospedale Maggiore, 3, 20162 Milan, Italy. [2] Department of Burn/Intensive Care, Ospedale Metropolitano Niguarda Ca' Granda, Milan, Italy.

Competing interests

The authors declare that they have no competing interests.

References

1. Knowles SR, Shapiro LE, Shear N. Anticonvulsant hypersensitivity syndrome: incidence, prevention and management. Drug Saf. 1999;21(6):489–501.
2. Wang X, Wang HF, Hang X, Au S, Huang X, Zhang JT, Tian CL, Lang SY. Lamotrigine induced DIHS/DRESS: manifestations, treatment, and outcome in 57 patients. Clin Neurol Neurosurg. 2015;138:1–7.
3. Nanau RM, Neuman MG. Adverse drug reactions induced by valproic acid. Clin Biochem. 2013;46(15):1323–38.
4. Blaszczyk B, Lason W, Czuczwar SJ. Antiepilectic drugs and adverse skin reactions: an update. Pharmacol Rep. 2015;67(3):426–34.
5. Armin S, Chavoshzadeh Z, Mohkam M, Rezaei N. Antiepileptic hypersensitivity and DRESS syndrome due to phenytoin in two pediatric cases. Turk J Pediatr. 2009;51(1):76–7.
6. Eginli A, Shah K, Watkins C, Krishnaswamy G. Stevens–Johnson syndrome and toxic epidermal necrolysis. Ann Allergy Asthma Immunol. 2017;118(2):143–7.
7. Bocquet H, Bagon M, Roujeau JC. Drug-induced pseudolymphoma and drug hypersensitivity syndrome (DrugRash with Eosinophilia and Systemic Symptoms: DRESS). Semin Cutan Med Surg. 1996;15(4):250–7.
8. Chan HL, Stern RS, Arndt KA, Langlois J, Jick H, Walker AM. The incidence of erythema multiforme, Stevens–Johnson syndrome, and toxic epidermal necrolysis. A population-based study with particular reference to reactions caused by drugs among outpatients. Arch Dermatol. 1990;126(1):43–7.
9. Knowles SR, Shear NH. Anticonvulsant hypersensitivity syndrome: an update. Expert Opin Drug Saf. 2012;11(5):767–78.
10. Paul C, Wolkenstein P, Adle H, Wechsler J, Garchon HJ, Revuz J, Roujeau JC. Apoptosis as a mechanism of keratinocyte death in toxic epidermal necrolysis. Br J Dermatol. 1996;134:710.
11. Chung WH, Hung SI, Hong HS, Hsih MS, Yang LC, Ho HC, et al. Medical genetics: a marker for Stevens–Johnson syndrome. Nature. 2004;28(6982):486.
12. Tassaneeyakul W, Tiamkao S, Jantararoungtong T, Chen P, Lin SY, Chen WH. Association between HLA-B*1502 and carbamazepine-induced severe cutaneous adverse drug reactions in a Thai population. Epilepsia. 2010;51:926.
13. Nguyen DV, Chu HC, Nguyen DV, Phan MH, Craig T, Baumgart K, van Nunen S. HLA-B*1502 and carbamazepine-induced severe cutaneous adverse drug reactions in Vietnamese. Asia Pac Allergy. 2015;5(2):68–77.
14. McCormack M, Alfirevic A, Bourgeois S, Farrell JJ. HLA-A*3101 and carbamazepine-induced hypersensitivity reactions in Europeans. N Engl J Med. 2011;364(12):1134–43.
15. Genin E, Chen DP, Hung SI, Sekula P, Schumacher M, Chang PY, Tsai SH, Wu TL, Bellòn T, Tamouza R, Fortier C, Tounbert A, Charon D, Hovnanian A, Wolkenstein P, Chung WH, Mockenhaupt M, Roujeau JC. HLA-A*31:01 and different types of carbamazepine-induced severe cutaneous adverse reactions: an international study and meta-analysis. Pharmacogen J. 2014;14:281–8.
16. Chang CC, Ng CC, Too CL, Choon SE, Lee CK, Chung WH, Hussei SH, Lim KS, Murad S. Association of HLA-B*15:13 and HLA-B*15:02 with phenytoin-induced severe cutaneous adverse reactions in a Malay population. Pharmacogen J. 2017;17:170–3.
17. Pichler WJ, Hausmann O. Classification of drug hypersensitivity into allergic, p-1, and pseudo-allergic forms. Int Arch Allergy Immunol. 2016;171:166–79.
18. Demoly P, Adkinson NF, Brockow K, Castells M, Chiriac AM, Greenberger PA, Khan DA, Lang DM, Park HS, Pichler W, Sanchez-Borges M, Shiohara T, Thong BY. International consensus on drug allergy. Allergy. 2014;69:420–37.
19. Kardaun SH, Sekula P, Valeyrie-Allanore L, Liss Y, Chu Y, Creamer D, Sidoroff A, Naldi L, Mockenhaupt M, Roujeay JC. Drug reaction with eosinophilia and systemic symptoms (DRESS): an original multisystem adverse drug reaction. Results from the prospective RegiSCAR study. Br J Dermatol. 2013;169:1071–80.
20. Papay J, Yueu N, Powell G, Mockenhaupt M, Bogenrieder T. Spontaneous adverse event reports of Stevens–Johnson syndrome/toxic epidermal necrolysis: detecting associations with medications. Pharmacoepidemiol Drug Saf. 2012;21:289–96.
21. Cacoub P, Musette P, Descamps V, Meyer O, Speirs C, Finzi L, Roujeau JC. The DRESS syndrome: a literature review. Am J Med. 2011;124(7):588–97.
22. Sassolas B, Haddan C, Mockenhaupt M, Dunat A, Liss Y, Bork K, Haustein UF, Vieluf D, Roujeau JC, Le Louet H. ALDEN, an algorithm for assessment of drug causality in Stevens–Johnson Syndrome and toxic epidermal necrolysis: comparison with case-control analysis. Clin Pharmacol Ther. 2010;88:60–8.
23. Mockenhaupt M, Viboud C, Dunand A, Naldi L, Halevy S, Bouwer Bavinck HN, Sidoroff A, Schneck J, Roujean JC, Flahault A. Stevens–Johnson syndrome and toxic epidermal necrolysis: assessment of medication risks with emphasis on recently marketed drugs. The EuroSCAR-study. J Invest Dermatol. 2008;128:35–44.

24. Arif H, Burchsbaum R, Weintraub D, Koyfman S, Salas-Humara C, Bazil CW, Resor SR Jr, Hirsvh LJ. Comparison and predictors of rash associated with 15 antiepileptic drugs. Neurology. 2007;68(20):1701–9.
25. Pichler WJ. Delayed drug hypersensitivity reactions. Ann Intern Med. 2003;139(8):683–93.
26. Ye YM, Thong BY, Park HS. Hypersensitivity to antiepileptic drugs. Immunol Allergy Clin N Am. 2014;34:633–43.
27. Schiohara T, Inaoka M, Kano Y. Drug-induced hypersensitivity syndrome (DIHS): a reaction induced by a complex interplay among herpes viruses and antiviral and anti drug immune responses. Allergol Int. 2006;55:1–8.
28. Posadas SJ, Pichler WJ. Delayed drug hypersensitivity reactions—new concepts. Clin Exp Allergy. 2007;37(7):989–99.
29. Brockow K, Romano A, Blanca M, Ring J, Pichler W, Demoly P. General considerations for skin test procedures in the diagnosis of drug hypersensitivity. Allergy. 2002;57(1):45–51.
30. Barbaud A. Skin testing and patch testing in non-IgE mediated drug allergy. Curr Allergy Asthma Rep. 2014;14:442.
31. Barbaud A, Collet E, Milpied B, Assier H, Staumont D, Avenel-Audran M, Grange A, Amarger S, Girardin P, Guinnepain MT, Truchetet F, Lasek A, Waton J, Toxidermies group of the French Society of Dermatology. A multicentre study to determine the value and safety of drug patch tests for the three main classes of severe cutaneous adverse drug reactions. Br J Dermatol. 2013;168(3):555–62.
32. Roujeau JC, Stern RS. Severe adverse cutaneous reactions to drugs. New Engl J Med. 1994;331:1272–85.
33. Chave TA, Mortimer NJ, Sladden MJ, Hall AP, Hutchinson PE. Toxic epidermal necrolysis: current evidence, practical management and future directions. Br J Dermatol. 2005;153(2):241–53.
34. Kano Y, Shiohara T. The variable clinical picture of drug-induced hypersensitivity syndrome/drug rash with eosinophilia and systemic symptoms in relation to the eliciting drug. Immunol Allergy Clin N Am. 2009;29:481–501.
35. Gentile I, Talamo M, Borgia S. Is the drug-induced hypersensitivity syndrome (DIHS) due to human herpes virus 6 infection or to allergy-mediated viral reactivation? Report of a case and literature review. BMN Infect Dis. 2010;10:49.
36. Avancini J, Maragno L, Santi CG, Criado PR. Drug reaction with eosinophilia and systemic symptoms/drug-induced hypersensitivity syndrome: clinical features of 27 patients. Clin Exp Dermatol. 2015;40(8):851–9.
37. Sachs B, Ronnau AC, Ruzicka T, Gleichmann E, Schuppe HC. Lamotrigine and toxic epidermal necrolysis (TEN) in Germany. Lancet. 1996;348:1041.
38. Alvestad S, Lydersen S, Brodtkorb E. Cross-reactivity pattern of rash from current aromatic antiepileptic drugs. Epilepsy Res. 2008;80:194–200.
39. Zaccara G, Franciotta D, Perucca E. Idiosyncratic adverse reactions to antiepileptic drugs. Epilepsia. 2007;48(7):1223–44.
40. Lin YF, Yang CH, Sindy H, Lin JY, Rosaline Hui CY, Tsai YC, Wu TS, Huang CT, Kao KC, Hu HC, Chiu CH, Hung SI, Chung WH. Severe cutaneous adverse reactions related to systemic antibiotics. Clin Infect Dis. 2014;58(10):1377–85.
41. Pichler WJ, Daubner B, Kawabata T. Drug hypersensitivity: flare-up reactions, cross-reactivity and multiple drug hypersensitivity. J Dermatol. 2011;38(3):216–21.
42. Schneck J, Gafot JP, Sekula P, Sassolas B, Roujeay JC, Mockenhaupt M. Effects of treatments on the mortality of Stevens–Johnson syndrome and toxic epidermal necrolysis: a retrospective study on patients included in the prospective EuroSCAR Study. J Am Acad Dermatol. 2008;58:33–40.
43. Husain Z, Reddy BY, Schwartz RA. DRESS syndrome: part II. Management and therapeutics. J Am Acad Dermatol. 2013;68(5):1–9.
44. Aihara M, Kano Y, Fujita Hm Kambara T, Matsukura S, Katayama I, Azukizawa H, Miyachi Y, Endo Y, Asada H, Miyagawa F, Morita E, Kaneko S, Abe R, Ochiai T, Sueki H, Watanabe H, Nagao K, Aoyama Y, Sayama K, Hashimoto K, Shiohara T, SJS/TEN Study Group. Efficacy of additional i.v. immunoglobulin to steroid therapy in Stevens–Johnson syndrome and toxic epidermal necrolysis. J Dermatol. 2015;42:768–77.
45. Faye O, Roujeay JC. Treatment of epidermal necrolysis with high dose intravenous immunoglobulin (IVIg): clinical experience to date. Drugs. 2005;65:2085–90.

10

Chitinase 3-like-1 is produced by human Th17 cells and correlates with the level of inflammation in juvenile idiopathic arthritis patients

Manuela Capone[1], Laura Maggi[1], Veronica Santarlasci[1], Maria Caterina Rossi[1], Alessio Mazzoni[1], Gianni Montaini[1], Rolando Cimaz[2], Matteo Ramazzotti[3], Marie Pierre Piccinni[1], Giusi Barra[4], Raffaele De Palma[4,5], Francesco Liotta[1], Enrico Maggi[1], Sergio Romagnani[1], Francesco Annunziato[1,6*] and Lorenzo Cosmi[1]

Abstract

Background: CHI3L1 is a chitinase-like protein without enzymatic activity, produced by activated macrophages, chondrocytes, neutrophils. Recent studies on arthritis, asthma, and inflammatory bowel diseases suggest that chitinases are important in inflammatory processes and tissue remodeling, but their production by human T cells, has never been reported.

Methods: A microarray analysis of gene expression profile was performed on Th17 and classic Th1 cell clones and CHI3L1 was found among the up-regulated genes on Th17 cells. Different types of helper T cell clones (TCCs) were then evaluated by Real Time PCR (RT-PCR) for CHI3L1 mRNA expression; protein expression was investigated in cell lysates by western blotting and in cultures supernatants by ELISA. ELISA was also used to measure CHI3L1 in the serum and in the synovial fluid (SF) of juvenile idiopathic arthritis (JIA) patients.

Results: At mRNA level CHI3L1 was highly expressed by Th17, Th17/Th1, non classic Th1 and even in Th17/Th2 cell clones, whereas it was virtually absent in CD161− classic Th1 and Th2 TCCs. CHI3L1 was also detected in cell culture supernatants of Th17 and Th17-derived cells but not of classic Th1. Moreover CHI3L1 was higher in the SF than in serum of JIA patients, and it positively correlated with the frequency of Th17 and non-classic Th1 cells in SF. CHI3L1 in SF also positively correlated with the C reactive protein (CRP) serum levels, and with the levels of some proinflammatory cytokines, such as IL-6 and p40, which is the common subunit of IL12 and IL23.

Conclusions: Here we describe for the first time CHI3L1 production by T cells owing the Th17 family. Moreover the positive correlation found between the frequency of Th17 and Th17-derived cell subsets and CHI3L1 levels in SF of JIA patients, in agreement with the suggested role of these cells in inflammatory process, candidates CHI3L1 as a possible biological target in JIA treatment.

Keywords: CHI3L1, Th17 cells, CD161, SF, JIA, CRP

Background

Chitinases belong to a family of hydrolases, the glycosyl hydrolase 18 proteins (GH18), characterized by the ability to cleave the environmental polysaccharide chitin, present in the coating of many pathogens including protozoan parasites, fungi, and nematodes. Although mammals do not synthesize chitin, they do synthesize chitinases and chitinase-like proteins (CLPs), that, due to mutations in their active domain, don't have chitinolytic enzyme activity. Members of this family include chitinase 3-like-1 (also known as YKL-40 or HC-gp39)

*Correspondence: f.annunziato@dmi.unifi.it
[6] Department of Internal Medicine, University of Florence, Viale Pieraccini 6, 50134 Florence, Italy
Full list of author information is available at the end of the article

[1], chitotriosidase [2], YKL-39 [3], Ym1 [4], acidic mammalian chitinase (AMCase) [5], oviduct-specific glycoprotein [6], and stabilin-1-interacting chitinase-like protein [7]. The physiological role of these secretory proteins remains unclear and debated, even if recent findings strongly support the concept that chitinases and CLPs are induced at sites of infection as part of an innate anti-pathogen response: in that context they are described to act by controlling tissue injury and specific innate immune response such as those induced by chitin fragments and augmenting adaptive immune responses, ensuring pathogen eradication [8]. The majority of the glycosyl 18-hydrolase family member are CLPs and among them chitinase 3-like-1 (CHI3L1) is the most studied: it is endogenously expressed by several cell types including macrophages, neutrophils, chondrocytes, fibroblasts, endothelial cells and colonic, ductal, and airway epithelial cells [1, 8]. CHI3L1 expression is upregulated during inflammatory conditions when it is essential for mounting Th2-type immune responses, stimulating dendritic cell accumulation/activation and recruitment of macrophages but also for inhibiting eosinophils, macrophages and T cells death-receptor mediated, apoptosis [9]. CHI3L1 has been also shown to stimulate proliferation of human connective tissue cells through a MAPK/AKT dependent pathway [10]. In agreement with these evidences on CHI3L1 activities, KO mice have been generated that developed less severe inflammatory responses at the acute phase of bacterial infectious colitis [11] as well as suppressed Th2-type immune responses, characterized by lower tissue inflammation, fibrosis and higher immune cell apoptosis [9]. Increased levels of CHI3L1 protein and/or mRNA have been shown in patients with a broad spectrum of diseases including asthma [9, 12], inflammatory bowel disease (IBD) [13, 14] and arthritis [15, 16] where they reflect the activity and natural history of the disease. In fact, genetic variation of CHI3L1 gene associated with its higher expression in serum and with exacerbation of asthma and airways tissue remodelling [17]. Finally CHI3L1 has been proposed as a candidate autoantigen in rheumatoid arthritis (RA) [18] due to its different expression in cartilage and synovial tissues, and to a possible link with the human leukocyte antigen (HLA)-DR4 shared epitope [19]. As a result of this knowledge CHI3L1 is already considered a prognostic biomarker for several immune mediated diseases and has been proposed to be a therapeutic target in conditions characterized by fibrosis, extracellular matrix remodeling and acute or chronic inflammation [12, 14–16].

It is already well described that T helper populations, in addition to their protective role, are involved in several chronic inflammatory immune-mediated disorders. CD4+ T helper (Th) cells can be classified into lineages on the basis of the cytokines production, the specific transcription factors expression and the immune-physiological function they mediate. Th1 cells, which express the transcription factor T-box expressed in T cells (T-bet) and secrete IFN-γ, protect the host against intracellular infections; Th2 cells, which express GATA-3 and secrete IL-4, IL-5 and IL-13, mediate host defense against helminths [20, 21]. Recently, additional subsets that preferentially produce distinct cytokines have been described. The most studied subset includes cells that selectively produce IL-17A (Th17 cells), express the transcription factor RAR-related orphan receptor (ROR)γt, the IL-23 receptor (IL-23R), the chemokine receptor CCR6 and the lectin receptor CD161 and protect the host against extracellular pathogens infections [22–24]. Human Th17 cells originate from CD161+ precursors present in umbilical cord blood (UCB) and new born thymus, and maintain CD161 expression, that is detectable on memory circulating and tissue-infiltrating Th17 lymphocytes [24–26]. Th17 lymphocytes, beyond their protective role in the clearance of extracellular pathogens, also play a role in the pathogenesis of several autoimmune and inflammatory diseases [27]. In particular, a determinant role for Th17 cells has been proposed in multiple sclerosis, RA and IBDs, but also in psoriasis and contact dermatitis [28, 29], under-evaluating the contribution of Th1 cells [30], previously shown to be crucial. Although classically viewed as distinct lineages, recent evidence indicate that Th17 cells are more plastic than previously thought. It is not fully understood how often such plasticity occurs in the course of physiologic responses to pathogens and what its importance is in protective immunity, but in inflammatory conditions Th17 lymphocytes, that have shifted towards a Th1 or Th2 phenotype maintaining CD161 and RORc expression and acquiring the ability to produce IFN-γ or IL-4, seem to be particularly aggressive and more pathogenic than the unshifted ones [31, 32]. In a recent study, we found that Th17 cells are rare in the SF of patients with JIA whereas Th1 cells were highly predominant, which was at least partially due to the property of Th17 cells to shift into Th1 cells in presence of IL-12, and/or TNF-α [33, 34]. The Th17-derived Th1 cells expressed CD161, while the other Th1 cells present in the SF did not, and we named the former cells as non-classic, as compared with classic CD161− Th1 cells [33]. Moreover, we found an accumulation of Th17 and non-classic CD161+ Th1 lymphocytes in fistula curettage of patients suffering of fistulising Crohn's disease [35, 36]. Another evidence of the high plasticity of human Th17 cells also emerges by the recent finding of the existence of a subset of human circulating memory CD4 T cells that produce both IL-17A and IL-4 [31]. This previously unknown population of Th17/Th2 lymphocytes maintains CD161 membrane expression, is more represented in the circulation of patients with allergic asthma than in healthy donors, and is enriched in cells specific for the sensitizing allergen, suggesting a possible role in the pathogenesis of the disease [31]. In the present study, we found that human Th17, and non-classic Th1 cells are able to produce CHI3L1, whereas classic Th1 cells are not. In agreement with the suggested role in inflammatory processes we also found CHI3L1 in the SF of JIA patients, which positively correlated to the inflammatory status. These data open new insights about the possible involvement of CHI3L1 in those chronic inflammatory disorders in which Th17 subsets play a pathogenic role.

Methods

Reagents

The culture media used was RPMI 1640 (Seromed) supplemented with 2 mM L-glutamine, 1% non-essential amino acids, 1% sodium pyruvate, 2×10^{-5} M 2-mercaptoethanol (2-ME; all from Invitrogen), and 10% FBS HyClone (Gibco Laboratories, Grand Island, NY). Unlabeled or fluorochrome-conjugated anti- CD3, CD4, CD8, CD161, CCR6, IFN-γ, and isotype-matched control mAb were purchased from BDBiosciences (San Jose, CA, USA). The fluorochrome-conjugated anti-IL-17 mAb was obtained from eBioscience (San Diego, CA, USA) and the fluorochrome-conjugated anti-CXCR3 mAb was obtained from R&D Systems (Minneapolis, MN, USA). PMA, ionomycin and brefeldin A were purchased from Sigma Chemical Co. (St. Louis, MO, USA). Activating mAb anti-CD3 and -CD28 were purchased from BDBiosciences (San Jose, CA, USA).

Establishment of T cell clones and their characterization

CD4+ T cells, derived from PBMNC of healthy donors by using the CD4 isolation kit II (Miltenyi Biotec, Bergisch Gladbach), were further divided into CD161+ and CD161− T-cell fractions by a staining with an anti-CD161–PE mAb, followed by incubation with an anti-PE microbead mAb (Miltenyi Biotec). Then the two cell subsets CD4+CD161+ and CD4+CD161− were cultured under limiting dilution (0.3 cell/well) in presence of 10^5 irradiated (9000 rad) allogeneic PBMCs as feeder cells, 1% PHA (vol/vol), and 50 U/ml rIL-2 (Proleukin, Prometheus, Inc. San Diego, USA), in order to obtain T cell clones. Recovered CD4+ T cell clones were classified on the basis of their ability to produce IFN-γ and/or IL-17 and to express surface marker CD161, as previously described [24]. Briefly, T cells were polyclonally stimulated with PMA plus ionomycin, fixed in formaldehyde and then analyzed for intracellular cytokines production on a BDLSR II flow cytometry (BDBiosciences). Selected T-cell clones of each phenotype were further analysed by flow cytometry for surface expression of CXCR3A and CCR6. Seven Th17, non-classic -Th1 and classic Th1 clones were stimulated at a culture concentration of 10^6 cells/ml for 72 h in presence of medium or mAbs anti-anti-CD3-CD28 (5 μg/ml each), then cultures supernatants were collected and stored at −30 °C for further analysis.

Microarray

Gene expression profiles on human Th17, classic and non-classic Th1 clones were assessed by cDNA microarray technique using the Human Genome Survey Microarray (Applied Biosystems). In brief, RNA from different samples was amplified and labeled with Digoxigenin-UTP (DIG-UTP; Applied Biosystems). 10 μg of DIG-labeled cRNA was hybridized to the Human Genome Survey Microarray and read using the 1700 Chemiluminescent Microarray Analyzer (Applied Biosystems). Expression Array System software (Applied Biosystems) was used to analyze the microarrays images. Only microarrays showing a normalized signal intensity >5000 and a median background <600 were analyzed and normalized using Spotfire and Intergomics software (Spotfi re Inc.). Class comparisons expressed as Benjamini–Hochberg false discovery rates were done using parametric tests (LIMMA) after log transformation. Each sample was analyzed three times. Microarray data are available from the Gene Expression Omnibus database (http://www.ncbi.nlm.nih.gov/gds) under the accession number GSE30664.

Real-time quantitative RT-PCR

Taq-Man RT-PCR was performed, as described elsewhere [24]. Quantitative PCR analysis of CHI3L1 was performed by using primers and probes purchased from Applied Biosystems (Warrington, UK). Quantification was performed on cell number.

Western Blot analysis

T Cell lysates were prepared in lysis buffer (RIPA buffer: 25 mM Tris–HCl pH 7.6, 150 mM NaCl, 1% NP-40, 1% sodium deoxycholate, 0.1% SDS and 5 mM EDTA) containing a protease- and phosphatase-inhibitor mixture (Pierce). Proteins were quantified by Bradford Assay before equivalent amounts were separated by SDS-PAGE were run on a 4–20% polyacrylamide gel (Bio-Rad, USA) for 2 h at 120 V, transferred to a nitrocellulose membrane for 16 h at 30 V, blocked in 5% milk for 1 h at room temperature. CHI3L1 protein expression was detected by anti-human CHI3L1 rabbit-pAb (ab88847; Abcam) administered for 18 h followed by incubation with horseradish peroxidase–conjugated anti-rabbit pAb

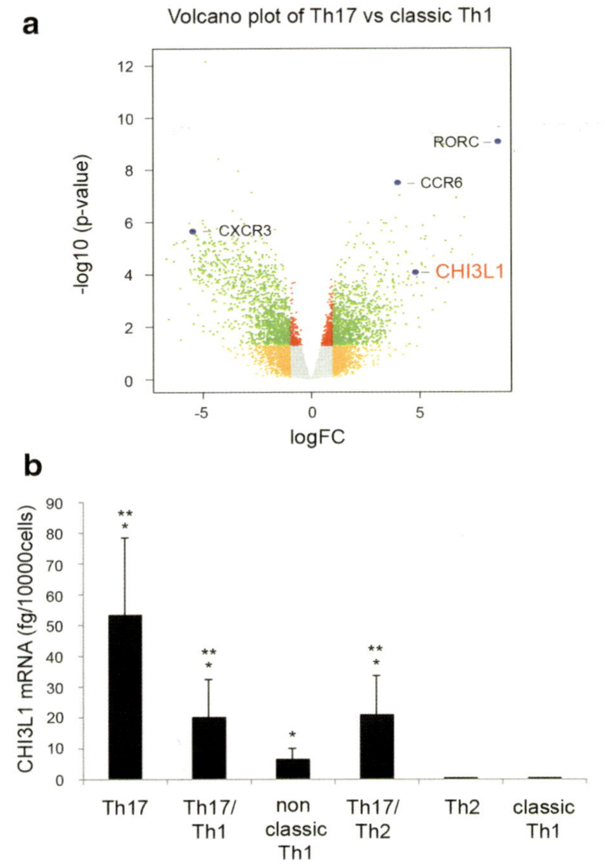

Fig. 1 CHI3L1 is expressed by Th17 and Th17-derived cells. **a** Volcano plot representation (log fold change vs. −log 10 p value) of Th17 and classic Th1 cells gene expression profiles. **b** CHI3L1 mRNA expression was evaluated by real time quantitative RT-PCR on Th17 (n = 14), Th17/Th1 (n = 7), non classic Th1 (n = 9), Th17/Th2 (n = 8), Th2 (n = 5) and classic Th1 (n = 15) clones. *Columns* represent mean values (±SE). *$p \leq 0.05$ compared to classic Th1 column; **$p \leq 0.05$ compared to Th2 column

(Santa-Cruz biotechnology) for 1 h at room temperature. An enhanced chemiluminescent substrate (GE Healthcare) for detection of HRP was used for visualization.

Subjects

Samples of PB and SF were obtained from 25 children, 15 average aged, with oligoarticular-onset JIA, whose diagnosis was made in accordance with the International League of Associations for Rheumatology classification criteria for JIA [37]. Patients with systemic-onset disease, polyarticular JIA, or enthesitis-related arthritis were excluded, in order to assess a homogeneous patient group. The C-reactive protein (CRP) serum levels (normal values up to 0.5 mg/dl), assessed using the particle-enhanced turbidimetric immunoassay method, were evaluated by staff in the service laboratory of the Anna Meyer Pediatric Hospital in Florence, Italy.

The procedures followed in the study were in accordance with the ethics standards of the Regional Committee on Human Experimentation. Informed consent was obtained by parents or guardians.

Quantitative detection of CHI3L1

CHI3L1 levels in the culture supernatants, sera and SF of JIA patients were assessed using a commercially available ELISA kit by R&D Systems. Assays were performed following manufacturer's instructions.

Enzyme-linked immunosorbent assays (ELISAs)

All the cytokines analyzed in the sera and SF of JIA patients were assessed using a Custom LEGENDplex ELISA kit from BioLegend whereas the detection of IL12p40 levels was done by an ELISA kit from Invitrogen.

Statistical analysis

A non-parametric Mann–Whitney test, performed by Origin Pro 2015 software, was used for statistical analysis. p values less than or equal to 0.05 were considered significant. Pearson's correlation coefficients were used to calculate the correlations.

Results

CHI3L1 is produced by non-classic Th1 and Th17 clones

In previous studies, we generated a series of classic Th1 and Th17 clones from circulating CD4+ T cells obtained from healthy donors. In order to identify the differences in the gene expression profile between Th17 and classic Th1 clones, a microarray analysis was performed [24, 26, 38, 39]. Among genes that fulfilled the criteria described in the Methods section as up- or down-regulated genes in Th17 versus classic Th1 clones, in addition to those expected on the basis of previous knowledge, such as, *RORγt, CCR6, CXCR3, CD161, IL-17, IL-23R and IL4I1* [40, 41], there was also *CHI3L1* (Fig. 1a). Therefore, CHI3L1 expression was analysed by quantitative-RT PCR and extended to a new panel of human Th17, Th17/Th1, non-classic Th1, Th17/Th2 and Th2 clones, derived from healthy subjects. As shown in Fig. 1b, Th17, Th17/Th1, non-classic Th1 and Th17/Th2 clones expressed significantly higher levels of CHI3L1 mRNA than classic Th1 and Th2 clones.

Based on the results obtained at mRNA level, we first assessed CHI3L1 expression at protein level by western blot analysis on resting TCCs lysates, confirming that Th17 and non-classic Th1 clones express CHI3L1 while classic Th1 did not (Fig. 2a). Then, in order to understand if Th17 and Th17-derived T cells, like non-classic Th1 clones were also able to secrete CHI3L1, TCCs of

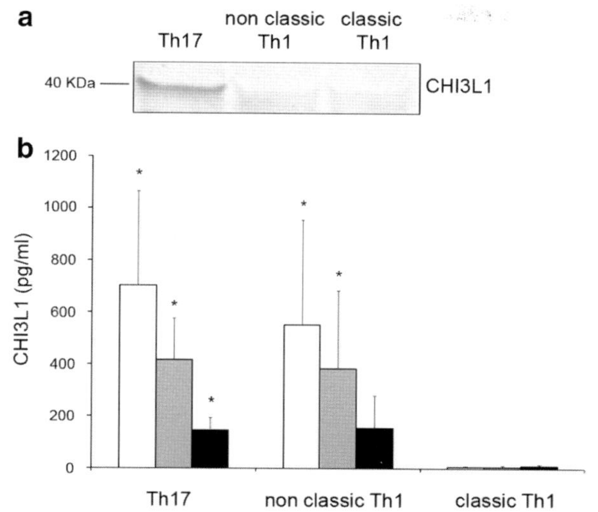

Fig. 2 CHI3L1 protein is secreted by Th17 and non-classic Th1 cells. **a** CHI3L1 protein (40 kDa) expression was evaluated on cell lysates of Th17, non classic-Th1 and classic-Th1 clones by western blot analysis. **b** Secreted CHI3L1 was measured on cell culture supernatants of Th17 (n = 7), non classic Th1 (n = 7) and classic Th1 (n = 7) clones after 72 h stimulation with medium (*white columns*), anti-CD3/CD28 mAbs (*grey columns*) or PMA plus Ionomycin (black columns) by ELISA. Columns represent mean values (±SE). *p ≤ 0.05

each phenotype were cultured in vitro for 72 h in the absence or presence of anti-CD3 plus anti-CD28 mAbs or PMA plus ionomycin and the cell culture supernatants collected. As shown in Fig. 2b, Th17 and non-classic Th1 clones produced comparable amounts of CHI3L1 independently of anti-CD3 plus anti-CD28 mAbs or PMA ionomycin stimulation, whereas, accordingly to mRNA data expression, classic Th1 cells did not produce CHI3L1. Interestingly we observed a reduction in CHI3L1 production by both Th17 and non-classic Th1 cells in the stimulating conditions (Fig. 2b).

The amount of CHI3L1 present in the SF of JIA patients positively correlates with the frequency of Th17 cells

It has been shown that, in RA patients serum, CHI3L1 levels positively correlated with levels of C reactive protein (CRP) [42, 43]. We have recently shown that the frequency of CD4+CD161+, found among CD4+ T cells present in the SF of JIA patients, positively correlates with the levels of two inflammatory parameters, such as the erythrocytes sedimentation rate (ESR) and the CRP, measured in the sera of the same patients [33]. In order to understand if CHI3L1 produced by Th17 cells may play a role in JIA pathogenesis, we evaluated both the CHI3L1 levels and the frequencies of the different T helper cell populations in the synovial fluid of a cohort of 25 JIA patients. As shown in Fig. 3a, the CHI3L1 amounts present in the SF were significantly higher than those observed in the sera of the same patients. Moreover, and more importantly, the CHI3L1 amounts present in the SF of JIA patients positively correlated with the frequencies of Th17 (Fig. 3b) and non-classic Th1 (Fig. 3c) cells, but not with the classic Th1 (Fig. 3d) cells. Finally CHI3L1 quantity in the SF of JIA patients positively correlated with the CRP levels present in the sera of the same patients (Fig. 3e). To further strengthen the association between CHI3L1 levels and the inflammatory status, we checked if these levels correlate also with inflammatory cytokines, in SF. To this end we firstly compared the levels of inflammatory cytokines in peripheral blood and SF of JIA patients (Fig. 3f). Among the inflammatory cytokines that resulted to be more expressed in SF than PB, we found a positive correlation of CHI3L1 levels with both IL6 and the p40 chain (Fig. 3g).

Discussion

In this paper we detected for the first time the expression of CHI3L1 in human T cells. As a result of a gene expression profile microarray analysis on T cell clones we unexpectedly found that CHI3L1 was one of the most up-regulated genes, together with other described (i.e. CCR6 and RORc), in resting Th17 clones when compared to classic Th1. We and others already assessed that the frequencies of CD161+ Th17-derived Th1, Th17/Th1 and Th17/Th2, cells, positively correlated with severe phenotype of different chronic inflammatory disorders such as JIA, IBDs and asthma, respectively [31–36]. In the same pathological conditions higher levels of CHI3L1 have been detected in patients' serum respect to healthy donors [14–16]. Based on this knowledge CHI3L1 mRNA expression was evaluated confirming the microarray data. We found that CHI3L1 mRNA was selectively expressed by human Th17, Th17/Th1, non-classic Th1, and Th17/Th2, cells but not by their CD161− counterparts. This finding means that CHI3L1 is expressed only by CD161+ cells. Of note, mRNA amounts of CHI3L1 were highest on pure Th17 cells and showed a trend to decrease in the other CD161+ subsets, suggesting that it could represent a sort of marker of Th17 lymphocytes. The finding that Th17/Th2 cells express high levels of CHI3L1 is in agreement with the possible pathogenic role of these cells in neutrophilic steroid-resistant asthma since both Th17/Th2 and serum levels of CHI3L1 result to be increased in such disease [42–44].

In the second part of the study, we focused on the three cell subsets Th17, non-classic Th1, as the main example of Th17-derived phenotype, and classic Th1 cells, performing western blot analysis of CHI3L1 protein expression on resting T cell lysates. Results showed an evident expression of CHI3L1 on Th17 cells even if on

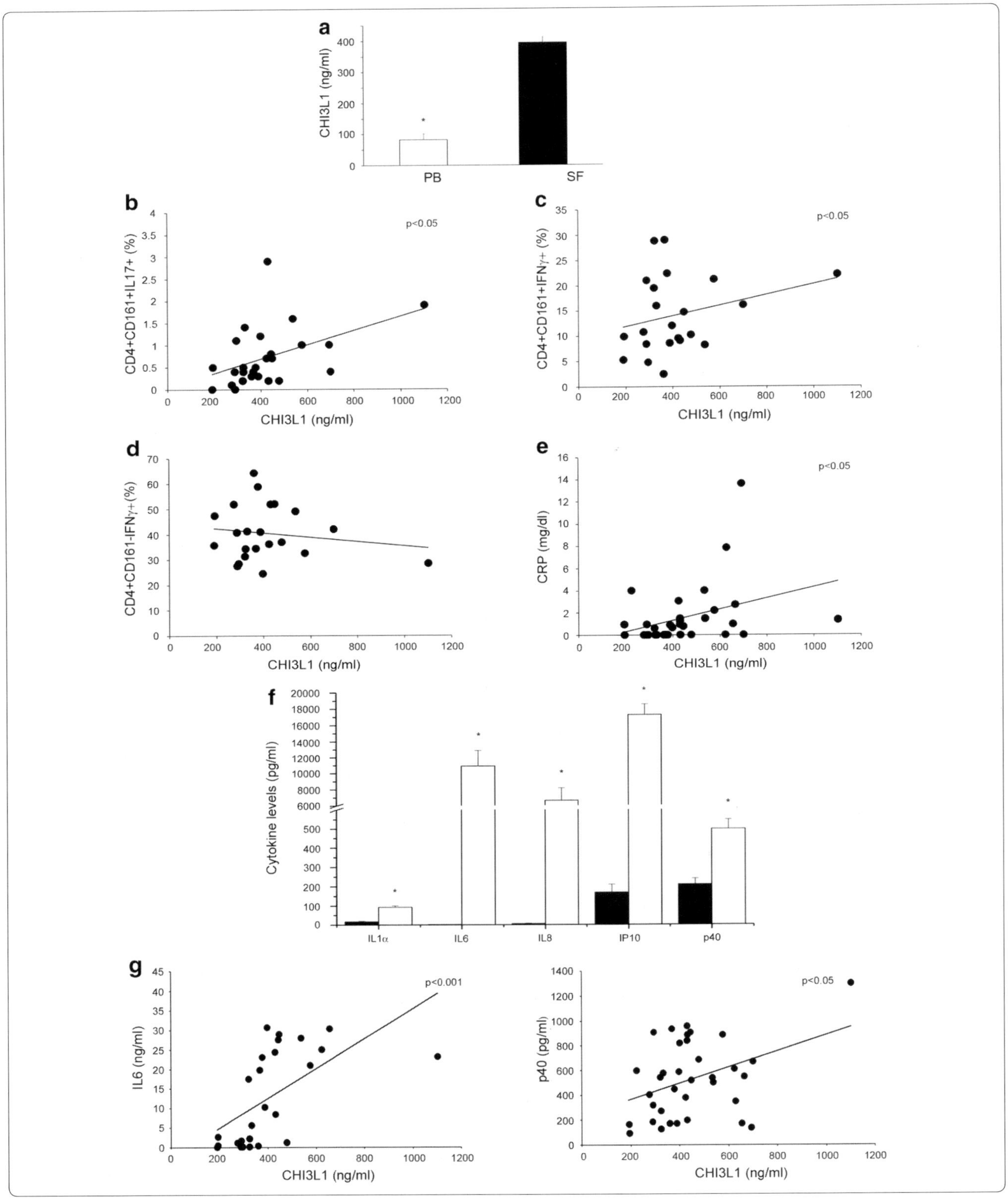
a
CHI3L1 (ng/ml)
PB
SF
b
CD4+CD161+IL17+ (%)
p<0.05
CHI3L1 (ng/ml)
c
CD4+CD161+IFNγ+ (%)
p<0.05
CHI3L1 (ng/ml)
d
CD4+CD161-IFNγ+(%)
CHI3L1 (ng/ml)
e
CRP (mg/dl)
p<0.05
CHI3L1 (ng/ml)
f
Cytokine levels (pg/ml)
IL1α
IL6
IL8
IP10
p40
g
IL6 (ng/ml)
p<0.001
CHI3L1 (ng/ml)
p40 (pg/ml)
p<0.05
CHI3L1 (ng/ml)

(See figure on previous page.)
Fig. 3 CHI3L1 levels positively correlate with the frequency of CD161+ cells in the SF of JIA. PB and SF from 25 JIA patients were evaluated: sera from peripheral blood (*white columns*) and SF (*black columns*) were obtained and CHI3L1 amounts evaluated by ELISA (**a**). *Columns* represent mean values (±SE). *$p \leq 0.05$. MNC cells obtained from SF were characterized by flow cytometry and correlation between CHI3L1 levels in SF and frequency of CD4+CD161+IL17+ cells (**b**), CD4+CD161+IFNγ+ cells (**c**) and CD4+CD161−IFNγ+ cells (**d**), in SF, was represented. **e** Correlation between CHI3L1 levels in SF and CRP serum levels in the same group of patients. **f** The indicated cytokines were assessed in the sera (*white columns*) and SF (*black columns*) from 25 JIA patients. *Columns* represent the mean values (±SE). *$p \leq 0.05$. **g** Correlation between CHI3L1 levels in SF and IL6 (*left panel*) or p40 (*right panel*) SF levels in the same group of patients, was represented

non-classic and classic Th1 it seemed virtually absent. This was apparently in contrast with the data obtained at mRNA level and in order to explain this discrepancy we moved to investigate CHI3L1 level cultures supernatants. CHI3L1 levels were measured by ELISA on supernatants obtained by culturing Th17, non-classic Th1 and classic Th1 clones in presence or absence of two types of polyclonal stimulus (mAbs anti-CD3/CD28 or PMA plus ionomycin). As expected CHI3L1 was produced only by Th17 and non-classic Th1 cell cultures whereas in classic Th1 ones it was not detected. This discrepancy between western blot analysis and ELISA, could be due to the fact that CHI3L1 is a secreted protein. Probably in Th17 cells it is anyway detectable, because it is stored in the intracellular compartment, whereas the same did not occur in non-classic Th1 cells where the amounts are lower. Recent studies demonstrated that increased levels of CHI3L1 in synovial fluid and serum have been found in patients with active RA compared to patients with inactive RA and healthy subjects, and changes in serum CHI3L1 during drug therapy reflect changes in disease activity. Moreover, in patients with early RA, a continuously elevated serum CHI3L1 is associated with progression of joint destruction [15, 16]. Given this literature we deepened our results on TCCs and considering our previous evidences on the involvement of Th17 and Th17-derived Th1 cells in JIA pathogenesis [33] we searched for any possible correlation between them and CHI3L1 expression. To this end we first assessed CHI3L1 levels on sera and synovial fluids from several JIA patients and showed that they are significantly higher at the inflamed tissue when compared to the periphery, thus confirming literature data on rheumatoid arthritis [45, 46]. Moreover we characterized SF for the presence of CD161-expressing cells and found that the frequencies of CD161+IL17− or IFNγ− producing cells positively correlated to CHI3L1 levels. This led us to hypothesize that CHI3L1 production by Th17 and non-classic-Th1 cells may be somehow related to their pathogenic role in JIA. Accordingly, in the same patients CHI3L1 levels in the synovial fluid were also positively correlated with the inflammatory status evaluated by CRP. Moreover, also the levels of proinflammatory cytokines, such as IL6 and the p40 chain, positively correlated with CHI3L1 in SF. The p40 chain is the common subunit of IL12 and IL23, whose role in the induction of the Th1 (both classic and non-classic) and Th17 effectors has been clearly shown [24]. In this view the finding of p40 overexpression in SF was not surprising, and in agreement with the proposed role of these T cell subset in JIA pathogenesis.

Our data are in agreement with the most accepted concept of CHI3L1 as a marker of disease activity and inflammation in several immune-mediated disorders. The previously unknown information that CHI3L1 is produced by Th17 and Th17-derived cells, open new insights on the possible role of this molecule in those inflammatory diseases in which these T cell subsets play a pathogenic role.

Conclusion

CHI3L1 is produced by Th17 and non-classic Th1 cells, already demonstrated to exert a role in the pathogenesis of JIA. CHI3L1 levels on SF from JIA patients positively correlated with frequencies of Th17-derived cells, with CRP levels and with the levels of IL6 and the p40 IL12/IL23 subunit in SF. These findings suggest a possible involvement of CHI3L1 in mediating joint inflammation in JIA. Based on these findings CHI3L1 could be considered a possible biological target for medical treatment of JIA.

Abbreviations

CHI3L1: chitinase 3-like-1; CLPs: chitinase-like proteins; IBD: inflammatory bowel diseases; RA: rheumatoid arthritis; JIA: juvenile idiopathic arthritis; SF: synovial fluid; CRP: reactive protein C.

Authors' contributions

MC, AM, MCR, MPP and GM performed the experiments and collected the data, MC, LM, VS, MCR, GM, MR and AM analysed data, MC, LM, VS and LC wrote the manuscript. FA, RC, LC, FL and RDP supervised the manuscript. FA, SR, EM and LC gave the final approval of the version of the manuscript. All authors read and approved the final manuscript.

Author details

[1] Department of Experimental and Clinical Medicine and DENOTHE Center, University of Florence, 50134 Florence, Italy. [2] Anna Meyer Children's Hospital and University of Florence, 50134, Florence, Italy. [3] Dept. of Biomedical Experimental and Clinical Sciences "Mario Serio", University of Florence, 50134 Florence, Italy. [4] Dept. of Clinical & Experimental Medicine, Second University of Naples, 80131 Naples, Italy. [5] Institute of Protein Biochemistry, CNR, 80131, Naples, Italy. [6] Department of Internal Medicine, University of Florence, Viale Pieraccini 6, 50134 Florence, Italy.

Acknowledgements

The experiments reported in this paper have been supported by funds of the Italian Ministry of Education (PRIN), the Ente Cassa di Risparmio di Firenze, Associazione Italiana Ricerca sul Cancro (AIRC).

Competing interests

The authors declare that they have no competing interests.

References

1. Hakala BE, White C, Recklies AD. Human cartilage gp-39, a major secretory product of articular chondrocytes and synovial cells, is a mammalian member of a chitinase protein family. J Biol Chem. 1993;268:25803–10.
2. Boot RG, Renkema GH, Strijland A, et al. Cloning of a cDNA encoding chitotriosidase, a human chitinase produced by macrophages. J Biol Chem. 1995;270:26252–6.
3. Hu B, Trinh K, Figueira WF, et al. Isolation and sequence of a novel human chondrocyte protein related to mammalian members of the chitinase protein family. J Biol Chem. 1996;271:19415–20.
4. Jin HM, Copeland NG, Gilbert DJ, et al. Genetic characterization of the murine Ym1 gene and identification of a cluster of highly homologous genes. Genomics. 1998;54:316–22.
5. Boot RG, Blommaart EF, Swart E, et al. Identification of a novel acidic mammalian chitinase distinct from chitotriosidase. J Biol Chem. 2001;276:6770–8.
6. Buhi WC. Characterization and biological roles of oviduct-specific, oestrogen-dependent glycoprotein. Reproduction. 2002;123:355–62.
7. Kzhyshkowska J, Mamidi S, Gratchev A, et al. Novel stabilin-1 interacting chitinase-like protein (SI-CLP) is up-regulated in alternatively activated macrophages and secreted via lysosomal pathway. Blood. 2006;107:3221–8.
8. Lee CG, Da Silva CA, Dela Cruz CS, et al. Role of chitin and chitinase/chitinase-like proteins in inflammation, tissue remodeling, and injury. Annu Rev Physiol. 2011;73:479–501.
9. Lee CG, Hartl D, Lee GR, et al. Role of breast regression protein 39 (BRP-39)/chitinase 3-like-1 in Th2 and IL-13-induced tissue responses and apoptosis. J Exp Med. 2009;206:1149–66.
10. Recklies AD, White C, Ling H. The chitinase 3-like protein human cartilage glycoprotein 39 (HC-gp39) stimulates proliferation of human connective-tissue cells and activates both extracellular signal-regulated kinase- and protein kinase B-mediated signalling pathways. Biochem J. 2002;365(Pt 1):119–26.
11. Tran HT, Lee IA, Low D, et al. Chitinase 3-like 1 synergistically activates IL6-mediated STAT3 phosphorylation in intestinal epithelial cells in murine models of infectious colitis. Inflamm Bowel Dis. 2014;20(5):835–46.
12. Chupp GL, Lee CG, Jarjour N, Shim YM, Holm CT, et al. A chitinase-like protein in the lung and circulation of patients with severe asthma. N Engl J Med. 2007;357:2016–27.
13. Mizoguchi E. Chitinase 3-like-1 exacerbates intestinal inflammation by enhancing bacterial adhesion and invasion in colonic epithelial cells. Gastroenterology. 2006;130:398–411.
14. Vind I, Johansen JS, Price PA, Munkholm P. Serum YKL-40, a potential new marker of disease activity in patients with inflammatory bowel disease. Scand J Gastroenterol. 2003;38:599–605.
15. Vos K, Steenbakkers P, Miltenburg AM, et al. Raised human cartilage glycoprotein-39 plasma levels in patients with rheumatoid arthritis and other inflammatory conditions. Ann Rheum Dis. 2000;59:544–8.
16. Baeten D, Steenbakkers PGA, Rijnders AMW, et al. Detection of major histocompatibility complex/human cartilage of MHC/HC gp-39 complexes in rheumatoid arthritis synovitis as a specific and independent histological marker. Arthritis Rheum. 2004;50:444–51.
17. Gomez JL, Crisafi GM, Holm CT, et al. Genetic variation in chitinase 3-like 1 (CHI3L1) contributes to asthma severity and airway expression of YKL-40. J Allergy Clin Immunol. 2015;136(1):51–58.e10.
18. Verheijden GF, Rijnders AW, Bos E, Coenen-de Roo CJ, van Staveren CJ, et al. Human cartilage glycoprotein-39 as a candidate autoantigen in rheumatoid arthritis. Arthritis Rheum. 1997;40:1115–25.
19. van Lierop MJ, den Hoed L, Houbiers J, et al. Endogenous HLADR-restricted presentation of the cartilage antigens human cartilage gp-39 and melanoma inhibitory activity in the inflamed rheumatoid joint. Arthritis Rheum. 2007;56:2150–9.
20. Mosmann TR, Coffman RL. TH1 And TH2 cells: different patterns of lymphokine secretion lead to different functional properties. Annu Rev Immunol. 1989;7:145–73.
21. Romagnani S. Lymphokine production by human T cells in disease states. Annu Rev Immunol. 1994;12:227–57.
22. Harrington LE, Hatton RD, Mangan PR, Turner H, Murphy TL, Murphy KM, Weaver CT. Interleukin-17-producing CD4+ effector T cells develop via a lineage distinct from the T helper type 1 and 2 lineages. Nat Immunol. 2005;5:1123–32.
23. Park H, Li Z, Yang XO, Chang SH, Nurieva R, Wang YH, Wang Y, et al. A distinct lineage of CD4 T cells regulates tissue inflammation by producing interleukin 17. Nat Immunol. 2005;5:1133–41.
24. Cosmi L, De Palma R, Santarlasci V, Maggi L, Capone M, Frosali F, Rodolico G, et al. Human interleukin-17-producing cells originate from a CD161+CD4+ T-cell precursor. J Exp Med. 2008;205:1903–16.
25. Kleinschek MA, Boniface K, Sadekova S, Grein J, Murphy EE, Turner SP, Raskin L, et al. Circulating and gut-resident human Th17 cells express CD161 and promote intestinal inflammation. J Exp Med. 2009;206:525–34.
26. Maggi L, Santarlasci V, Capone M, Peired A, Frosali F, Crome SQ, Querci V, et al. CD161 is a marker of all human IL-17-producing T-cell subsets and is induced by RORC. Eur J Immunol. 2010;40:2174–81.
27. Oukka M. Th17 cells in immunity and autoimmunity. Ann Rheum Dis. 2008;67:26–9.
28. Fouser LA, Wright JF, Dunussi-Joannopoulos K, Collins M. Th17 cytokines and their emerging roles in inflammation and autoimmunity. Immunol Rev. 2008;226:87–102.
29. van Beelen AJ, Teunissen MB, Kapsenberg ML, de Jong EC. Interleukin-17 in inflammatory skin disorders. Curr Opin Allergy Clin Immunol. 2007;7:374–81.
30. Chen Z, O'Shea JJ. Th17 cells: A new fate for differentiating helper T cells. Immunol Res. 2008;41:87–102.
31. Cosmi L, Maggi L, Santarlasci V, Capone M, Cardilicchia E, Frosali F, Querci V, et al. Identification of a novel subset of human circulating memory CD4(+) T cells that produce both IL-17A and IL-4. J Allergy Clin Immunol. 2010;125:222–30.
32. Nistala K, Adams S, Cambrook H, Ursu S, Olivito B, de Jager W, Evans JG, Cimaz R, Bajaj-Elliott M, Wedderburn LR. Th17 plasticity in human autoimmune arthritis is driven by the inflammatory environment. Proc Natl Acad Sci USA. 2010;107:14751–6.
33. Cosmi L, Cimaz R, Maggi L, Santarlasci V, Capone M, Borriello F, Frosali F, et al. CD4+CD161+ T cells showing transient nature of the Th17 phenotype are present in the synovial fluid from patients with juvenile idiopathic arthritis. Arthritis Rheum. 2011;63:2504–15.
34. Maggi L, Cimaz R, Capone M, Santarlasci V, Querci V, Simonini G, Nencini F, Liotta F, Romagnani S, Maggi E, Annunziato F, Cosmi L. Brief report: etanercept inhibits the tumor necrosis factor α-driven shift of Th17 lymphocytes toward a nonclassic Th1 phenotype in juvenile idiopathic arthritis. Arthritis Rheumatol. 2014;66(5):1372–7.
35. Maggi L, Capone M, Giudici F, Santarlasci V, Querci V, Liotta F, Ficari F, Maggi E, Tonelli F, Annunziato F, et al. CD4+CD161+ T lymphocytes infiltrate Crohn's disease-associated perianal fistulas and are reduced by anti-TNF-α local therapy. Int Arch Allergy Immunol. 2012;161:81–6.
36. Giudici F, Maggi L, Santi R, Cosmi L, Annunziato F, Nesi G, Barra G, Bassotti G, De Palma R, Tonelli F. Perianal Crohn's disease and hidradenitis suppurativa: a possible common immunological scenario. Clin Mol Allergy. 2015;13(1):12.

37. Petty RE, Southwood TR, Baum J, Bhettay E, Glass DN, Manners P, et al. Revision of the proposed classification criteria for juvenile idiopathic arthritis: Durban, 1997. J Rheumatol. 1998;25:1991–4.
38. Santarlasci V, Maggi L, Capone M, Querci V, Beltrame L, Cavalieri D, D'Aiuto E, Cimaz R, Nebbioso A, Liotta F, et al. Rarity of human T helper 17 cells is due to retinoic acid orphan receptor-dependent mechanisms that limit their expansion. Immunity. 2012;36:201–14.
39. Maggi L, Santarlasci V, Capone M, Rossi MC, Querci V, Mazzoni A, Cimaz R, De Palma R, Liotta F, Maggi E, et al. Distinctive features of classic and non-classic (Th17 derived) human Th1 cells. Eur J Immunol. 2012;42:3180–8.
40. Lee YK, Turner H, Maynard CL, Oliver JR, Chen D, Elson CO, Weaver CT. Late developmental plasticity in the T helper 17 lineage. Immunity. 2009;30:92–107.
41. Kurschus FC, Croxford AL, Heinen AP, Wörtge S, Ielo D, Waisman A. Genetic proof for the transient nature of the Th17 phenotype. Eur J Immunol. 2010;40:3336–46.
42. Nezgovorova V, Liu Q, Hu B, et al. Sputum gene expression of IL-13 receptor α2 chain correlates with airflow obstruction and helper T-cell Type 2 inflammation in asthma. Ann Am Thorac Soc. 2016;13(Suppl 1):S96–7.
43. Cosmi L, Liotta F, Annunziato F. Th17 regulating lower airway disease. Curr Opin Allergy Clin Immunol. 2016;16(1):1–6.
44. Cosmi L, Liotta F, Maggi E, Romagnani S, Annunziato F. Th17 cells: new players in asthma pathogenesis. Allergy. 2011;66(8):989–98.
45. Baeten D, Boots AM, Steenbakkers PG, et al. Human cartilage gp-39+, CD16+ monocytes in peripheral blood and synovium: correlation with joint destruction in rheumatoid arthritis. Arthritis Rheum. 2000;43:1233–43.
46. Johansen JS, Stoltenberg M, Hansen M, Florescu A, Horslev-Petersen K, Lorenzen I, et al. Serum YKL-40 concentrations in patients with rheumatoid arthritis: relation to disease activity. Rheumatology. 1999;38:618–26.

11

Guidelines for the use and interpretation of diagnostic methods in adult food allergy

Donatella Macchia[1], Giovanni Melioli[2], Valerio Pravettoni[3], Eleonora Nucera[4], Marta Piantanida[3], Marco Caminati[5*], Corrado Campochiaro[6], Mona-Rita Yacoub[6], Domenico Schiavino[4], Roberto Paganelli[7], Mario Di Gioacchino[8] and On behalf of the Food Allergy Study Group (ATI) of the Italian Society of Allergy, Asthma and Clinical Immunology (SIAAIC)

Abstract

Food allergy has an increasing prevalence in the general population and in Italy concerns 8 % of people with allergies. The spectrum of its clinical manifestations ranges from mild symptoms up to potentially fatal anaphylactic shock. A number of patients can be diagnosed easily by the use of first- and second-level procedures (history, skin tests and allergen specific IgE). Patients with complex presentation, such as multiple sensitizations and pollen-food syndromes, frequently require a third-level approach including molecular diagnostics, which enables the design of a component-resolved sensitization profile for each patient. The use of such techniques involves specialists' and experts' skills on the issue to appropriately meet the diagnostic and therapeutic needs of patients. Particularly, educational programs for allergists on the use and interpretation of molecular diagnostics are needed.

Keywords: Food allergy diagnosis, Skin prick test, Molecular allergens, Molecular-based diagnosis, Challenge test, Basophil activation test

Background

Food Allergy (FA) is an increasingly recognized problem in relation to its prevalence in the general population. In Italy, it corresponds to 8 % of all patients with allergies [1–3] and the broad spectrum of its clinical manifestations, ranging from mild symptoms up to potentially fatal anaphylactic shock (Table 1). FA significantly affects the quality of life of patients and their families [4]. In adults, FA may persist from childhood or may develop at an older age. In the latter case, once established, FA is maintained throughout life, while paediatric FA frequently disappears during adolescence. FA may be responsible for signs and symptoms that occur shortly after consumption of the culprit food (from a few minutes to a few hours). The earlier they arise, the more serious they are. At times, symptoms appear after physical exercise (food dependent exercise induced anaphylaxis, FDEIA) and the ingestion (about 3 h before) of a specific food, which is safely eaten in the absence of exercise [5].

FA most commonly affects the skin (atopic dermatitis, urticaria, angioedema, eczema and various skin rashes) [6, 7]. Frequently, gastrointestinal manifestations are associated with cutaneous symptoms. The gut is rarely the only organ affected by food allergy. Symptoms range from dyspepsia and meteorism to colic, diarrhoea (rarely constipation), vomiting, gastroesophageal reflux, up to the most complex malabsorption syndromes, generally due to the infiltration of inflammatory cells in the gastrointestinal mucosa [8–10]. In some cases, mainly in pollen-allergic patients sensitive to molecules homologous to those contained in specific foods, symptoms appear in the form of itching and burning of the oral mucosa, papules or vesicles in the mouth, swelling of the lips and difficulty in swallowing, being defined as oral allergy syndrome [11]. Rhinitis, conjunctivitis, asthma and laryngeal edema are all possible FA manifestations independent from sensitization to inhalant allergens [12].

Each year 4–5/100,000 patients experience an anaphylactic shock, with a cumulative risk equal to 0.5–2 % [13].

*Correspondence: ma.caminati@gmail.com
[5] Allergy Unit, Verona University and General Hospital, Verona, Italy
Full list of author information is available at the end of the article

Table 1 Main food allergy symptoms

Organs and systems	Clinical manifestations
Respiratory	Oculorhinitis
	Bronchial asthma
	Oedema of the glottis
Skin and subcutaneous tissue	Erythematous rash
	Itching without rash
	Urticaria-angioedema
	Atopic dermatitis
	Eczema
Gastro-enteric	Oral Allergy Syndrome
	Abdominal pains
	Vomiting
	Diarrhoea
Cardiovascular system	Hypotension
	Cardiac arrest
	Anaphylactic shock

Foods are the main cause of anaphylactic shock for children and young adults, whereas for older people, insect stings are mainly responsible. This syndrome is due to the involvement of the cardiovascular system with a drop in blood pressure due to vasodilation and leakage of fluids from the circulation, with systemic consequences [14]. The term anaphylaxis (without shock) is referred to a reaction involving multiple organs, usually the skin, gastrointestinal tract and respiratory system.

There is no consensus on allergy due to food contaminant and additives. Clinicians sometimes report the disappearance of the characteristic symptoms of food allergy after an additive-free diet, despite the fact that there is no scientific evidence on their actual role in causing symptoms [15–17]. In any case, reactions are not mediated by an immunological mechanism and are classified as non-allergic hypersensitivity reactions. There is a possibility that food reactions also stem from some non-protein food component or from other mechanisms, for example, cell-mediated mechanisms. These include reactions to orally ingested nickel, the so-called Systemic Nickel Allergy Syndrome, which is characterized by the appearance of gastrointestinal symptoms (typically meteorism, colic and diarrhoea) and skin manifestations (eczema, urticaria and angioedema) in sites without nickel contact in patients with nickel contact dermatitis, and responds positively to a low-nickel diet [18].

Diagnostic efforts are directed to the identification of the food(s) involved in triggering and/or maintaining the symptoms. This can be achieved by using all available diagnostic methods applied in an appropriate sequence, avoiding non-standardized ones.

The purpose of this document is to define guidelines for the use and interpretation of scientifically validated and recognized diagnostic methods for food allergy.

Basic concepts of FA

Primary forms of FA are due to a sensitization process caused by ingestion. In the secondary forms, the patient is sensitized by inhalation to allergens containing molecules homologous to those contained in certain foods, whose ingestion may cause symptoms usually in the oral cavity, in the frame of an oral allergy syndrome [19]. Several molecules with different characteristics act as food allergens. Some of them are stable, enduring heating, cooking, storage and digestion (linear epitopes), while others are less stable (conformational epitopes) losing their allergenicity in cooking and preservation [20]. The patient with FA can be sensitized to both labile and stable components. The stability/lability to physical agents (heat, gastric pH, enzymes like protease, pepsin and so on) is a requisite for an allergen to interact with the IgE antibody. Thus, a component sensitive to heat will be virtually absent in a cooked food, while a determinant resistant to heat, pH and peptidase (for example, Lipid Transfer proteins–LTP) will reach the bowel practically intact despite cooking and passage through the gastric and pancreatic digestion [21]. A particular situation arises with the use of antacid drugs that do not allow (or partially allow) the denaturation of acid sensitive proteins, thus resulting in unpredictable symptoms [22]. Other substances can act as "co-factors", increasing the likelihood of anaphylaxis from food allergens. They include alcohol, non-steroidal anti-inflammatory drugs (NSAIDs), hormonal influences, bacterial or viral or parasitic infections [23] and chemicals [24–26].

The large variety of clinical manifestations (Table 1) and the complexity of allergens often make the diagnosis of FA difficult. A component-specific profile, other than extract-specific, should be used for an optimal definition of the sensitization. In addition, in the specific field of food allergy, it is crucial to discriminate between cross-reactions and co-sensitization, particularly for members of the plant kingdom ("pollen food allergy"), and to more accurately estimate the risk of severe reactions. The sensitization to cross-reactive molecules is relatively rare in childhood but tends to appear during adolescence and remains stable in adults. The recent adoption of individual allergenic molecules (Molecular-Based Diagnosis, MBD) in diagnosis allows for the definition of a more precise IgE profile for the patient, e.g. adding prognostic information related to the possible risk profile of the reaction. Understanding the fine relationships between the results of in vivo and in vitro tests and the patient's clinical picture is the key for any further clinical decisions.

Diagnostic methods for food allergy

A correct diagnosis of FA requires an established diagnostic procedure. The first step is always the patient's history aimed at identifying the suspected relevant food(s) and the relationship between the ingestion of a specific food and the occurrence of symptoms. Then, the dependence of clinical manifestations from an immune mediated reaction must be assessed. This can be done by both in vivo and in vitro tests.

The standardized diagnostic methods are classified into first, second and third level.

Table 2 Food panel for Prick test

Egg	Peach
Peanut	Apple
Beta-lactoglobulin	Cod
Banana	Hazelnut
Carrot	Walnut
Casein	Fish
Bean	Pea
Wheat flour	Chicken
Shrimp	Tomato
Lactalbumin	Rice
Pork	Celery
Corn	Soybeans
Almond	Egg yolk

First-level methods

Medical history

Medical history is essential in every field of medicine because it allows one to obtain all the information and data that can help to move towards the diagnosis of a certain disease. It comprises the physiological, family (investigating all possible genetic risk factors or any family predisposition) and the past and current medical history. The latter investigates the disorder for which the patient consulted a doctor. In suspected FA, repeated clinical manifestations related to the ingestion of given meals are highly indicative. Medical history should be addressed to clarify (a) the presence or absence of similar symptoms in other people when they consumed the same food(s); (b) the ingested food(s) in the 2–4 h before the onset of symptoms; (c) the allergens that may contaminate food preparation (for example, casein, latex, ovomucoid); (d) the cooking and storage of food; (e) the presence of triggering factors; (f) the existence of other allergies (such as respiratory or skin allergy) or other diseases [27]. A correct diagnostic approach also requires a complete physical examination. When too much time has elapsed from the appearance of symptoms, it could be difficult to identify the offending food, in particular, if the allergen is not easily identifiable or "hidden". Medical history can be re-evaluated starting from the results of in vitro and in vivo tests, which could demonstrate sensitizations to foods that were initially not considered [28, 29].

Skin tests

Skin prick test (SPT) The SPT is a well-standardized, simple, cheap and low-risk diagnostic test. It should be the first step performed and both inhalant and food allergens should be tested. Table 2 shows a panel of food allergens to be tested, supplemented, where appropriate, by foods chosen according to patient's history and dietary diaries, and Table 3 shows the technical procedure to be used. The SPTs to foods have a low specificity with a low positive predictive value. Thus, a positive result, unless confirmed by the clinical data, does not allow for a definitive diagnosis of FA [28–30]. In children, cut-off values for the SPT reaction diameter for certain food allergen (milk: 8 mm, egg: 7 mm, peanut: 8 mm) have been identified but are not universally acknowledged. However, oral food challenges were always positive (100 % specificity) in children with cutaneous reactions of this diameter or above [31, 32]. In general, SPT have an excellent sensitivity with high negative predictive value (>90 %), thus a negative result generally rules out the possibility of an IgE-mediated sensitization. However, this is true only for foods containing stable proteins, such as casein from cow's milk, egg ovomucoid, albumin and peanut vicilins, which are well represented in the extract. The SPT performed with allergenic extracts containing thermolabile molecules, such as pathogenesis-related-10 (PR-10) proteins have a low negative predictive value. For these allergens, the prick + prick (P + P) procedures with fresh foods can be useful.

The major limitations of allergen extracts for SPT are represented by (a) the content, because each extract is a heterogeneous mixture composed of major and minor allergenic proteins, and other biologically inactive components such as non-allergenic proteins, glycoproteins and carbohydrates, (b) the production process, because some allergens may undergo partial degradation during the extraction, (c) the cross-reactions, as different biological sources may contain cross-reactive allergens.

An in vivo MBD approach (available in vitro for many molecules, shown in Table 4) is also possible with extracts containing high concentrations of LTP (a gastro- and thermo-stable protein from *Rosaceae*) and palm profilins (Pho d 2, an ubiquitous gastro- and heat labile plant protein). Their use, to complete the diagnostics performed with extracts from whole sources, allow for a

Table 3 Technical procedure for SPT

Apply one drop for each allergen extract to be tested, maintaining a minimum distance of 3 cm between drops on the volar part of the patient's forearm (5 cm from wrist and 3 cm from the antecubital fossa)
Apply pressure, through a sterile, disposable lancet, to each single allergen, pricking to a depth of 1 mm for each drop, perpendicular to the skin's surface
Hold for about 3 s with moderate pressure without moving the hand or turning to avoid bleeding
Carefully remove the allergen solution with blotting paper
The same procedure is to be followed to test histamine (10 mg/ml) as a positive control and physiological glycerine as a negative control
Reading of the results: after 15 min from the performance of the test
Interpretation of the test: a positive result is defined by the appearance of a wheal of at least 3 mm in average diameter. Responses to histamine and the negative control should be carefully considered. The latter verifies that the patient does not suffer from dermographism and the former demonstrates a "normal response" to histamine (with no negative interference from drugs or other conditions, such as hypo-reactivity of the skin)

Table 4 Native or recombinant molecules available for SPT

Molecule	Source
Lactalbumin	Cow's milk
Beta-lactoglobulin	Cow's milk
Casein	Cow's milk
Ovalbumin	Egg white
Ovomucoid	Egg white
LTP (Pru p 3)	Peach
Profilin (Pho d 2)	Palm tree
PR10 (Mal d 1)	Apple (not available in Italy)

more precise assessment of the ingestion risk of the suspected food [33].

Prick + prick (P + P) P + P is performed with fresh food, in particular vegetables, when the commercial extract is negative (or unavailable) but the clinical history is suggestive. When the food is solid, the technique involves firstly puncturing the fresh food (some allergens are located just under the skin of the fruit) and then the patient's skin with a lancet according to the SPT standard procedure [34]. When the food is liquid, the technique is the same as in SPT.

P + P has a good diagnostic reliability [35] with high predictive negative values. In the case of a positive result, it must be always taken into account that some foods are rich in histamine and lectins and can produce false positives. Obviously, the use of skin P + P with fresh food is not entirely risk-free and highly sensitive subjects may suffer systemic adverse reactions [36].

Atopy patch test (APT)

The APT is performed through the same technique used for common patch testing to identify the responsible hapten in contact dermatitis, and is aimed at assessing the delayed cell-mediated hypersensitivity to foods that may especially occur in children with atopic dermatitis or gastrointestinal reactions to foods. In 2010, the APT was considered an emerging test, like BAT and MBD [37], but subsequent studies did not confirm its diagnostic role to be as important as the other two techniques.

Second-level methods

In vitro assays for total serum IgE (tIgE) and specific IgE (sIgE) to foods

Like SPT and P + P, in vitro tests only certify a sensitization and the interpretation of results is the allergist's task. Thus, measuring tIgE may be useful in grading allergy conditions, but only when used in combination with other tests. Indeed, tIgE alone has no predictive value in relation to the diagnosis of FA. The assay of sIgE for food extracts is a second-level test in the view of costs. Thus, it should be requested only after skin tests. However, it may still be exceptionally considered a first-level test in those conditions in which SPT cannot be performed (e.g. very young paediatric patients, concomitant antihistamine therapy or skin alterations, risk of systemic reactions). Importantly, an in vivo test is able to detect the biological effects (revealed by wheal, redness, itching, etc.) caused by the presence of sIgE bound to skin mast cells, while the serum test only detects the presence of circulating IgE specific to a particular allergen. It is therefore possible that the results of the two tests are different [38].

Nowadays, quantitative methods with extracts have levels of sensitivity (and negative predictive values) comparable to APT, with high specificity and positive predictive value [37]. The test is suitable to detect the IgE specific for a given allergen, in a quantitative way, in a range between 0.10 and 100 kU/L. As for the SPT reaction diameter, specific IgE levels exceeding a certain value ("diagnostic cut-off") showed a predictive value of 95 % for a symptomatic allergy [32, 39] (Table 5). Thus, in the presence of a compatible clinical history, sIgE can confirm the diagnosis of FA without requiring further challenge tests. However, the predictive values vary from one study to another. The results are influenced by many variables such as the patient's age, duration of food allergen avoidance at the time of testing, selection of patients

Table 5 Sensitivity, specificity, positive (PPV) and negative (NPV) predictive value of tests for the detection of specific IgE in vitro for the most common food allergens

Allergen	Sensitivity (%)	Specificity (%)	PPV (%)	VPN (%)	Diagnostic cut-off (kUA/l)
Egg	61	95	98	38	6
Milk	57	94	95	53	15
Peanut	57	100	100	36	14
Codfish	63	91	56	93	3
Soybean	44	94	73	82	30
Wheat	61	92	74	87	26

and clinical disorders, and have been validated on non-European test subjects. It is also important to stress that the values of specific IgE <0.10 kU/L does not exclude the possibility of an IgE-mediated allergic reaction and that the confirmation of a negative test, in the case of strong clinical suspicion, can only be achieved with negative SPTs and negative challenge tests.

In vitro MBD

Diagnostics based on allergenic extracts allow for the identification of the allergen source (e.g. fish, egg, milk, etc.) but not the molecular component to which a patient is sensitized, which can be studied instead through in vitro MBD and therefore used to improve the result of a sIgE test [20]. In vitro MBD uses molecular allergens isolated from a given allergen source (purified or native allergens) or produced by recombinant DNA technology (recombinant allergens) (Tables 6, 7). This approach improves the description of the IgE repertoire against food allergens or their molecular components and explains cross-reactions and their role in FA.

The MBD approach should be used to distinguish patients with genuine sensitization towards a food (with high risk of accidental ingestion) from those with co-sensitization, i.e. sensitization to ubiquitous proteins present in pollen (which act as primary sensitizing) and also common in food (with a much lower risk of adverse reaction). Again, it is possible to identify patients characterized by sensitization to food independently by a sensitization to aeroallergens (primary sensitization) and patients with a "pollen-food syndrome", where the first sensitization occurs via inhalation and the great homology between the allergen of the "first sensitizer" and some food allergens is responsible for the patient's symptoms presenting as an oral allergy syndrome [40, 41].

Identifying cross-reactions is a further benefit of MBD. The allergist is able to understand whether a single, a few closely related or several widely different food allergen sources should be considered in a dietary approach. The allergist will also be able to assess the risk of a given FA identifying, by in vitro MBD, patients sensitized to "relatively harmless" or potentially very dangerous components [20] that need the prescription of life-saving drugs such as auto-injectable adrenaline together with a strict allergen avoidance. The use of MBD requires allergists to acquire new skills.

Primarily, they need to learn the new allergen nomenclature [42, 43]. International classification ranks the allergenic source first by its scientific name, from which it takes the first three letters of the generic name and the first letter of the species (or two letters when confusion is possible): e.g. apple is scientifically called "*Malus domestica*": therefore Mal d indicates the allergen source. Adding a number (1, 2, 3 etc.) indicating the chronological order of the identification allows for the classification any allergenic molecules: e.g. for apple the identified molecules are named Mal d 1, Mal d2, Mal d 3, and Mal d 4.

It is also important to know the molecular allergenic content of foods. Some molecules are specific for a given food, allowing the identification of the primary sensitizer, others share common epitopes (antibody binding sites) and the same IgE can induce an immune response to allergenic molecules with similar structures from different allergen sources [33]. In the example of apple, Mal d 3 is an LTP molecule homologous to the LTP of peach, nuts, apricot, cherry, etc. and an exclusion diet should prohibit all these foods, but only according to the patient's history [44]. Indeed, Mal d 1 is highly homologous to the birch pollen allergen Bet v 1 and characteristically induces an oral allergic reaction [45].

The molecular structure and physiochemical properties of allergens are major determinants of their clinical relevance. For example, LTPs are particularly resistant to high temperature and enzymatic degradation, so cooking and digestive processes are unable to deactivate their allergenic capacity. For this reason, LTP exposure through the gastrointestinal tract may induce sensitization in predisposed individuals and may trigger severe reactions in sensitized patients [46]. The specific patient's sensitization profile is relevant in terms of risk assessment. In

Table 6 Major food allergens and components available for molecular diagnostics using ImmunoCAP (or ImmunoCAP ISAC)

Allergens (or allergen source)	Protein family
Cupin superfamily	
Vicilins	Ara h 1 (peanut)
Legumins	Ara h 3 (peanut), Cor 9 (hazelnut)
Prolamin superfamily	
2S albumin	Ber e 1 (brazil nut), Ara h 2 (peanut), Gly m 6
Lipid transfer protein (LTP)	Pru p 3 (peach), Cor 8 (hazelnut), Art v 3 (*Composite*) Jug r 3 (walnut)
Cereal prolamines	Tri 19 (wheat) Tri a 14
Pathogenesis-related (PR) proteins	
PR10: intracellular proteins	Pru p 1 (peach), Api g 1 (celery), Gly m 4 (soy)
PR3: chitinase Class 1	Hev b 11, Hev b 2.6 (latex, banana, avocado)
Profilins	Pru p 4 (peach) (Bet v 2, Phl p 12, Hev b 8)
Cross-reactive carbohydrate determinants	MUXF3 (celery, tomato)
Tropomyosins	Pen a 1 (shrimp)
Calcium binding proteins	
Parvalbumin	Gad c 1 (codfish)
Milk proteins	Bos d 4 (α-albumin), Bos d 5 (β-lactoglobulin), Bos d 8 (casein), Bos d lactoferrin (lactoferrin)
Egg protein	Gal d 1 (ovomucoide)
	Gal d 2 (ovalbumin)
	Gal d 3 (conalbumin)
	Gal d 4 (lysozyme)

Table 7 Families of protein carbohydrate molecules mainly involved in food allergy

Molecules associated with allergy to food source (or source allergen)
PR-10 proteins (homologous to Bet v 1)
Non-specific lipid transfer proteins (nsLTP)
Profilins
Storage proteins
Thaumatin-like-proteins (TLP)
Cross-reactive carbohydrate determinants (CCD)
Molecules associated with allergy to food of animal origin
Tropomyosins
Parvalbumins
Caseins
Lipocalin, Family of lysozyme, Family Transferrins, Ovomucoids

fact, the simultaneous sensitization to peach LTP Pru p 3, Pru p 1 and Pru p 4 in the same patient seems to exert a protective role in comparison with Pru p 3 sensitization alone, as it is associated with less severe symptoms [47]. Similarly, it has been recently shown that in peach-allergic patients with tomato hypersensitivity, sensitization to rPru p3 seems to be a surrogate biochemical marker for a severe tomato allergy, whereas the presence of anti-rPru p 1 IgE may be an indicator of a mild tomato allergy [48].

Profilins are pan-allergens (present in many plant species not botanically related) protease sensitive and less heat sensitive that mainly induce an oral allergy syndrome, while severe reactions are rare [49].

Therefore, the allergist approaching the MBD should know the chemical, physical and immunological characteristics of all allergenic families, their biodegradability, cooking/heat resistance/sensibility etc. The stability/lability of a molecule (along with the clinical history) helps the clinician to evaluate the risk of systemic versus local reactions. Stable allergens are generally associated with severe systemic reactions, whereas labile allergens are associated with low/mild reactions and cooked food is often tolerated.

Moreover, it is essential to know to which family the various molecules belong and their structural similarity within the family (generally characterized by a greater than 50–70 % sequence homology).

In the above-mentioned example of apple, MBD can distinguish between fruit allergy due to LTP sensitization and a pollen-related apple allergy. Sensitization to Mal d 3 (an LTP protein) indicates a fruit allergy where peach is often the primary sensitizer [50, 51]. Sensitization to Mal d 1 (a PR-10 protein) is seen in birch-pollen allergic patients and is caused by cross-reactivity with the main birch allergen Bet v 1 [52, 53]. The presence of IgE antibodies to profilin (e.g. Mal d 4, homologous of Phl p 12) is indicative of an apple allergy related to a grass-pollen sensitization [53, 54].

Patients with IgE antibodies to Mal d 2 and 3 (LTP stable proteins) are at higher risk of developing systemic reactions. IgE antibodies to Mal d 1 and/or profilin and not to Mal d 2 and 3 suggest that predominantly local oral symptoms may occur. Apple-allergic patients sensitized to Mal d 3 may tolerate peeled apples. Apple-allergic patients sensitized to Mal d 1 and/or profilin (that are labile proteins) may often tolerate cooked apples.

MBD is a complex area, but as it provides new and relevant information for the allergist, it will soon become a standard tool for the diagnosis of FA. Educational programs for allergists on the use and interpretation of MBD are needed [55].

In vitro MBD is defined as single or multi-plexed IgE assay microarray. By the single-plexed diagnostics the choice of the components to be tested is relies on the allergist's judgment, based on the patient's sIgE profile. In poly-sensitized patients, a complete recognition of the IgE profile might require a large number of assays. In these cases, it may be reasonable to use the multi-plexed allergen microarray (AMA) that allows for the detection of specific reactivity to over 100 allergen components. The most popular form (the Immuno-Sorbent Allergen Chip—ISAC) currently contains inhalants, foods, latex and insect venom. Despite AMA not being a quantitative assay, the correlation between the results of microarrays and the results of sIgE tests are largely super-imposable. Thus AMA is suitable in both paediatric and adult serum samples when the number of molecular components to be tested using single-plexed methods is too high to be cost-convenient or when the need for extensive research of sensitization is required [20]. This is particularly true in highly complex patients presenting symptoms of a cross-sensitization to inhalant and food and clinical evidence of food allergy. AMA is a powerful in vitro test that requires specific expertise but provides a very large amount of information to the allergist.

MBD diagnostics, especially microarray, are expensive compared with traditional tests, unless a single test is considered. Economic considerations may influence the decision of using a single or multiplex approach in individual patients. Using the microarray diagnostics allows for the performance of a broad-spectrum analysis of a patient's IgE profile with a small blood sample. It may reveal unanticipated sensitivities, possibly to potentially harmful molecules, making the interpretation of such sensitization difficult in the case of a clinically silent history, but giving the allergist the chance to investigate other hypersensitivities and to alert the patient towards possible risks. This clearly demonstrates that in vitro diagnostics, including MB, should be evaluated within the framework of a patient's clinical history, since allergen sensitization does not necessarily imply clinical responsiveness.

Third-level methods

Oral provocation test (OPT)

OPTs are the most reliable tests in the diagnosis of clinically relevant IgE associated food allergies once allergen specific IgE has been detected. The OPT remains the "gold standard" to establish or exclude the liability of a particular food in causing an adverse reaction [56–61]. The actual value of this method is its functional result. Indeed, only foods causing a clinical evidence of allergy are considered positive. When first and second-level methods have been unable to indicate the food that is responsible for the symptoms, the clinical relevance of a detected sensitization may also be investigated by a targeted elimination diet to perform before the OPT [28]. Furthermore, if multiple triggers are suspected, the elimination diet can help in selecting food to be tested through the OPT, which remains the most important diagnostic tool in food allergy diagnosis. Once the diagnostic work-up has been concluded, the elimination diet of the culprit food/s usually represents the treatment for known food allergies, as well as educating the patient about proper food preparations and the risks of occult exposure [28, 29]. Ongoing investigations are currently evaluating the role of food immunotherapy as a potential FA therapy, to be performed by highly skilled specialists in appropriate settings [29, 62].

The OPT is a third-level procedure that should be carried out when previous diagnostic levels were unable to give sufficient information for the clinical diagnosis [60]. During the patient follow-up, OPT is useful in detecting an acquired tolerance for the specific food. The functional identification of the causative food allows one to avoid its assumption as well as the establishment of unnecessary rigid diets. Due to the potential risk of severe adverse events, the test has to be performed in a hospital setting with personnel trained in resuscitation procedures and the availability of emergency drugs.

The indications of OPT [61, 63–65] are: (a) to identify the food responsible for acute reactions, or to monitor the unexpected tolerance in case of a history of allergy; (b) to determine the offending food in chronic conditions such as atopic dermatitis or eosinophilic esophagitis; (c) to expand the diet in subjects with multiple dietary restrictions; (d) to establish the degree of tolerance to cross-reactive foods and to establish possible acquisition of a spontaneous tolerance to food.

The contraindications are: (a) previous severe anaphylactic reactions (especially recent); (b) level of specific IgE exceeding the cut-off for which there is a high probability that the oral test is positive; (c) reactivity to individual molecules identified with the MBD that indicate a possible severe reaction; (d) reactions occurred during the performance of the SPT and (e) a progressive systemic disease, in particular when the patient is taking medications that could mitigate (antihistamines, corticosteroids) or amplify (β-blockers, ACE inhibitors, NSAIDs, etc.) the reaction [63, 64].

The test consists of gradually increasing doses of the appropriately diluted food, starting from the lowest dose and checking the presence of relevant symptoms. The test can be performed in three different settings [63]:

Open OPT is used for immediate reactions when the risk of severe reaction is reduced. It can be performed on an outpatient basis with a simplified protocol of administration and an observation time of about 2 h. It can be strongly influenced by the age and by the subject's psychological behaviour. If negative, the food can be reintroduced into the diet. In the case of suspected positive reaction, it should be checked in a double-blind OPT setting.

Single-blind placebo OPT (SBP-OPT) it consists of two sessions, one with placebo and one with the suspected food. When a strong psychological component is suspected, the placebo should be tested first. The patient undergoing the SPB-OPT is informed that the food may or may not be present in the administered dose. If the answer is negative or positive symptoms are observed, it is not necessary to continue the investigation. Repeated sessions with placebo or suspected food are useful for the confirmation of vague symptoms. In the case of positivity with placebo, a DBP-OPT will be necessary. In the case of a negative result, the tolerated food must be ingested in its natural form 2 h after or on the day after the test. The tolerance should be checked with follow-up.

Double–blind placebo controlled test (DBPCT) the gold standard. The foods to be tested are prepared by professional personnel not involved in the clinical examination. Placebo and food must have a very similar look and taste. Only when the test is completed can the doctor and patient know the pattern of administration and discuss the results [66].

Fourth-level methods

Basophil activation test (BAT)

The BAT can be used in the study of IgE (and non-IgE) mediated allergic reactions [67, 68]. The rationale of this test is the change in the phenotype of activated basophils after in vitro incubation of the patient's whole blood with the allergen. The BAT is a useful complementary tool to the in vitro diagnosis of FA caused by milk, egg, peanut and wheat [69, 70] when IgE may be involved. Interestingly, a recent study of 20 peanut-allergic children showed that when basophils were stimulated with decreasing doses of allergens until threshold sensitivity was reached, 19 were negative to peanut but 17 were positive to rAra h 8, suggesting that the children sensitized to Ara h 8 but not peanut storage proteins may be at risk of systemic allergic reactions, especially when eating large amounts of peanuts [70].

Reactions unrelated to IgE may also be assessed by BAT, as evidenced for wine and beef [71, 72]. Recently it was also used in the decision-making process for the reintroduction of milk in children allergic to casein [73]. Today, BAT is the only assay that mimics, in the test tube, what happens in vivo. After an extensive validation, BAT should distinguish sensitization from a clinical allergy. The method still suffers some critical issues that can make it a routine test only in specialized laboratories (Fig. 1).

Complementary alternative tests

Frequently, patients undergo complementary/alternative tests after a negative response to a common diagnostic work-up or when non specific symptoms predominate (e.g. migraine, abdominal discomfort, chronic urticaria or other skin abnormalities, chronic fatigue, weight gain or lack of success in weight loss diets), which are erroneously classified as "food allergy" [74]. It represents a common diagnostic label suggested by physicians without specific expertise in the field of FA mechanisms and food-related disorders [75, 76].

The most common (not validated) alternative diagnostic techniques are:

In vivo:

- Electrodermal tests: they measure the change in the skin's electrical conductance once the subject has been exposed to an allergenic substance through specific devices [75].
- Kinesiology: it registers the decreased strength of muscular contraction related to contact with an allergen [75].
- Provocation/neutralization testing: it identifies the onset of "untoward effects" provoked by the administration (intradermal or sublingual) of allergenic substances [76]. The same technique is used as a therapeutic tool.

In vitro:

- Leukocytotoxic tests: they detect the shape/volume abnormalities of peripheral leukocytes when an allergen in a solid and not measurable phase comes into contact with them [77].

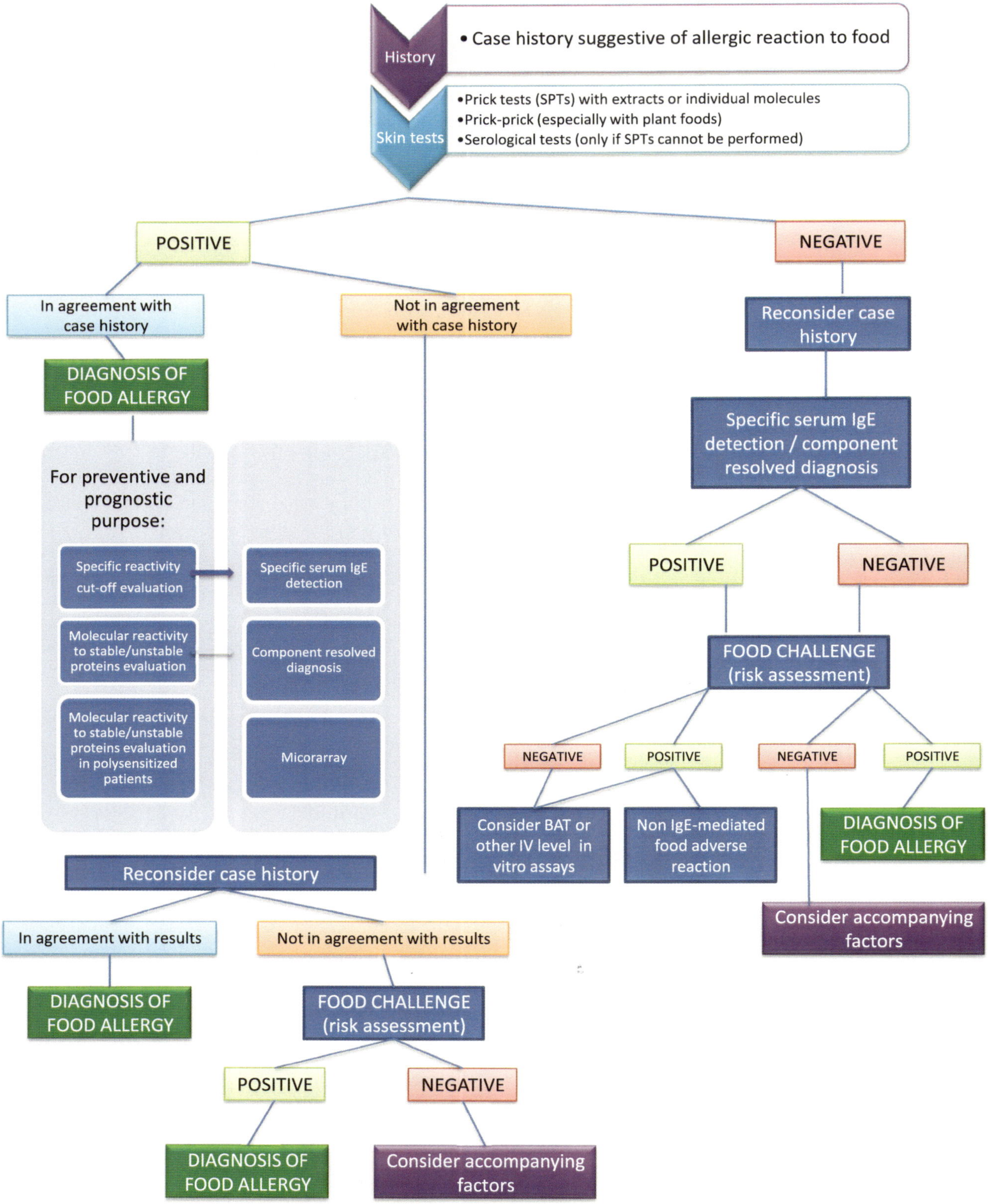

Fig. 1 Flow chart for the diagnosis of food allergy

A direct comparison between such tests and gold standard methods has so far failed in all cases to demonstrate their validity [78]. Their use is strongly discouraged.

Conclusion

The diagnosis of FA is an integrated procedure that can be carried out in different steps (Fig. 1). Some patients can be diagnosed easily by the use of first- and second-level tests, while complex patients, with poly-sensitization and pollen-food syndromes, frequently require a third-level approach. In recent years, the diagnostic assays for FA have been significantly expanded and standardized tools and procedures are now available to the allergist.

Currently, demanding issues are related to FA diagnosis: (1) Identified food(s) should be excluded from the diet; (2) the patient must be properly informed about the relative risk of ingesting the sensitizing foods, even inadvertently as hidden foods in different preparations; (3) the allergist should explain all preventive and curative measures to be taken in case of allergic reactions, including potential medical urgency. In particular, the patient must be informed of the possibility that certain concurrent conditions could favour the onset of FA. This involves a great deal of renewed research specialists and experts on the subject to be able to respond appropriately to the diagnostic and therapeutic needs of patients.

Abbreviations

AMA: allergen microarray; APT: atopy patch test; BAT: basophil activation test; DBPCT: double-blind placebo-controlled test; FA: food allergy; FDEIA: food dependent exercise induced anaphylaxis; ISAC: immuno-sorbent allergen chip; LTP: lipid transfer protein; MBD: molecular-based diagnosis,; NSAIDs: non-steroidal anti-inflammatory drugs; OPT: oral provocation test; PR-10: pathogenesis-related-10; P + P: prick + prick; SBT-OPT: single-blind placebo oral provocation test; sIgE: specific IgE; SPT: skin prick test; tIgE: total IgE.

Authors' contributions

DM conceived the review and coordinated the other contributors; DM, GM, VP, EN, MP, MC, CC, MRY, DS, RP contributed to literature review process and to the final version of the manuscript. MDG provided the final revision of the manuscript. All authors read and approved the final manuscript.

Authors' information

DM is the current Food Allergy Study Group (ATI-Area Tematica di Interesse) Chairperson of the Italian Society of Allergy, Asthma and Clinical Immunology (SIAAIC). VP is the current Food Allergy Study Group (ATI-Area Tematica di Interesse) Secretary of the Italian Society of Allergy, Asthma and Clinical Immunology (SIAAIC). MC is the current Junior Members Chairperson of the Italian Society of Allergy, Asthma and Clinical Immunology (SIAAIC). RP is the current Immunodeficiencies Study Group (ATI-Area Tematica di Interesse) Chairperson of the Italian Society of Allergy, Asthma and Clinical Immunology (SIAAIC). MDG is the current vice-President of the Italian Society of Allergy, Asthma and Clinical Immunology (SIAAIC).

Author details

[1] SS Allergology and Clinical Immunology, S. Giovanni di Dio Hospital, Florence, Italy. [2] Respiratory Diseases and Allergy, University of Genoa, IRCCS AOU S. Martino-IST, Genoa, Italy. [3] Allergology and Immunology Unit, IRCCS Ca' Granda, Osp. Maggiore Policlinico, Milan, Italy. [4] Servizio di Allergologia, Policlinico Gemelli, Rome, Italy. [5] Allergy Unit, Verona University and General Hospital, Verona, Italy. [6] Department of Allergy and Clinical Immunology, IRCCS San Raffaele Hospital, Milan, Italy. [7] Department of Medicine and Science of Ageing, G. d'Annunzio University, Chieti, Italy. [8] Unit of Allergy and Immunotoxicology, CeSi, "G. d'Annunzio" University Foundation, Chieti, Italy.

Acknowledgements

The authors would like to thank all the members of the Food Allergy Study Group (ATI-Area Tematica di Interesse) of the Italian Society of Allergy, Asthma and Clinical Immunology: Giovanna Alaimo, Valerio Beltrami, Elisa Boni, Maria Bova, Luciana Broccucci, Alessandro Buonomo, Maria Filomena Caiaffa, Stefania Capretti, Mario Caringi, Gloria Castiglioni, Maria Rosaria Cavaluzzo, Michele Cipullo, Pasquale Comberiati, Giovanni Coniglio, Mariaelisabetta Conte, Simona D'Alò, Corrado Danzi, Tiziana De Pasquale, Maria Distaso, Vito Ditta, Maria Pia Dolcher, Paola Fantini, Carmelo Genovese, Paolo Giaccone, Claudio Giagnoni, Davide Grataroli, Ilenia Illuminati, Selene Imbesi, Marco Ispano, Maria Stefania Leto Barone, Fabio Lodi Rizzini, Michela Maggioletti, Diomira Magliacane, Roberto Manetti, Irene Martignago, Ilaria Massaro, Marina Mauro, Valerie Melli, Paolo Meloni, Francesca Mero, Elisa Meucci, Sabrina Mietta, Manlio Milanese, Michela Mineni, Ambra Modiano, Paolo Morandi, Franco Nebiolo, Elisa Olivieri, Angelo Passaleva, Giampiero Patriarca, Giuseppe Pingitore, Alessio Pirino, Celestino Pucci, Cristina Quecchia, Francesca Racca, Erminia Ridolo, Marco Saletti, Gilda Varricchi, Maria Teresa Ventura, Alice Vignoli.

The authors also would like to thank Helen Farrel who provided medical writing services.

References

1. Lack G. Epidemiologic risks for food allergy. J Allergy Clin Immunol. 2008;121:1331–6.
2. de Blok BM, Vlieg-Boerstra BJ, Oude Elberink JN, Duiverman EJ, DunnGalvin A, Hourihane JO, et al. A framework for measuring the social impact of food allergy across Europe: a EuroPrevall state of the art paper. Allergy. 2007;62:733–7.
3. Boyce JA, Assa'ad A, Burks AW, Jones SM, Sampson HA, Wood RA, et al. Guidelines for the diagnosis and management of food allergy in the United States: summary of the NIAID-sponsored expert panel report. Nutr Res. 2011;31:61–75.
4. DunnGalvin A, Dubois AE, Flokstra-de Blok BM, Hourihane JO. The effects of food allergy on quality of life. Chem Immunol Allergy. 2015;101:235–52.
5. Romano A, Di Fonso M, Giuffreda F, Papa G, Artesani MC, Viola M. Food-dependent exercise-induced anaphylaxis: clinical and laboratory findings in 54 Subjects. Int Arch Allergy Immunol. 2001;125:264–72.
6. Rowlands D, Tofte SJ, Hanifin JM. Does food allergy cause atopic dermatitis? Food challenge testing to dissociate eczematous from immediate reactions. Dermatol Ther. 2006;19:97–103.
7. Burks W. Skin manifestations of food allergy. Pediatrics. 2003;111:1617–24.
8. Chehade M, Sampson HA. The role of lymphocytes in eosinophilic gastrointestinal disorders. Immunol Allergy Clin North Am. 2009;29:149–58.
9. Nowak-Wegrzyn A, Sampson HA, Wood RA, Sicherer SH. Food protein-induced enterocolitis syndrome caused by solid food proteins. Pediatrics. 2003;111:829–35.
10. Furuta GT, Liacouras CA, Collins MH, Gupta SK, Justinich C, Putnam PE, et al. Eosinophilic esophagitis in children and adults: a systematic review and consensus recommendations for diagnosis and treatment. Gastroenterology. 2007;133:1342–63.
11. Kondo Y, Urisu A. Oral allergy syndrome. Allergol Int. 2009;58:485–91.
12. James JM. Respiratory manifestations of food allergy. Pediatrics. 2003;111:1625–30.

13. Sicherer SH, Leung DY. Advances in allergic skin disease, anaphylaxis, and hypersensitivity reactions to foods, drugs, and insects in 2014. J Allergy Clin Immunol. 2015;135:357–67.
14. Sampson HA, Munoz-Furlong A, Bock SA, Schmitt C, Bass R, Chowdhury BA, et al. Symposium on the definition and management of anaphylaxis: summary report. J Allergy Clin Immunol. 2005;115:584–91.
15. Nettis E, Colanardi MC, Ferrannini A, Tursi A. Sodium benzoate-induced repeated episodes of acute urticaria/angio-oedema: randomized controlled trial. Br J Dermatol. 2004;151:898–902.
16. Park HW, Park CH, Park SH, Park JY, Park HS, Yang HJ, et al. Dermatologic adverse reactions to 7 common food additives in patients with allergic diseases: a double-blind, placebo-controlled study. J Allergy Clin Immunol. 2008;121:1059–61.
17. Jones SM. The spectrum of allergic reactions to foods. In: Metcalfe DD, Sampson HA, Simon RA, editors. Food allergy: adverse reactions to foods and food additives, vol. 4. Malden: Wiley-Blackwell; 2008. p. 101–9.
18. Braga M, Quecchia C, Perotta C, Timpini A, Maccarinelli K, Di Tommaso L, Di Gioacchino M. Systemic nickel allergy syndrome: nosologic framework and usefulness of diet regimen for diagnosis. Int J Immunopathol Pharmacol. 2013;26:707–16.
19. Ballmer-Weber BK. Food allergy in adolescence and adulthood. Chem Immunol Allergy. 2015;101:51–8.
20. Canonica GW, Ansotegui IJ, Pawankar R, Schmid-Grendelmeier P, van Hage M, Baena-Cagnani CE, et al. A WAO–ARIA–GA2LEN consensus document on molecular-based allergy diagnostics. World Allergy Organ J. 2013;6:17.
21. Asero R. In patients with LTP syndrome food-specific IgE show a predictable hierarchical order. Eur Ann Allergy Clin Immunol. 2014;46:142–6.
22. Pali-Schöll I, Herzog R, Wallmann J, Szalai K, Brunner R, Lukschal A, et al. Antacids and dietary supplements with an influence on the gastric pH increase the risk for food sensitization. Clin Exp Allergy. 2010;40:1091–8.
23. Ciprandi G, Cavallucci E, Cuccurullo F, Di Gioacchino M. Helminthic infection as a factor in new-onset coffee allergy in a father and daughter. J Allergy Clin Immunol. 2008;121:773–4.
24. Muñoz-Cano R, Pascal M, Bartra J, Picado C, Valero A, Kim DK, et al. Distinct transcriptome profiles differentiate nonsteroidal anti-inflammatory drug-dependent from nonsteroidal anti-inflammatory drug-independent food-induced anaphylaxis. J Allergy Clin Immunol. 2015;. doi:10.1016/j.jaci.2015.05.042.
25. Ben-Shoshan M, Soller L, Harrington DW, Knoll M, La Vieille S, Fragapane J, et al. Eczema in early childhood, sociodemographic factors and lifestyle habits are associated with food allergy: a nested case-control study. Int Arch Allergy Immunol. 2015;166:199–207.
26. Stelmach I, Majak P, Jerzynska J, Podlecka D, Stelmach W, Polańska K, et al. The effect of prenatal exposure to phthalates on food allergy and early eczema in inner-city children. Allergy Asthma Proc. 2015;36:72–8.
27. Wüthrich B. History of food allergy. Chem Immunol Allergy. 2014;100:109–19.
28. Sampson HA, Aceves S, Bock SA, James J, Jones S, Lang D, et al. Food allergy: a practice parameter update-2014. J Allergy Clin Imm. 2014;134:1016–25.
29. Sicherer SH, Sampson HA. Food allergy: epidemiology, pathogenesis, diagnosis, and treatment. J Allergy Clin Immunol. 2014;133:291–307.
30. de Silva D, Geromi M, Panesar SS, Muraro A, Werfel T, Hoffmann-Sommergruber K, et al. Acute and long term management of food allergy: systematic review. Allergy. 2014;69:159–67.
31. Sporik R, Hill DJ, Hosking CS. Specificity of allergen skin testing in predicting positive open food challenges to milk, egg and peanut in children. Clin Exp Allergy. 2000;30:1540–6.
32. Du Toit G, Santos A, Roberts G, Fox AT, Smith P, Lack G. The diagnosis of IgE-mediated food allergy in childhood. Pediatr Allergy Immunol. 2009;20:309–19.
33. Valenta R, Hochwallner H, Linhart B, Pahr S. Food allergies: the basics. Gastroenterology. 2015;148:1120–31.
34. Vlieg-Boerstra BJ, van de Weg WE, van der Heide S, Dubois AE. Where to prick the apple for skin testing? Allergy. 2013;68:1196–8.
35. Henzgen M, Ballmer-Weber BK, Erdmann S, Fuchs T, Kleine-Tebbe J, Lepp U, et al. Skin testing with food allergens. Guideline of the German Society of Allergology and Clinical Immunology (DGAKI), the Physicians' Association of German Allergologists (ADA) and the Society of Pediatric Allergology (GPA) together with the Swiss Society of Allergology. J Dtsch Dermatol Ges. 2008;6:983–8.
36. Cantani A, Micera M. Can skin prick tests provoke severe allergic reactions? Eur Rev Med Pharmacol Sci. 2000;4:145–8.
37. Lieberman JA, Sicherer SH. The diagnosis of food allergy. Am J Rhinol Allergy. 2010;24(6):439–43.
38. Rancé F, Juchet A, Brémont F, Dutau G. Correlations between skin prick tests using commercial extracts and fresh foods, specific IgE, and food challenge. Allergy. 1997;52:1031.
39. Sampson HA. Utility of food-specific IgE concentrations in predicting symptomatic food allergy. J Allergy Clin Immunol. 2001;107:891–6.
40. Katelaris CH. Food allergy and oral allergy or pollen-food syndrome. Curr Opin Allergy Clin Immunol. 2010;10:246–51.
41. Price A, Ramachandran S, Smith GP, Stevenson ML, Pomeranz MK, Cohen DE. Oral allergy syndrome (Pollen-food allergy syndrome). Dermatitis. 2015;26:78–88.
42. Allergome Database. http://www.allergome.org/script/search_step2.php?action=all_allergen. Accessed 30 Aug 2015.
43. Radauer C, Nandy A, Ferreira F, Goodman RE, Larsen JN, Lidholm J, et al. Update of the WHO/IUIS Allergen Nomenclature Database based on analysis of allergen sequences. Allergy. 2014;69:413–9.
44. Gomez F, Aranda A, Campo P, Diaz-Perales A, Blanca-Lopez N, Perkins J, et al. High prevalence of lipid transfer protein sensitization in apple allergic patients with systemic symptoms. PLoS One. 2014;9:e107304.
45. Kollmann D, Geroldinger-Simic M, Kinaciyan T, Huber H, Ebner C, Lidholm J, Bohle B. Recombinant Mal d 1 is a reliable diagnostic tool for birch pollen allergen-associated apple allergy. J Allergy Clin Immunol. 2013;132:1008–10.
46. Ruiter B. Shreffler WG Innate immunostimulatory properties of allergens and their relevance to food allergy. Semin Immunopathol. 2012;34:617.
47. Pastorello EA, Farioli L, Pravettoni V, Scibilia J, Mascheri A, Borgonovo L, et al. Prup p3–sensitized Italian peach–allergic patents are less likely to develop severe symptoms when also presenting IgE Antibodies to Pru P1 and Pru P 4. Int Arch Allergy Immunol. 2011;156:362–72.
48. Mascheri A, Farioli L, Pravettoni V, Piantanida M, Stafylaraki C, Scibilia J, et al. Hypersensitivity to tomato (Lycopersicon esculentum) in peach-allergic patients: rPrup 3 and rPrup 1 are predictive of symptom severity. J Investig Allergol Clin Immunol. 2015;25:183–9.
49. Santos A, Van Ree R. Profilins: mimickers of allergy or relevant allergens? Int Arch Allergy Immunol. 2011;155:191–204.
50. Fernandez-Rivas M, Bolhaar S, González-Mancebo E, Asero R, van Leeuwen A, et al. Apple allergy across Europe: how allergen sensitization profiles determine the clinical expression of allergies to plant foods. J Allergy Clin Immunol. 2006;118:481–8.
51. Asero R. Lipid transfer protein cross-reactivity assessed in vivo and in vitro in the office: pros and cons. J Investig Allergol Clin Immunol. 2011;21:129–36.
52. Cudowska B, Kaczmarski M, Restani P. Lipid transfer protein in diagnosis of birch-apple syndrome in children. Immunobiology. 2008;213:89–96.
53. van Ree R, Fernández-Rivas M, Cuevas M, van Wijngaarden M, Aalberse RC. Pollen-related allergy to peach and apple: an important role for profilin. J Allergy Clin Immunol. 1995;95:726–34.
54. Asero R, Mistrello G, Roncarolo D, Amato S, Zanoni D, Barocci F, et al. Detection of clinical markers of sensitization to profilin in patients allergic to plant-derived foods. J Allergy Clin Immunol. 2003;112:427–32.
55. Melioli G, Spenser C, Reggiardo G, Passalacqua G, Compalati E, Rogkakou A, Riccio AM, Di Leo E, Nettis E, Canonica GW. Allergenius, an expert system for the interpretation of allergy microarray results. World Allergy Organ J. 2014;7(1):15.
56. Beyer K, Teuber SS. Food allergy diagnostics: scientific and unproven procedures. Curr Opin Allergy Clin Immunol. 2005;5:261–6.
57. Sicherer SH. Food allergy: when and how to perform oral food challenges. Pediatr Allergy Immunol. 1999;10:226–34.
58. Franxman TJ, Howe L, Teich E, Greenhawt MJ. Oral food challenge and food allergy quality of life in caregivers of children with food allergy. J Allergy Clin Immunol Pract. 2015;3:50–6.
59. O'Keefe AW, De Schryver S, Mill J, Mill C, Dery A, Ben-Shoshan M. Diagnosis and management of food allergies: new and emerging options: a systematic review. J Asthma Allergy. 2014;7:141–64.
60. Macchia D, Capretti S, Cecchi L, Colombo G, Di Lorenzo G, Fassio F, et al. Position statement: in vivo and in vitro diagnosis of food allergy in adults. It J Allergy Clin Immunol. 2011;21:57–72.

61. Mori F, Pucci N, Rossi ME, de Martino M, Azzari C, Novembre E. Oral desensitization to milk: how to choose the starting dose. Pediatr Allergy Immunol. 2010;21:e450–3.
62. Wood RA. Diagnostic elimination diets and oral food provocation. Chem Immunol Allergy. 2015;101:87–95.
63. Bindslev-Jensen C. Standardization of double-blind, placebo-controlled food challenges. Allergy. 2001;56(Suppl 67):75–7.
64. Sabato V, van Hengel AJ, De Knop KJ, Verweij MM, Hagendorens MM, Bridts CH, et al. Human basophils: a unique biological instrument to detect the allergenicity of food. J Investig Allergol Clin Immunol. 2011;21:179–84.
65. Hoffmann HJ, Santos AF, Mayorga C, Nopp A, Eberlein B, Ferrer M, et al. The clinical utility of basophil activation testing in diagnosis and monitoring of allergic disease. Allergy. 2015. doi:10.1111/all.12698.
66. Vassilopoulou E, Karathanos A, Siragakis G, Giavi S, Sinaniotis A, Douladiris N, et al. Risk of allergic reactions to wine, in milk, egg and fish-allergic patients. Clin Transl Allergy. 2011;1:10.
67. Santos AF, Du Toit G, Douiri A, Radulovic S, Stephens A, Turcanu V, et al. Distinct parameters of the basophil activation test reflect the severity and threshold of allergic reactions to peanut. J Allergy Clin Immunol. 2015;135:179–86.
68. Glaumann S, Nilsson C, Johansson SG, Asarnoj A, Wickman M, Borres MP, et al. Evaluation of basophil allergen threshold sensitivity (CD-sens) to peanut and Ara h 8 in children IgE-sensitized to Ara h 8. Clin Mol Allergy. 2015;13:5.
69. Rolland JM, Apostolou E, Deckert K, de Leon MP, Douglass JA, Glaspole IN, et al. Potential food allergens in wine: double-blind, placebo-controlled trial and basophil activation analysis. Nutrition. 2006;22:882–8.
70. Kim JH, An S, Kim JE, Choi GS, Ye YM, Park HS. Beef-induced anaphylaxis confirmed by the basophil activation test. Allergy Asthma Immunol Res. 2010;2:206–8.
71. Nucera E, Pecora V, Buonomo A, Rizzi A, Aruanno A, Pascolini L, et al. Utility of basophil activation test for monitoring the acquisition of clinical tolerance after oral desensitization to cow's milk: Pilot study. United European Gastroenterol J. 2015;3:272–6.
72. Senna G, Bonadonna P, Schiappoli M, Leo G, Lombardi C, Passalacqua G. Pattern of use and diagnostic value of complementary/alternative tests for adverse reactions to food. Allergy. 2005;60:1216–7.
73. Heffler E, Minciullo PL, Fassio F, Rossi FW, Patafi M, Mondino M, et al. Pertinence of requested allergy consultations for suspected food allergy/intolerance. A Junior Members working group of Italian Society of Allergy and Clinical Immunology (SIAIC) multicenter study. J Allergy Clin Immunol. 2011;21:18–24.
74. Semizzi M, Senna G, Crivellaro M, Rapacioli G, Passalacqua G, Canonica WG, et al. A double-blind, placebo-controlled study on the diagnostic accuracy of an electrodermal test in allergic subjects. Clin Exp Allergy. 2002;32:928–32.
75. Garrow JS. Kinesiology and food allergy. Br Med J (Clin Res Ed). 1988;296:1573–4.
76. Jewett DL, Fein G, Greenberg MH. A double-blind study of symptom provocation to determine food sensitivity. N Engl J Med. 1990;323:429–33.
77. Terr AI. The cytotoxic test. West J Med. 1983;139:702–3.
78. Senna G, Passalacqua G, Lombardi C, Antonicelli L. Position paper: controversial and unproven diagnostic procedures for food allergy. Eur Ann Allergy Clin Immunol. 2004;36:139–45.

12

How to fit allergen immunotherapy in the elderly

Erminia Ridolo[1*], Anti Rogkakou[2], Maria Teresa Ventura[3], Irene Martignago[1], Cristoforo Incorvaia[4], Gabriele Di Lorenzo[5] and Giovanni Passalacqua[2]

Abstract

Asthma, allergic rhinitis (AR) and atopic dermatitis are very common in young people, but in the latest decades it was increasingly recognized that also individuals of higher ages, including the population over 65 years, are concerned. Actually, it is now acknowledged the aging does not considerably alter the immune response to allergens. Allergen immunotherapy (AIT) is the only treatment that works on the causes of allergy, but elderly people are commonly excluded from AIT, except the cases of insect sting allergy. A number of recent studies showed that aged individuals also successfully respond to AIT for respiratory allergy. Therefore, there is no reason to exclude elder patients from AIT. Anyhow, clinical conditions that are considered absolute or relative contraindications are quite frequent in this aged population, thus the risk/benefit ratio must be carefully evaluated for each patient, taking into account that the more frequent occurrence of co-morbidities and the consequent need of daily-based multidrug regimen can favor adverse effects. An important issue concern the ability of AIT, and particularly of sublingual immunotherapy, to significantly improve the quality of life, that often is particularly impaired in the elderly, reducing symptoms and drugs consumption.

Keywords: Allergy, Elderly, Immunosenescence, Allergen immunotherapy

Background

Asthma, allergic rhinitis (AR) and other atopic diseases (e.g. food allergy or atopic dermatitis) are very common in young people, but it is now recognized they can also affect individuals of higher ages. For instance, AR was reported to affect up to 5–10% of the population over 65 years [1]. However, a global decline of the prevalence of allergic disorders in elderly, at least on epidemiological basis has been repeatedly claimed. This might be ascribed to the expected decrease in serum IgE antibodies due to an unbalance of cytokines and soluble factors involved in its production. However, in studying non-allergic individuals aged 20–93 years, assessing serum IgE, sCD23 and Th2 type cytokine production, IgE levels were not significantly different between young and old subjects [2]. This was confirmed in another similar study [3]. These results suggest that the type 2 cytokine pattern is not necessarily defective in older age. Data also confirmed that IL-13, a key cytokine in IgE regulation, is not impaired in old subjects. Although IL-4 has been considered the most critical cytokine linked to allergic responses and immunity against parasites, recent observations indicate that IL-13 has equal or even greater importance in those processes. IL-4 and IL-13 share several functional properties, however IL-13 can independently induce class switching and IgE secretion from human B cells. In addition, IL-13 enhances expression of CD23 and of the major histocompatibility complex class II antigens, and may act as a monocyte chemoattractant [4, 5]. The clinical findings indicating that the allergic reactivity could decrease with age [6, 7] make ageing an interesting in vivo model to study the waning of allergic response. Yet, there is not sufficient information to establish that the frequency of onset of allergic symptoms, as well as their severity, declines with aging. According to the aforementioned aspects, the clinical use of allergen specific immunotherapy (AIT) has been so far considered of little interest in

*Correspondence: erminia.ridolo@unipr.it
[1] Medicine and Surgery Department, University of Parma, Via Gramsci 14, 43126 Parma, Italy
Full list of author information is available at the end of the article

the elderly, since AIT is commonly used in young people, with a well-defined TH2-high immunological phenotype. We review herein the main immunologic aspects of aging, according to the presence of allergic diseases, and the current evidence on the use of AIT in elderly patients.

Aging and the immune system

Immunosenescence is a complex process in which genetic and environmental factors are involved, characterized by a "remodeling" more than a "decline" of the immune system, and associated to various factors: oxidative stress, apoptotic phenomena, increased production of pro-inflammatory lymphokines [8]. This results in a state of chronic, low-grade, inflammation described by some authors as "inflamm-aging" [9]. The cells of the immune system are constantly renewed by the hematopoietic stem cells, but during senescence this activity declines and the overall amount of hematopoietic tissue decreases. This event also seems related to the shortening of telomeres [10]. Thymic involution process in the elderly goes along with the reduction of naïve T cells, although the total number of T cells does not undergo large displacements due to the increase in population of non-regulatory cells CD8+ CD45RO+ CD25+, that represent a promising biomarker of immune competence in old age. In the elderly a reduced response of T cells to growth factors and specific antigens can be documented [11]. The compartment of B cells is also affected by ageing and this influences the efficiency of cooperation between T and B lymphocytes. Even if the total B cells does not change, the number of memory B lymphocytes, becoming less sensitive to apoptosis, increases. At the same time, the naïve B cells are reduced [12]. All these changes may result in an enhancement of monoclonal serum immunoglobulins. The role of regulatory T cells (Treg), a cell subsets with regulatory function, including CD4+ and CD8+ Treg, deserves special attention in the elderly. CD4+ Tregs are involved in suppressing the activation, proliferation, and cytokine production, as well as the function of dendritic cells. The Tregs are characterized by the expression of IL-2R α-chain (CD25) and CTLA-4. The transcription factor FoxP3 (Forkhead box P3) plays an important role in the function of Tregs. The naturally occurring CD4+ and CD8+ Treg increase in the elderly and have equivalent expression of CTLA-4 and equivalent regulatory function with cytokine production after polyclonal T cell stimulation compared to younger subjects, while the number of inducible CD4+ and CD8+ Treg decreases with advancing years [13]. The relevance of these cells in the elderly is not yet fully clarified in relation to immunosenescence. In particular, the Tregs induce down-regulation of mast cells, basophils and eosinophils through the production of IL-10 and TGF-β and may also induce reduction of Th2 cells and their cytokines. In turn, IL-10 and TGF-β elicit the suppression of IgE by B lymphocytes and, in particular, IL-10 causes the switch towards IgG4 producing plasma cells and consequently to an increased synthesis of allergen-specific IgG4 isotype blocking antibodies [14, 15]. Recently, it was identified in the senescence an immunological risk phenotype (IRP) characterized by inversion of the CD4/CD8 ratio, increase in $CD8^+CD28^-$ lymphocyte population, identified as memory/effector cells and reduction of B lymphocytes. In addition, patients with IRP manifested a marked serum positivity for cytomegalovirus and the increase of proinflammatory cytokines, including in particular IL-6, IL-1β, tumor necrosis factor (TNF)-α and acute phase proteins [16]. An interesting research in elderly patients has shown not only an enhancement of the type 1 cytokines such as IL-1, interferon (IFN)-γ and TNF-α, whose role is of great importance for the increase of cancer and chronic infections, but also of type 2 such as IL-4, IL-5, IL-10, which constitutes the substrate for the development of allergic diseases [2]. In particular, in cytokine cultures stimulated with PHA, the production of T-helper 2 cytokines does not appear to be significant different in young and elderly subjects. As it is well known that in allergic patients there is an overproduction of Th2 cytokines, that can induce the isotopic switch of B cells toward IgE isotype immunoglobulins and recall on-site cells responsible for the allergic inflammation (mast cells and eosinophils), the authors concluded that there is no valid justification for the statement that allergic diseases decline in the elderly. Moreover, the same authors showed that IL-13, that plays a key role in the regulation of IgE, is not affected in the elderly [2] thus confirming that the occurrence of allergic reactions in the elderly is supported by high serum levels of IgE and type 2 cytokines. However, data on the production of IgE in the literature are contradictory. In fact, in opposition to the claim that the levels are reduced in the elderly [17], in the most recent literature there is increasing evidence that in the allergic disease IgE levels are perfectly comparable to those found in young subjects [2, 18]. We must remember that an efficient IgE response requires both the presence of IL-4 or IL-13 and also a physical interaction between T and B-cells, involving a number of surface and adhesion molecules [19, 20], that include the CD40/CD40L interaction that is defective in old subjects [21]. However, these studies analyzed young and old non-allergic individuals, while it would be of greater interest to compare these parameters in allergic young and old subjects.

Alterations of innate immunity have an essential role and the studies on the issue have identified a separate trend in the field of immunogerontology, beginning with the reduction of epithelial barriers in the skin and mucous membranes, both at respiratory and gastrointestinal tract [22]. As regards the immunoglobulins of IgA type at the mucosal level, significant changes can be found with a marked increase of monomeric IgA1, both in serum and in saliva. Some changes, especially in the functional aspects related to chemotaxis, phagocytosis and oxidative burst are shown both in the compartment of neutrophils and macrophages. In addition, it is possible to observe reductions in the level of macrophage-derived chemokines, including macrophage inflammatory protein (MIP)-1α, MIP-1β and eotaxin. The natural killer (NK) cells do not decrease in number, indeed their absolute number was found to increase in geriatric patients. However, the reduced production of IL-2, of critical importance in the processes of lymphocyte activation and killing, induces a deficiency of cytotoxic function in which the numerical increase may occur for a mere compensatory mechanism [23]. Also, dendritic cells play an important role, both in the innate and adaptive immunity. These cells have the role to start the immune response with the function of antigen presenting cells (APC), becoming able to process the antigen and to secrete cytokines. The prolonged administration of allergen as occurs during AIT promotes the production of high levels of IL-12 and IL-27, favouring allergen-specific switches from the Th2 to the Th1 and Th17 phenotype and the expression of NK and NKT cells which in turn induce the increased levels of IFN-γ and activation of APC [24]. The role of vitamins and trace elements, including iron and zinc should be also considered, especially in the light of the frequent conditions of malnutrition in geriatric patients. Vitamin D, and especially its active form, is very important in both innate and adaptive immunity. In particular calcitriol is able to act on APCs and on T lymphocytes by determining inhibition of inflammatory responses through induction of T reg [25].

Allergen sensitizations and AIT in the elderly

Elderly spend most of their time indoors and consequently the most frequent allergen sensitizations are towards indoor allergens, such as house dust mites, cockroaches, furred pets [26]. AIT is an important guideline-approved therapy for AR and asthma, which can modify the disease's natural history, with a long lasting effect on symptoms after its cessation [27]. Indeed, IgE positivities reveal sensitization, but clinical allergy has to be confirmed on the ground of evidence of a relationship between results of IgE test and occurrence of symptoms from exposure to the specific allergen, as well as by demonstration of concomitant inflammation in the airways as assessed by the presence of eosinophils in nasal smears and increase of FeNO [28]. These investigations can be easily performed and are mandatory for the AIT indication in these conditions. A large number of studies confirmed the efficacy and safety of AIT in AR and asthma [29], which is especially related to the mechanism of action itself [15]. Of note, only few studies were designed for AIT in the elderly. Therefore, specific indications and contraindications for AIT in old people are not yet available. Currently, allergists can rely, their everyday practice only on the general guidelines also for the elderly.

The GA^{2}LEN/EAACI pocket guide on AIT for AR and asthma points out that there is not an upper age limit for prescribing AIT [28], as also suggested by the recent EAACI (European Academy of Allergy and Clinical Immunology) position paper on the clinical contraindications to AIT [30], that gave no indication on the upper age limit. In the mentioned document, the only absolute contraindications to AIT were the presence of uncontrolled asthma, autoimmune disorders not responding to therapy, active immune-deficiency and active malignancies. These chronic diseases are frequent among elderly and it is, therefore, warranted to collect a detailed medical history before prescribing AIT. Uncontrolled asthma can depend on an inappropriate therapy and/or poor compliance by the patient. If adequate adjustment of therapy and careful education of the patient allows a good control of asthma symptoms, AIT can be administered.

Autoimmune diseases in remission phase are considered a relative contraindication. Concerning hymenoptera venom immunotherapy (VIT), the position paper states "VIT is a highly advised option in high-risk venom allergic patients" [30]. There are few data on the risk of developing autoimmune diseases. Only a Danish observational study on 18,841 patients treated with subcutaneous immunotherapy (SCIT) vs. 428,484 controls treated with drug therapy for over 10 years found that there was a lower incidence of autoimmune diseases in patients undergoing subcutaneous immunotherapy (SCIT) [31]. In a recent survey among American allergists, it was observed that AIT (VIT and pollen SCIT) performed in patients with stable autoimmune diseases had an high safety profile [32, 33]. Concerning cancer, there is currently no evidence of a new onset or relapse when administering AIT. The possibility that the immunomodulation stimulated with AIT may have a negative effect on the natural history of cancer is the real concern about prescribing AIT [34]. A study from Austria study analyzed the use of AIT in six patients with cancer [35]. One of them received SCIT after 14 years of melanoma diagnosis without presenting relapse of the malignancy during AIT for house dust mites, while another patient interrupted SCIT for grass-pollen because the diagnosis was made few months after AIT initiation. Another patient undergoing VIT had a relapse of breast cancer 3 months after having reached the maintenance dose of immunotherapy, but she ended the 5 years course of VIT while maintaining the neoplastic disease under control. No immunologic mechanisms able to account for a negative effect of AIT on cancer were detected thus far.

Cardiovascular diseases, such as unstable angina, recent myocardial infarction, significant arrhythmia, and uncontrolled systemic hypertension, are very common in old people. The EAACI document considers them as a relative contraindication for inhalant AIT and advises to accurately evaluate the current status of the disease before starting AIT [30]. In fact, the Danish observational study cited above pointed out that SCIT was associated with a lower incidence of acute myocardial infarction and a lower risk of developing ischemic heart disease, compared to medical conventional therapy [31]. Also the presence of chronic pulmonary diseases (not only asthma) that reduce lung function must be evaluated in elderly patients before administering AIT [36].

A daily-based multidrug regimen is widely diffuse in population over 60 years and antihypertensive drugs are among the medications most frequently taken. In everyday practice the allergist often encounters patients who take β-blockers and ACE-inhibitors. In a study on murine models, Nassiri et al. stated that the use of β-blockers slightly aggravates an anaphylactic reaction, while the combined therapy with β-blockers and ACE-inhibitors synergistically could worsen anaphylaxis, due to their action on reducing the mast-cell activation threshold [37]. Clinically, β-blockers use is considered a relative contraindication for VIT, because the block of β1 and β2-receptors decreases the epinephrine action in case of anaphylaxis. However, β-blockers may be replaced by other kind of drugs in case of hypertension but not in case of arrhythmia or ischemic disease. Also ACE-inhibitors use is controversial in patients undergoing VIT, but do not represent a contraindication for inhalant AIT [30]. Importantly, the possible contraindications to use β-blockers and ACE-inhibitors concern only SCIT and not sublingual immunotherapy (SLIT).

Other chronic diseases are common in the elderly and must be evaluated before prescribing AIT. Patients with psychiatric or mental disorders could be not enough compliant or can be unable to report early symptoms of AIT side-effects. Concerning drug treatment of such disorders, the use of monoamine oxidase inhibitors is not a contraindication for AIT, but it must be considered that their action combined with epinephrine could cause severe hypertension and tachycardia [38].

On the other hand, AIT has an important outcome in reducing the risk of side effects to anti-allergic drugs, such as oral corticosteroids (diabetes, osteoporosis, hypertension, etc.), and anti-histamines (sedation, anticholinergic effects).

According to the available data there are not real limitations in administering AIT to elderly people if we consider only age as a limit, but thus far studies on AIT in the elderly are rare, because they are often excluded (mainly for concomitant diseases requiring daily drug-regimen) or present in a small number. Another limit concern defining the elderly age: in developed countries people over 65 of age is usually considered as elderly [39], but often the inclusion age criteria to participate to an AIT trial is 60 years or less. The first study about efficacy and safety of AIT in old patients was performed in 1993 by Armentia et al. [40] on 22 geriatric patients treated with AIT, in whom a significant clinical improvement and a decrease in drug use was achieved. In 2000 Eidelman et al. demonstrated for the first time that AIT was effective in elderly as much as in the younger, treating with SCIT otherwise healthy patients over 60 years of age. In this case the authors chose, as control group, patients with similar allergic history before AIT, but aged $\leq$ 60 years, obtaining a similar good response in both groups of patients [41]. In 2004 Asero investigated whether SCIT could be safely performed in elderly sensitized to seasonal allergens (birch and ragweed); 39 subjects (aged between 55 and 70 years) with a disease's duration of less than 10 years were included. Patients underwent AIT for 1–5 years, achieving a lower use of cetirizine ($p < 0.001$) and/or salbutamol ($p < 0.05$), compared to controls [42].

In recent years an increasing number of studies addressed the safety and efficacy of SLIT [43]. The first study investigating SLIT in elderly population was conducted in 2008 by Marogna et al. In the overall study population of 167 patients (including subjects aged 18–65 years) with AR and mild asthma due to dust mite allergy, 40 patients were aged more than 55 years [44]. The patients underwent SLIT with a dust mite extract and the results were compared to a control group treated with standard drug treatment. The end points were symptoms and drug scores every month, respiratory function tests, metacholine challenge and eosinophils counts at the start and at the end of the study. The authors found in the SLIT group an improvement in all examined variables ($p < 0.001$), achieving also a lower number of new allergen sensitizations ($p = 0.03$), compared to the control group. The results were similar in both young and elderly patients as long as the disease had started fairly recently. However, it is needed to underline that no elderly subject was included, according to the common accepted limit age stated above [39]. The same limit is present in the trial by Baptistella et al. who treated 104 patients with AR over 55 of age (55–74 years) with SLIT for dust mites for 1 year, but there was no information on the number of patients aged more than 65 years [45]. Moreover, patients undergoing any kind of treatment for any comorbidity were excluded. The authors demonstrated the efficacy and the safety of SLT in their patients, with clinical improvement on rhinitis symptoms and absence of side effects. The critical issue regarding these SLIT studies is that they were not blinded.

The first two double-blind placebo-controlled trials were performed recently on a population over 60 years of age. In the initial trial, Bozek et al. recruited 106 patients between 60 and 75 years of age with demonstrated AR due to dust mites [46]; 51 subjects underwent SLIT and the other 57 were included in the placebo group. After 3 years of treatment the patients treated with SLIT had a significant improvement of 44% ($p < 0.05$) in symptoms and of 35% for the medication scores ($p < 0.05$). No side effect was reported. The same authors examined the safety and the efficacy of SLIT for grass pollen allergy in a population aged over 60 years [47]; 78 subjects between 60 and 70 years of age were included in the trial and divided in two groups: 41 patients were treated with SLIT and 37 were in the placebo group. At the end of AIT (3 years), the total nasal symptom score and the total medication score in the SLIT group improved significantly, obtaining a decrease of 64 and 51%, respectively ($p < 0.05$ for both). Only three patients had common local side effects, such as oral itching and facial flushing, while no systemic reaction was observed. Recently, these authors also investigated the safety and efficacy of preseasonal SCIT for grass pollen allergy in 62 patients older than 65 years with seasonal AR. It was demonstrated that the total nasal symptom score decreased by 76% and that the total medication score of the active group decreased by a maximum of 62% in the active group after 3 years of AIT. Moreover, no adverse systemic reactions were reported during therapy [48]. Studies about AIT in elderly are summarized in Table 1.

Conclusions

The older age per se does not preclude the prescription of AIT, that should be considered in elderly individuals when there is a clear indication. Anyhow, clinical conditions that are considered absolute or relative contraindications are quite frequent in this age population and can interfere with AIT effectiveness and safety. The risk/benefit ratio must be carefully evaluated for each patient, taking into account that in the elderly the frequent occurrence of co-morbidities and the consequent need of daily-based multidrug regimen can favor adverse effects as well as drug interactions [49]. An important issue concern the ability of AIT, particularly SLIT, to significantly improve the quality of life, reducing symptoms and drugs consumption [43]. Actually, a study stated that in patients with AR the impairment of quality of life is significantly higher in elderly than in young people [50]. In older patients, this may result in altered cognitive functions giving rise to a vicious circle with unremitting worsening, that warrants to be broken by treatment with significant effectiveness and particularly with persistence over time also following its stopping, thus ensuring to patients

Table 1 AIT studies in elderly

Study	N. patients	AR/AA	Allergen	SCIT/SLIT	Length (years)
Armentia et al. [40]	22	NA	NA	SCIT	1
Eidelman et al. [41]	26	AR and AA	NA	SCIT	NA
Asero [42]	39	AR and AA	Birch and ragweed	SCIT	1–5
Marogna et al. [44]	40	AR and AA	HDM	SLIT	NA
Baptistella et al. [45]	104	AR and AA	HDM	SLIT	1
Bozek et al. [46]	106	AR	HDM	SLIT	3
Bozek et al. [47]	78	AR	Grass pollen	SLIT	3
Bozek et al. [48]	62	AR	Grass pollen	SLIT	3

AR allergic rhinitis, *AA* allergic asthma, *SCIT* subcutaneous immunotherapy, *SLIT* sublingual immunotherapy, *HDM* house dust mites, *N.A.* not available data

a good control of allergic symptoms with no or minimal use of symptomatic drugs. Such requirement is fulfilled by the therapeutic performances of AIT.

Abbreviations

AIT: allergen specific immunotherapy; APC: antigen presenting cells; AR: allergic rhinitis; EAACI: European Academy of Allergy and Clinical Immunology; FeNO: fractional exhaled nitric oxide; IFN: interferon; IRP: immunological risk phenotype; MIP: macrophage inflammatory protein; NK: natural killer; SLIT: sublingual immunotherapy; SCIT: subcutaneous immunotherapy; TNF: tumor necrosis factor; Treg: regulatory T cells; VIT: hymenoptera venom immunotherapy.

Authors' contributions

GDL, MTV, IM wrote and coordinated the draft of the manuscript. ER, CI, AR, GP carried out the bibliographic search, contributed to the draft of the manuscript and made substantial contribution to the revision of the article. All authors read and approved the final manuscript.

Author details

[1] Medicine and Surgery Department, University of Parma, Via Gramsci 14, 43126 Parma, Italy. [2] Allergy and Respiratory Diseases Clinic, DIMI, University of Genoa, IRCCS AOU San Martino-IST, Genoa, Italy. [3] Department of Interdisciplinary Medicine, University of Bari, Bari, Italy. [4] Cardiac/Pulmonary Rehabilitation, ASST Pini/CTO, Milan, Italy. [5] Dipartimento BioMedico di Medicina Interna e Specialistica (Di.Bi.M.I.S), Università di Palermo, Palermo, Italy.

Funding

No sources of funding were used to conduct this study or prepare this manuscript.

References

1. Cardona V, Guilarte M, Luengo O, et al. Allergic diseases in the elderly. Clin Transl Allergy. 2011;1:11.
2. Di Lorenzo G, Pacor ML, Esposito Pellitteri M, Listì F, Colombo A, Candore G, Mansueto P, Lo Bianco C, Ditta V, Battista Rini G, Caruso C. A study of age-related IgE pathophysiological changes. Mech Ageing Dev. 2003;124:445–8.
3. Moro-García MA, Alonso-Arias R, López-Larrea C. Molecular mechanisms involved in the aging of the T-cell immune response. Curr Genomics. 2012;13:589–602.
4. Caramori G, Groneberg D, Ito K, Casolari P, Adcock IM, Papi A. New drugs targeting Th2 lymphocytes in asthma. J Occup Med Toxicol. 2008;3(Suppl 1):S1–6.
5. Walford HH, Doherty TA. STAT6 and lung inflammation. JAKSTAT. 2013;2:e25301.
6. Di Lorenzo G, Leto-Barone MS, La Piana S, Ditta V, Di Fede G, Rini GB. Clinical course of rhinitis and changes in vivo and in vitro of allergic parameters in elderly patients: a long-term follow-up study. Clin Exp Med. 2013;13:67–73.
7. Marone G, Poto S, Giugliano R, Bonini S. Studies on human basophil releasability. Int Arch Allergy Appl Immunol. 1985;77:103–6.
8. Franceschi C, Capri M, Monti D, Giunta S, Olivieri F, Sevini F, Panourgia MP, Invidia L, Celani L, Scurti M, Cevenini E, Castellani GC, Salvioli S. Inflammaging and anti-inflammaging: a systemic perspective on aging and longevity emerged from studies in humans. Mech Ageing Dev. 2007;128:92–105.
9. Cavanagh MM, Weyand CM, Goronzy JJ. Chronic inflammation and aging: DNA damage tips the balance. Curr Opin Immunol. 2012;24:488–93.
10. Maicher A, Kastner L, Dees M, Luke B. Deregulated telomere transcription causes replication-dependent telomere shortening and promotes cellular senescence. Nucleic Acids Res. 2012;40:6649–59.
11. Schwaiger S, Wolf AM, Robatsher P, Jenewein B, Grubeck-Loebenstein B. Il-4-producing CD8 + T cells with a CD62L ++(bright) phenotype accumulate in a subgroup of older adults and are associated with the maintenance of intact humoral immunity in old age. J Immunol. 2003;170:613–9.
12. Weksler ME, Szabo P. The effect of age on the B-cell repertoire. J Clin Immunol. 2000;20:240–9.
13. Jagger A, Shimojima Y, Goronzy JJ, Weyand C. Regulatory T cells and immune aging process. A mini review. Gerontology. 2014;60:130–7.
14. Radulovic S, Jacobson MR, Durham SR, Nouri-Aria KT. Grass pollen immunotherapy induces Foxp3-expressing CD4+ CD25+ cells in the nasal mucosa. J Allergy Clin Immunol. 2009;121:1467–72.
15. Akdis CA, Akdis M. Mechanisms of immune tolerance to allergens: role of IL-10 and T regs. J Clin Invest. 2014;124:4678–80.
16. Wikby A, Ferguson F, Forsey R, Thompson J, Strindhall J, Löfgren S, Nilsson BO, Ernerudh J, Pawelec G, Johansson B. An immune risk phenotype, cognitive impairment, and survival in very late life: impact of allostatic load in Swedish octogenarian and nonagenarian humans. J Gerontol A Biol Sci Med Sci. 2005;60:556–65.
17. Jakola DR, Pierson-Mullant LK, Daniels LR, Rosenberg AQ, Blumental R. Robustness into advanced age of atopy-specific mechanism in atopy-prone family. A Boil Sci Med Sci. 2003;58:99–107.
18. Ventura MT, Gelardi M, D'Amato A, Buquicchio R, Tummolo R, Misciagna G, Canonica GW, Passalacqua G. Clinical and cytologic characteristics of allergic rhinitis in elderly patients. Ann Allergy Asthma Immunol. 2012;108:41–4.
19. Hänel KH, Cornelissen C, Lüscher B, Baron JM. Cytokines and the skin barrier. Int J Mol Sci. 2013;14:6720–45.
20. Bunyavanich S, Rifas-Shiman SL, Platts-Mills TA, Workman L, Sordillo JE, Camargo CA Jr, Gillman MW, Gold DR, Litonjua AA. Peanut, milk, and wheat intake during pregnancy is associated with reduced allergy and asthma in children. J Allergy Clin Immunol. 2014;133:1373–82.
21. Blaeser A, McGlauchlen K, Vogel LA. Aged B lymphocytes retain their ability to express surface markers but are dysfunctional in their proliferative capability during early activation events. Immun Ageing. 2008;5:15.
22. Gomez CR, Boehmer ED, Kovacs EJ. The aging innate immune system. Curr Opin Immunol. 2005;17:457–62.
23. Borrego F, Alonso MC, Galiani MD, Carracedo J, Ramirez R, Ostos B, Peña J, Solana R. NK phenotypic markers and IL2 response in NK cells from elderly people. Exp Gerontol. 1999;34:253–65.
24. Maggi E. T cell response induced by allergen specific therapy. Clin Exp Immunol. 2010;161:10–8.
25. Chambers ES, Hawrylowicz CM. The impact of vitamin D on regulatory T cells. Curr Allergy Asthma Rep. 2011;11:29–36.
26. Yáñez A, Cho SH, Soriano JB, et al. Asthma in the elderly: what we know and what we have yet to know. World Allergy Organ J. 2014;7:8.
27. Demoly P, Calderon MA, Casale TB, Malling HJ, Wahn U. The value of pre- and co-seasonal sublingual immunotherapy in pollen-induced allergic rhinoconjunctivitis. Clin Transl Allergy. 2015;4(5):18.

28. Zuberbier T, Bachert C, Bousquet PJ, Passalacqua G, Walter Canonica G, Merk H, Worm M, Wahn U, Bousquet J. GA2LEN/EAACI pocket guide for allergen-specific immunotherapy for allergic rhinitis and asthma. Allergy. 2010;65:1525–30.
29. Passalacqua G, Canonica GWC. Allergen immunotherapy: history and future developments. Immunol Allergy Clin North Am. 2016;36(1):1–12.
30. Pitsios C, Demoly P, Bilò MB, et al. Clinical contraindications to allergen immunotherapy: an EAACI position paper. Allergy. 2015;70:897–909.
31. Linneberg A, Jacobsen RK, Jespersen L, Abildstrøm SZ. Association of subcutaneous allergen-specific immunotherapy with incidence of autoimmune disease, ischemic heart disease, and mortality. J Allergy Clin Immunol. 2012;129(2):413–9.
32. Calabria CW, Hauswirth DW, Rank M, Sher L, Larenas-Linnemann D. American Academy of Asthma, Allergy & Immunology membership experience with venom immunotherapy in chronic medical conditions and pregnancy, and in young children. Allergy Asthma Proc. 2017;38(2):121–9.
33. Larenas-Linnemann DE, Hauswirth DW, Calabria CW, Sher LD, Rank MA. American Academy of Allergy, Asthma & Immunology membership experience with allergen immunotherapy safety in patients with specific medical conditions. Allergy Asthma Proc. 2016;37(5):112–22.
34. Ridolo E, Montagni M, Bonzano L, Senna G, Incorvaia C. Arguing the misconceptions in allergen-specific immunotherapy. Immunotherapy. 2014;6(5):587–95.
35. Wöhrl S, Kinaciyan T, Jalili A, Stingl G, Moritz KB. Malignancy and specific allergen immunotherapy: the results of a case series. Int Arch Allergy Immunol. 2011;156(3):313–9.
36. Scichilone N, Ventura MT, Bonini M, et al. Choosing wisely: practical considerations on treatment efficacy and safety of asthma in the elderly. Clin Mol Allergy. 2015;13:7.
37. Nassiri M, Babina M, Dölle S, et al. Ramipril and metoprolol intake aggravate human and murine anaphylaxis: evidence for direct mast cell priming. J. Allergy Clin Immunol. 2015;135(2):491–9.
38. Livingston MG, Livingston HM. Monoamine oxidase inhibitors. An update on drug interactions. Drug Saf. 1996;14:219–22.
39. Bernabei R, Gray L, Hirdes J, et al. International gerontology. In: Halter JB, Ouslander JG, Tinetti ME, Studenski S, High KP, Asthana S, editors. Hazzard's geriatric medicine and gerontology. New York City: McGraw-Hill; 2009. p. 69–96.
40. Armentia A, Fernández A, Tapias JA, et al. Immunotherapy with allergenic extracts in geriatric patients: evaluation of effectiveness and safety. Allergol Immunopathol (Madr). 1993;21(5):193–6.
41. Eidelman F, Darxentas N. Efficacy of allergy immunotherapy in the elderly. J Allergy Clin Immunol. 2000;105:s313.
42. Asero R. Efficacy of injection immunotherapy with ragweed and birch pollen in elderly patients. Int Arch Allergy Immunol. 2004;135(4):332–5.
43. Canonica GW, Cox L, Pawankar R, et al. Sublingual immunotherapy: World Allergy Organization position paper 2013 update. World Allergy Organ J. 2014;7:6.
44. Marogna M, Bruno ME, Massolo A, Falagiani P. Sublingual immunotherapy for allergic respiratory disease in elderly patients: a retrospective study. Eur Ann Allergy Clin Immunol. 2008;40:22–9.
45. Baptistella E, Maniglia S, Malucelli DA, et al. Allergen-specific immunotherapy in patients 55 years and older: results and review of literature. Int Arch Otorhinolaryngol. 2013;17:375–9.
46. Bozek A, Ignasiak B, Filipowska B, Jarzab J. House dust mite sublingual immunotherapy: a double-blind, placebocontrolled study in elderly patients with allergic rhinitis. Clin Exp Allergy. 2013;43(2):242–8.
47. Bozek A, Kolodziejczyk K, Warkocka-Szoltysek B, Jarzab J. Grass pollen sublingual immunotherapy: a double-blind, placebo-controlled study in elderly patients with seasonal allergic rhinitis. J Am J Rhinol Allergy. 2014;28(5):423–7.
48. Bozek A, Kolodziejczyk K, Krajewska-Wojtys A, Jarbaz J. Pre-seasonal, subcutaneous immunotherapy: a double-blinded, placebo-controlled study in elderly patients with an allergy to grass. Ann Allergy Asthma Immunol. 2016;116(2):156–61.
49. Ridolo E, Caminati M, Martignago I, et al. Allergic rhinitis: pharmacotherapy in pregnancy and old age. Expert Rev Clin Pharmacol. 2016;9(8):1081–9.
50. Ventura MT, Gelardi M, D'Amato A, Buquicchio R, Tummolo R, Misciagna G, et al. Clinical and cytologic characteristics of allergic rhinitis in elderly patients. Ann Allergy Asthma Immunol. 2012;108:141–4.

13

Eosinophilic disorders of the gastro-intestinal tract

Erminia Ridolo*, Valerie Melli, Gianluigi De' Angelis and Irene Martignago

Abstract

Eosinophilic diseases of the gastrointestinal tract, including eosinophilic esophagitis (EoE) and eosinophilic gastroenteritis (EGE), are rare chronic pathologies of the digestive system, with an immuno-mediated pathogenesis. Recent data suggest that, together with the "classic" IgE-response to allergens, also a delayed hypersensitivity mechanism could be involved in the development of eosinophilic disorders. EoE and EGE were studied only in the latest decades and as a consequence accurate data are not yet available, concerning not only pathogenesis, but also epidemiology, treatment and outcomes. The diagnosis of EoE is centered on endoscopic findings but the certainty is obtained by histological examination from biopsy samples, that has a sensitivity of 100% when based on five samples. The currently available treatments include topical corticosteroids, specific diets and endoscopic treatment. Concerning EGE, three subtypes (mucosal, muscular, and serosal) were identified. The diagnosis is based, as for EoE, on endoscopic and histological assessment, and the treatment includes pharmacological and dietetic approaches. Further studies are warranted in order to better define the etiology and pathogenesis of eosinophilic diseases of the gastrointestinal tract, and thus to develop more appropriate and specific therapies.

Keywords: Eosinophilic esophagitis, Eosinophilic gastroenteritis, Pathogenesis, Diagnosis, Therapy

Background

Primitive eosinophilic esophagitis (EoE) and eosinophilic gastroenteritis are part of a group of diseases first described in 1937 by Kaijser and called EGIDs (eosinophilic gastrointestinal diseases) [1]. These clinical entities are characterized by selective infiltration of gastrointestinal tract by eosinophils, in absence of other causes of known eosinophilia.

Interest in EGIDs dates back to the latest decades and, also due to the rarity of these disorders, the data about epidemiology, pathogenesis, therapy and outcomes thus far available are partial. There is an urgent need to better characterize EGIDs, to understand the etiology and to define a more precise therapeutic approach. In fact, current treatments are yet controversial and there is no consensus on how long the diet and/or steroid therapy should be maintained.

*Correspondence: erminia.ridolo@unipr.it
Department of Clinical and Experimental Medicine, University of Parma, via Gramsci, 14, 43100 Parma, Italy

Eosinophilic esophagitis

EoE is a chronic inflammatory disease of the esophagus with an immuno-allergic pathogenesis, characterized by eosinophilic infiltration ($\geq$15 Eo/high power field [HPF]) and secondary fibrosis [1]. EoE was once considered a rare clinical entity and in fact it was relatively unknown until the '90s, while now it is of increasing interest.

In United States and Europe epidemiological studies found a prevalence of EoE of 50 patients per 100.000 inhabitants [2].

EoE can affect any age, from infancy to old age, but diagnosis is more frequent in third/fourth decades [3]. Male subjects are more frequently affected than females, with a rate of 3:1 [2, 3]. The reason for this gender difference is not yet explained, but a single nucleotide polymorphism (SNP) in the gene for thymic stromal lymphopoietin (TSLP), was identified on chromosome Xp22.3 and also on chromosome Yp11.3. These findings can be a possible explanation for the prevalence of EoE in males [4]. Caucasian ethnicity is more commonly interested in EoE, with a reported predominance of 90% in some case studies. However, the disease can affect also

African American, Asian, Native American and Hispanic populations [5].

Pathogenesis

EoE pathogenesis is complex with many factors involved, particularly genetic and environmental, and the precise mechanism is still unknown. Environmental factors seems to play a significant role in development of EoE: in fact, though the heritability rate is about 70%, concordance between monozygotic twins is only 30%, suggesting a powerful role for environmental factors (81.0%) [6]. An important epidemiological study, conducted in Cincinnati (US) evaluated 6108 individuals from 1366 families of patients with EoE: the recurrence risk ratio was found to be increased 10- to 64-fold compared with the general population, with an incidence of EoE in relatives from 1.8 to 2.4%, depending on relationship and sex [6].

In literature, an association between EoE and some hereditary collagen alterations, such as Marfan and Enhlers-Danlos syndromes, was reported [7]. More recently another associated disease was reported: three patients with EoE suffered from hypertrophic cardiomyopathy, leading the Authors to suggest a possible genetic alteration underling both diseases [8].

Several genetic alterations have been identified in patients with EoE. The most common involved gene is the one for eotaxin-3, a chemokine active on eosinophils, that plays a fundamental role in EoE. In fact, it is expressed in esophageal mucosa 53 times more than in healthy subjects. The alteration is represented by SNP in the 3′ untranslated region of eotaxin-3 gene [5, 9].

Another important mutation concerns the gene for TSLP, and its risk alleles, such as rs3806932, present on chromosome 5q22. TLSP is a cytokine produced by epithelial cells, whose action consists of inducing a Th2 cell-mediated response in dendritic cells [10–12]. Also a SNP for TLSP-receptor seems to be involved and its presence on chromosome Y could be a possible cause of male prevalence for EoE [11].

A recent study suggested a possible mechanism underling the role of TLSP for development of EoE. According to these results specific food antigens (hen's egg ovalbumin) can trigger TSLP secretion by differentiated epithelial cells in esophagus [13].

While eotaxin-3 and TLSP are responsible for epithelial dysregulation, also the barrier function is altered in EoE. In this case other two proteins are involved: filaggrin and desmoglein-1.

A SNP of the gene for filaggrin (2282del4) was analyzed in a cohort of 365 patients with EoE compared to 165 healthy subjects, showing a significantly association with the disease (OR = 5.0) [11]. The hyperplasia of esophageal epithelial cells observed in patients with EoE is secondary to decreased expression of genes that regulate epidermal differentiation. One of these lacking proteins is desmoglein 1 (DSG1), whose action is important to maintain an effective barrier in the esophagus [14]. Moreover, downregulation of DSG1 promotes upregulation of periostin, an extracellular matrix protein that is involved in fibrosis of the esophagus tissue [15].

The eosinophils' role is unquestionable, due to the production of potent pro-inflammatory mediators, such as cytokines, GM-CSF, TGF-β and TNF-α, Th2 lymphocytes and their cytokines (IL-5, IL-4, IL-13) that are main actors in coordinating adaptive immunity in the pathogenesis of EoE. IL-5 is the most important mediator for eosinophilic activation and recruitment. Its action is confirmed by a study demonstrating its overexpression in esophageal biopsies from pediatric patients with EoE [16]. IL-13 is produced primarily by Th2 cells and its activation leads to an increased generation of eotaxin-3. High concentrations of IL-13 were detected in esophageal biopsies [17]. IL-4 stimulates, together with IL-13, the production of eotaxin-3 [12].

Recently a genome-wide genetic association of EoE was identified at 2p23 spanning, the calpain 14 (CAPN14) gene. CAPN14 is a gene induced by IL-13 that encodes for calpain 14, a cysteine-protease, which is overexpressed in esophageal biopsies of patient with EoE [12, 18]. The role of calpain 14 is not clearly defined, but its overexpression results also in loss of desmoglein 1 [18].

IL-13 is responsible to increase the expression of other genes involved in EoE pathogenesis, such as BANCR (BRAF-activated non-coding RNA) and NTRK1 (Neurotropic Tyrosine Kinase Receptor type 1). RNA sequencing in esophageal biopsies identified an overexpression of lcnRNA BANCR, that is responsible for local hypereosinophilia. BANCR is also related to the increase of periostin production [19]. NTRK1 is an early transcription target of IL-13 and its expression is higher in esophageal tissue of patients with EoE than in healthy subjects. Its increased concentration determines an augmented response to its ligand NGF (Neurotropic Tyrosine Kinase) that has a primary role in hyperplasia [20]. IL-13 is also responsible of inducing production of chemokines CCL11, CCL24 AND CCL26 from eotaxins [5]. Other genetic variants in the cluster of IL-5 and IL-13 regions have been identified, but their role is not clearly defined [12]. New actors of EoE pathogenesis were recently identified: mast cells and invariant natural killer T (iNKT).

Mast cells seem to contribute to EoE releasing prostaglandin D2 that is able to recruit eosinophils in esophagus [21]. In fact, in animal models of EoE, mast cells are increased in number after allergen stimulation, proportionally with time and dose of the stimulus [22].

iNKT are a subpopulation of T cells, whose concentration in esophageal biopsies of patients with EoE is increased compared to healthy subjects. These cells are able to recognize the glycolipid antigen and this may explain their role in development of EoE: iNKT cell-deficient CD1d-null mice were protected from food allergen-induced EoE, while in the same animals iNKT activation is sufficient to induce EoE. In fact, their activation induces the release of inflammatory cytokines, including IL-4, IL-5 and IL-13 [23]. Moreover, a recent study suggests that sphingolipids of milk may stimulate iNKT cells to produce these cytokines [24].

Another mediator released by eosinophils and implicated in EoE pathogenesis is TGF-β1. It mediates the epithelial cell proliferation and extracellular remodeling, through the upregulation of genes involved in fibrosis, i.e. matrix metalloproteinase 2 [12]. Also leukotriene C4 may contribute to worsen fibrosis through its metabolites LTD4 and LTE, that are able to stimulate smooth cells contraction [5].

The pathogenetic role of atopy was confirmed by experimental and epidemiological studies. EoE is associated with a condition of atopy in 75% of patients [5]. Sensitization regards inhalant and/or food allergens (in adults 86–93% towards inhalants and 50–82% towards food allergens). Sensitization is associated with allergic clinical presentations in 68% of adult patients: the most frequent symptoms are respiratory (allergic rhinitis 60% approximately, allergic asthma 39%) [25, 26]. In pediatric patients a family history of atopy was present in 73.5% [26]. The important effect of food allergy in patients affected by EoE is demonstrated indirectly by the improvement of symptoms after elimination of allergenic food from diet, as we will discuss below. In addition, development of EoE was described as a complication of oral tolerance induction for food allergens. Ridolo et al. reported how EoE occurred in a 10 year-old child after acquiring tolerance for egg with an oral protocol of induction. The patient presented dyspepsia and dysphagia 5 months after egg reintroduction in diet, with an endoscopic and histological demonstration of EoE. Symptoms disappeared persistently after elimination of egg from the diet [27]. Other cases were described after administration of oral specific immunotherapy for milk, egg or peanuts [28, 29]. Notably, only a small part of EoE patients with food IgE- sensitization presents with anaphylaxis. The protection mechanism underlying this aspect is not yet well defined, but a recent study highlighted the conceivable role of IgG4 in the development of EoE. In fact, an increase in production of IgG4 can be detected in lamina propria of esophagus in biopsies of patients with EoE [30]. This hypothesis was formulated after finding that omalizumab did not reduce nor symptoms of EoE neither tissue eosinophilia compared to placebo in a prospective trial. Moreover the Authors observed granular deposits of IgG4, plasma cells containing IgG4 and serum levels of IgG4 reactive to specific foods and suggested that EoE could be an IgG4-associated pathology [30]. Further studies are warranted to confirm these findings.

Regarding the role of inhalant allergens in development of EoE, the data in favor of their involvement are certain. In a study of Yamazaki et al. mononuclear cells from 25 patients with EoE were incubated with inhalant allergens (dust mites, *Aspergillus fumigatus*, *Alternaria alternata*, and ragweed pollen): significantly higher levels of IL-5 and IL-13 were detected in response to the allergens, compared than healthy controls, even in the absence of an evident IgE-mediated sensitization [31]. Another study on animal models demonstrated that intranasal exposure to inhalant allergen (*A. fumigatus*) in sensitized mice induced esophagus eosinophilia, eosinophilic degranulation and epithelial hyperplasia [32].

Furthermore, a study performed in patients with seasonal respiratory allergy established a correlation between esophageal eosinophilic infiltration and seasonal symptoms [33]. In fact a seasonal distribution of new diagnoses of EoE was demonstrated: a 1-year study highlighted that in 41 adults patients, a new EoE diagnosis was more frequent in spring months (44%, 18 of 41 patients) [10], while a 6-years-long retrospective analysis of a pediatric population confirmed that new diagnosis were significantly less frequent in winter than in other seasons [11]. A retrospective Australian study reported a higher recurrence of esophageal food bolus during the pollen season in patients with EoE [12].

Moreover patients with EoE presents an high prevalence of sensitizations to pan-allergens, responsible for cross-reactivity among inhalant and food allergens. In particularly, sensitization to PR-10, the birch allergen Bet v 1, seems to be very frequent: in a study of Van Rhijn 39% of patients presents sensitization to this molecule [34]. In a recent study the association between bolus as first symptom of EoE, more severe eosinophilic infiltration and sensitization to PR-10 has been established [35].

Of note, there are differences in the sensitization patterns among children and adult population affected by EoE, with a progressive increase in inhalant allergy with age and a parallel diminution in food sensitization. These differences, although not specific for EoE, are correlated with patient age and have important therapeutic implications, suggesting a predominant role of food allergens in children.

Clinical presentation

As mentioned above, EoE can affect any age, but clinical presentation differs between children and adult patients [26]. In adults the most common symptoms are dysphagia, food bolus, thoracic and epigastric pain, the onset being similar to a PPI (Pomp Proton Inhibitors)—not responding GERD [26]. In pediatric patients the most common manifestations are food refusal and growth retardation in infants, and vomit, nausea and abdominal pain in older children [4]. It is important to ascertain also the presence of coping mechanism that patients can apply during swallow in order to overcome symptoms [36].

Endoscopic findings

The possible macroscopic findings during gastroscopy are: mucosa edema, white exudates, longitudinal grooves, concentric rings ("trachealization" of the esophagus), and stenosis. In about 20% of cases esophagus may, however, appear macroscopically normal. A meta-analysis including 4678 patients with EoE and 2742 controls, estimated the following frequency of the endoscopic features: trachealization in 44%, linear grooves in 48%, white exudates in 27%, stenosis in 21% and reduction in caliber 9% [37]. None of these endoscopic features is pathognomonic of EoE: sensitivity is low, varying between 15% for stenosis and 48% for esophagus rings, while the specificity ranged between 90% for pale mucosa and 95% for stenosis [37] (Fig. 1).

Histology

Esophagus is the only gastrointestinal organ that does not present eosinophils in normal condition. The number of eosinophil present in mucosa increases progressively from stomach to cecum [38]. Even if finding eosinophils in esophagus is a pathologic sign, it is not pathognomonic of EoE. In fact, other clinical entities, such as gastroesophageal reflux disease (GERD), eosinophilic gastroenteritis, parasitosis, celiac disease, Crohn disease, drugs hypersensitivity, vasculitis, idiopathic hypereosinophilic syndrome, Graft vs Host disease, and scleroderma, can present eosinophilic infiltration in esophagus [39].

First of all, it is necessary to perform histology only after at least 8 weeks of therapy with PPI to make diagnosis of EoE. Then biopsy must present ≥15 eosinophils/HPF in at least one sample. Other characteristic findings are microabscesses, elongation of the papillae, hyperplasia of the basal layer, detachment of the surface layers, degranulation of eosinophils, increased number of mast cells and lymphocytes [40] (Figs. 2, 3).

Diagnosis

The symptoms mentioned above are not pathognomonic of EoE. Also sensibility, specificity and predictive value of the endoscopic features are insufficient to make a certain diagnosis [41]. Biopsy of esophagus is always necessary, even when the macroscopic appearance is normal. A study conducted on 66 adults patients confirmed that sensibility of histological examination was 100% when based on the analysis of five samples, while it was only 55% if even a single sample was withdrawn [42]. These data were validated also in pediatric population, in which sensibility was 73, 84, 95 and 100% for 1, 2, 3 and 6 biopsies, respectively [43]. Thanks to studies like these, also guidelines recommend to perform multiple biopsies in proximal, medium and distal esophagus [5]. It is also strongly suggested to perform biopsies also in stomach and duodenum in order to exclude eosinophilic gastroenteritis. At least 15 or more eosinophils/HPF must be found in case of EoE. As mentioned above, eosinophils are not present in esophagus in normal condition, but this finding is possible also in other pathologies. In particular two pathologies can present isolated eosinophilic esophagitis: GERD and PPI-responsive eosinophilic esophagitis. In order to distinguish them from EoE, a further biopsy after an 8-week-long therapy

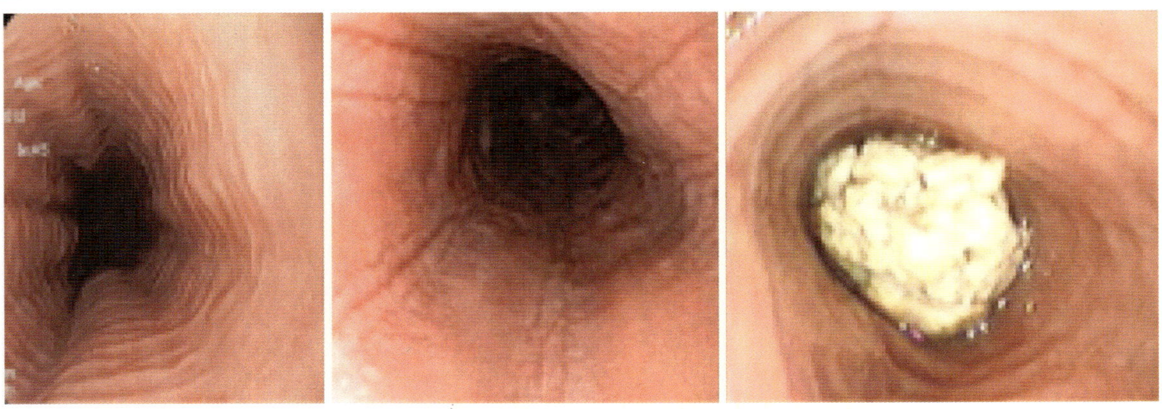

Fig. 1 EoE

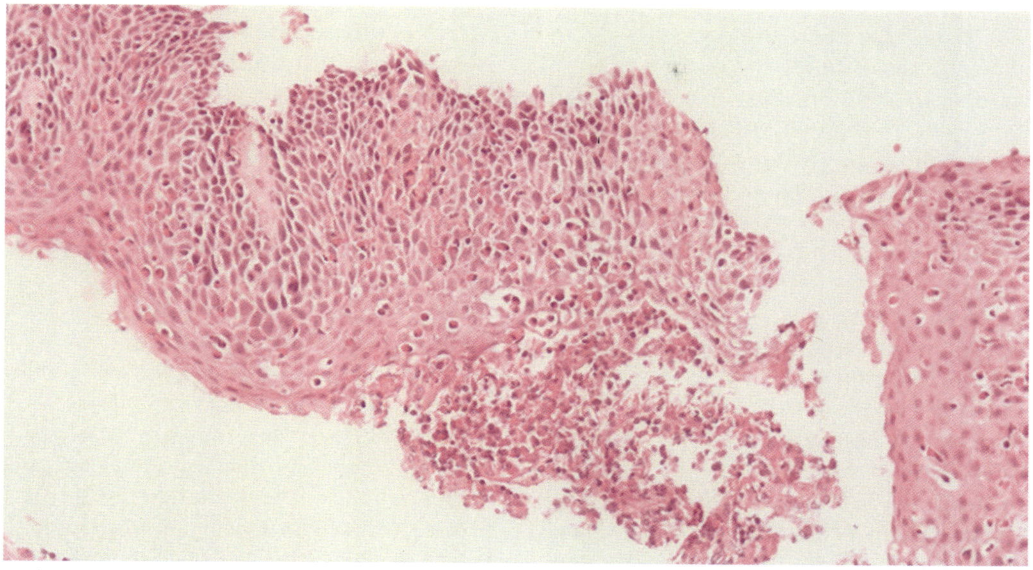

Fig. 2 Hematoxylin-eosin, 20× magnification: Frustule of esophageal mucosa with diffuse infiltration of eosinophils (Eo > 20/HPF), microabscesses, disruption of the epithelial barrier

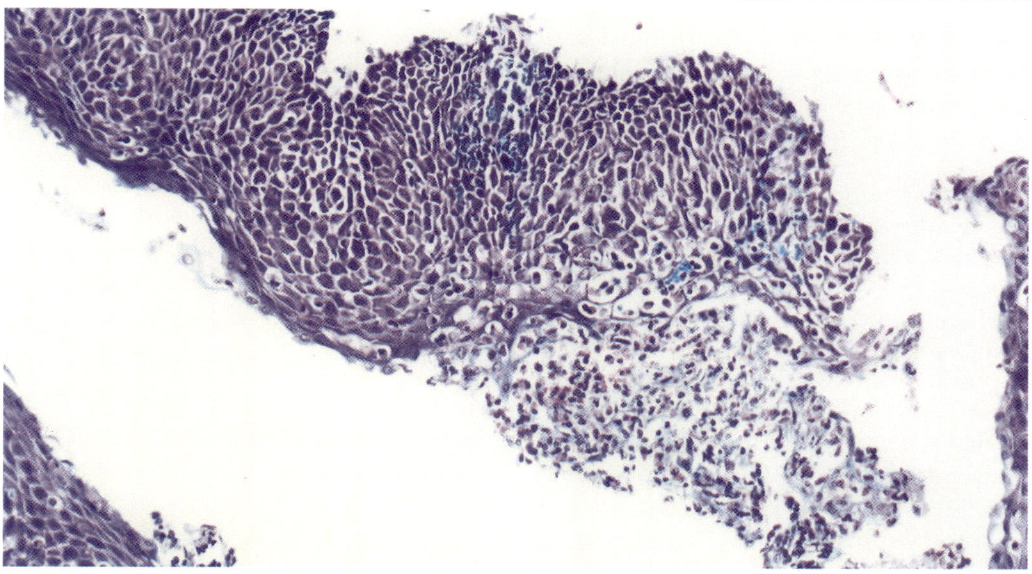

Fig. 3 Same sample of Fig. 2 in Giemsa, 20× magnification: diffuse eosinophilic infiltration with microabscesses, it can be appreciate also the intercellular edema and the acantholysis resulting from the eosinophils' degranulation

with PPI must be done. In case of absence of clinical and histological response, it is possible to set a diagnosis of EoE [40].

It is unclear whether the esophageal eosinophilia responsive to PPI is a variant of gastroesophageal reflux or a variant of EoE. A small series of four pediatric patients (mean age 9.5 years) with esophageal eosinophilia (mean 52 eosinophils/HPF), initially responsive to PPI, showed an evolution towards primitive EoE [44]. The reason of the initial response to PPI is unclear, though a possible anti-inflammatory activity, and for omeprazole also the capacity to block in vitro the secretion of eotaxin-3 from esophageal cells, should be involved [45].

Therapy

Treatment of EoE includes pharmacologic, dietetic and endoscopic therapy. The appropriate therapy must be evaluated according to symptoms and time of response with a step-up/step down process. Dietetic and pharmacologic treatments are often required for long periods as EoE is a chronic disease. No fixed timing is standardized and the duration must be customized to each single patient and his/her response.

Pharmacologic therapy

An 8-weeks-long therapy with PPIs is necessary to rule out GERD or eosinophilic esophagitis responsive to PPI, before an EoE diagnosis can be made.

First line therapy for EoE is represented by topical glucosteroids. A great part of patients presents both clinical and histological improvement with this treatment [46]. Topical treatment has an anti-inflammatory action thanks to ability in inducing some anti-inflammatory genes, such as FK-506 binding protein and miRs, and in reversing the eosinophilic transcriptome [5].

The molecules more frequently prescribed for EoE are budesonide and fluticasone. Industry does not provide specific formulation for EoE and then available devices for asthma must be prescribed to patients. Therefore, clinicians must educate subjects to swallow and not to inhale corticosteroids in order to have a topic action on esophagus.

Doses of fluticasone usually vary between 88 and 440 mcg/die in children and between 880 and 1760 mcg/die in adults, while budesonide is 1 mg in children and 2 mg/die in adults [1]. Only 1% of these swallowed steroids is absorbed and consequently systemic side effects are very rare. The most common unwanted effect is oral and esophageal candidosis, that can be prevented educating patients to rinse their mouth after therapy [47].

Occasionally, discrepancy between histological response and clinical improvement can be found. In fact, some patients continue to present symptoms even if endoscopic test is negative. This is probably secondary to the pre-existing fibrosis and muscle hypertrophy [5]. Pediatric patients are indeed more responsive to topical steroids because adults have already a significant remodeling of esophagus before diagnosis and treatment are performed [48].

Systemic steroids are also very effective to improve symptoms, but their use must be limited to the most severe cases (i.e. important weight loss secondary to dysphagia and/or esophagus stenosis). The recommended dose is 1–2 mg/kg (max 60 mg/24 h) for 7–15 days [44]. Recurrence of EoE is more frequent after withdrawal of systemic steroids [47].

Among the other drugs that were evaluated there are biological drugs such as monoclonal antibodies directed towards IL-5, IL-13, CRTH2 and IgE, immunomodulators and leukotriene inhibitors. Immunomodulators, such as azathioprine and 6-mercaptopurine were used in three patients with corticosteroid-dependence obtaining long-term remission of EoE, but their use is not currently recommended [49]. In contrast, montelukast improves clinical symptoms, but is not able to gain histological improvement [50].

Omalizumab, an antibody against IgE, failed in gaining both symptoms control and eosinophilic infiltration in esophageal biopsies [30]. Antibodies against IL-5 (mepolizumab and reslizumab) were selected to treat EoE patients due the fundamental role of this cytokine in development and activation of eosinophils, but only a limited number of patients have an acceptable response to them. Mepolizumab was administered to 11 adults [51] and to 45 children [52] in two different trials, obtaining decrease of eosinophilic infiltration, but not a significant improvement in clinical manifestations. A double-blind placebo controlled study on the use of reslizumab was performed on 226 children and adolescents, but the difference in improvements between treated and placebo groups was not statistically significant [53]. A recent trial studied the effectiveness of QAX576, anti-IL-13 antibody, in 23 adult patients, demonstrating a significantly decrease of intraepithelial esophageal eosinophilia and of the expression of EoE-relevant esophageal transcripts, such as eotaxin-3, inducing a sustained clinical improvement [12, 54].

Dietetic therapy

Dietetic therapy of EoE can be effective and it is usually prescribed initially together with pharmacologic treatment, even though it is often recommended after drugs discontinuation.

Three different treatments have been used during the last decades:

1. Elemental diet, during which patients are fed only with elemental amino-acid based formula;
2. IgE targeted diet, during which patients must eliminate only food to which they are sensitized.
3. SFED (Six Food Elimination Diet), in which patients must exclude the six more probable food allergens: milk and dairy products, egg, soy, tree nut/peanut, sea food (fish/shellfish);

The first type of diet seems to be very effective to induce clinical an histological remission, if given for at least 6 weeks [47]. In 1995 Kelly et al. was the first to demonstrate that a diet based almost exclusively on amino acids (only exceptions were corn, apple and clear liquids) was successful in obtaining a complete resolution of clinical manifestations in 8 of 10 children with EoE. The remaining two still achieved a significant clinical improvement, and children presented a complete histological remission [55]. Peterson et al. confirmed these data in an adult population of 18 patients: 13 obtained a full histological response and 4 presented a reduction of 50% of the eosinophilia in esophagus [56].

A recent meta-analysis confirmed the efficiency of the elemental diet in achieving histologic remission in both children and adults in about 90% of the cases [57]. The most important limitation of this diet is its strong impact on the quality of life. In fact, patients are required to drink great amount of liquid, unpalatable and very expensive formulas [5, 47].

The second dietetic approach is based on elimination of foods to which the patient is sensitized. A great variability in remission rates has been highlighted in a meta-analysis, so that the Authors stated that these data are likely to support the involvement of a cell-mediated delayed hypersensitivity reaction, instead of an IgE-mediated mechanism underlying EoE pathogenesis [57].

In another study, the foods that clinically caused symptoms to patients were compared to sensitizations identified towards food with skin prick test (SPT). In these patients SPT were able to identify the actual trigger food only in 13% of cases [58]. Anyway, a target diet with elimination of foods inducing positive results to SPT and atopy patch test was effective in 26 children with EoE. The foods most frequently positive to SPTs are milk, egg, peanuts, seafood, peas, rye, tomato and wheat, while the most common positivity to atopy patch tests were wheat, corn, beef, milk, soy, rye, chicken, oats and potato [58]. In adults, the effectiveness of this type of diet is not yet clearly demonstrated.

The third dietetic approach is SFED diet. In 2006 Kagalwalla proposed the empiric use of SFED, starting from foods most frequently involved in children allergy [59]. The efficacy of SFED was about 70% according to a meta-analysis. Such analysis documented that the most commonly causative foods involved in relapsing of symptoms after their reintroduction were cow's milk, wheat, eggs, and soy/legumes [57].

Endoscopic treatment

In case of severe stenosis (diameter < 10 mm), in patients not responsive to pharmacological and/or dietetic therapy, endoscopic dilatation leads to a rapid improvements of clinical manifestations. In some cases this remission can last several months, but multiple sessions are needed to achieve an optimal dilatation. At least an esophageal diameter of 15–18 mm must be reached to obtain symptoms relief. The risk of perforation after dilatation is low, about 0, 1%. Obviously this treatment does not have any effect on pathogenetic and inflammatory process [47].

Natural history

Knowledge on long-term prognosis of EoE is actually limited. Available data unfortunately indicate a progressive trend towards esophageal fibrosis/stenosis.

A retrospective study in 200 patients highlighted that diagnosis' delay is associated with a higher prevalence of fibrostenotic form (from 46.5% for diagnostic delay between 0 and 2 years to 87.5% for diagnostic delay >20 years) and is the only factor associated with an increased risk of stenosis [60]. These results were also confirmed by another recent retrospective analysis: Dellon et al. indicated that for every age increase of 10 years the risk of having a fibrostenotic form doubled [61]. Spergel et al. followed 620 pediatric patients for over 14 years, showing that EoE persisted in the vast majority of cases. Fortunately there was not even a case of progression to any other gastrointestinal disease [62]. In literature there are no reported cases of progression to neoplastic diseases. Actually we can state that, when the diagnosis is made during childhood, EoE seems to persist throughout adult life, but follow-up studies in the long term are not yet available.

Eosinophilic gastroenteritis

Eosinophilic Gastroenteritis (EGE) is a rare and idiopathic group of diseases characterized by eosinophilia in one or more tracts of gastrointestinal system. If eosinophilia is limited to stomach, it is defined as eosinophilic gastritis; if it is limited to colon, it is called eosinophilic colitis. Clinical manifestations are different and never specific of this spectrum of disease, also according to the interested tract [46].

The precise incidence is unknown, due to EGE rarity, but it is rising in the latest years, probably because of a better recognition and an increasing interest [63]. Nowadays, incidence is estimated about 1–30/100.000, but it is probably underestimated [46].

Adults seem to be more affected by EGE then children, with a maximum incidence in the fourth–fifth decades. Male are slightly more interested than woman (3:2), with the exception of serosal subtype. Even in this case, EGE is more common in Caucasians [46, 64].

About 70% of patients suffering from EGE present a personal or familiar history of atopy. The most common allergies presented by these patients are food sensitizations [65].

Pathogenesis

EGE etiology and pathogenesis are not clearly defined. Delayed type hypersensitivity to food is the most probable underlying mechanism, according to the current data. In these patients hypereosinophilia found in peripheral blood and in gastrointestinal tissue, increased serum levels of IgE, presence of elevated mediators produced by eosinophils in intestinal biopsies and response to steroids therapy are supporting this pathogenetic hypothesis [46].

Classification and clinical manifestations

Anatomic localization of eosinophilic inflammation influences clinical manifestations, that can vary from nausea to intestinal obstruction. As a consequence, EGE is classified according to the most infiltrated layer of the intestinal wall in [66]:

1. *Mucosal* the most common subtype. Patients have non-specific symptoms, such as nausea, vomiting, diarrhea, anemia due to chronic inflammation or iron deficiency, clinical manifestations secondary to malabsorption. In particular, in children weight loss and protein losing enteropathy are the most common manifestations [40, 63].
2. *Muscular* the second form for frequency. The interest of this layer often leads to intestinal obstruction secondary to the thickening of intestinal wall [67]. The most common is jejunal obstruction [38]. Colo-colonic intussusceptions are rare [68].
3. *Serosal* the most uncommon subtype, even though is the most frequent in females [40]. Clinical presentation begins usually with ascites, sometimes associated with symptoms of intestinal obstruction. Ascites is characterized by marked eosinophilia in ascitic fluid. Serosal subtype differs also for its consistent response to corticosteroids therapy [40, 63].

EGE subtypes, correlate with prognosis. Serosal pattern in fact does not present a continuous chronic course, but mostly single episodic flares up, with long disease-free periods. Instead, mucosal subtype is characterized by a persistent presence of symptoms and muscular pattern presents frequent relapses [69].

It must be noted anyway that it is difficult in everyday practice to distinguish which is the most involved layer for two reasons: overlap among 2 or 3 subtypes is very common and often only mucosal and submucosal biopsies are taken [69].

Endoscopic and histological aspects

Often, endoscopic aspects, either for stomach and for colon, can be normal or demonstrate non-specific aspects of chronic inflammation [70]. Mucosal erythema, friability, ulcerated mucosa, mucosal nodules or whitish specks can be also found [63] (Figs. 4, 5).

Diagnosis must be based on the finding of eosinophilic infiltration of mucosa. There is not a universally accepted threshold of eosinophils/HPF, in fact they are present in normal conditions in gastroenteric tract (only exclusion is esophagus). The most accepted definition is a count that exceeds 20 Eo/HPF [63, 70] in at least one sample. Besides eosinophils, a higher concentration of theirs mediator can be found in biopsies, in particularly metalloproteinases and eosinophilic cationic protease, IL-3, IL-5 and GMCSF [40, 63].

Since distribution of eosinophilic infiltration is not linear and can be present even in areas macroscopically normal, multiple biopsies are necessary [63].

Diagnosis

Establishing a diagnosis of EGE is not easy: in fact, single laboratory tests or procedures that allow to identify this disease are lacking. Certainly, patients must present chronic or recurrent gastrointestinal symptoms, with documented eosinophilic infiltration of one or more gastrointestinal areas. Then, other causes of gastrointestinal eosinophilia and eosinophilic infiltration in other organs must be excluded.

If EGE is suspected, a blood sample must be collected. In fact, up to 80% of these patients presents peripheral eosinophilia. It appears to be more severe in patients affected by serosal subtype of EGE [71]. Anyway, it does not correlate with the activity of disease and it must not be used for follow up during or after therapy [72].

Moreover, before setting the diagnosis, it must be included [63]:

- Endoscopic and histological evaluations, that must present the characteristic mentioned above.
- Exclusion of other causes of gastrointestinal eosinophilia, such as hypereosinophilic syndrome, eosinophilic granulomatosis with polyangiitis (EGPA), celiac disease, inflammatory bowel disease, polyarteritis nodosa, other connective tissue disorders, infections, and drug hypersensitivity, through the use of careful collected history, laboratory testing and histological examination.

Once diagnosis of EGE is established, allergy evaluation must be carried out. In fact, up to 70% of patients with EGE can present a personal or family history of atopy, especially food allergy is very common [73]. Food allergies may be a trigger of clinical manifestations and/or pathogenesis of EGE. Atopy's role is not yet well defined, also because EGE seems to be determined by both an IgE mediated mechanism and IgE-mediated- Th2 delayed

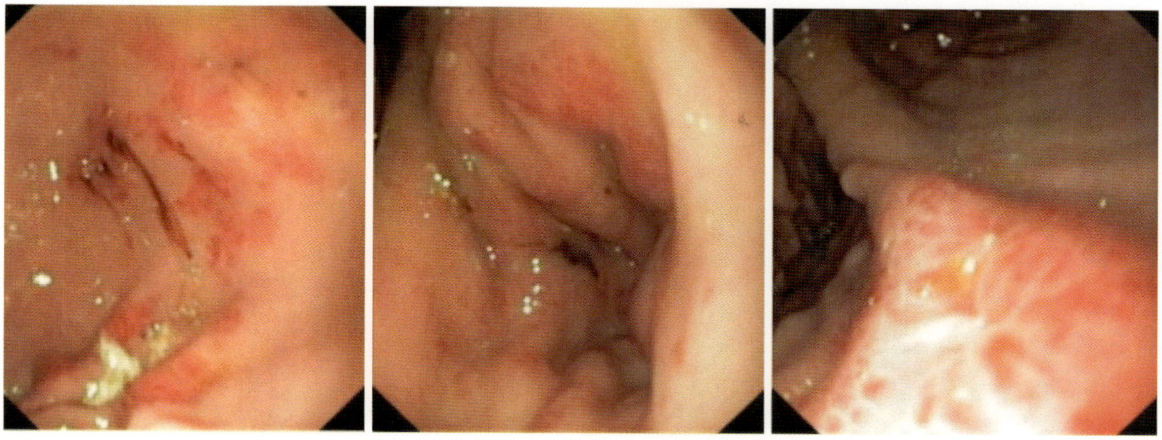

Fig. 4 Eosinophilic gastroduodenitis, bulb mucosa

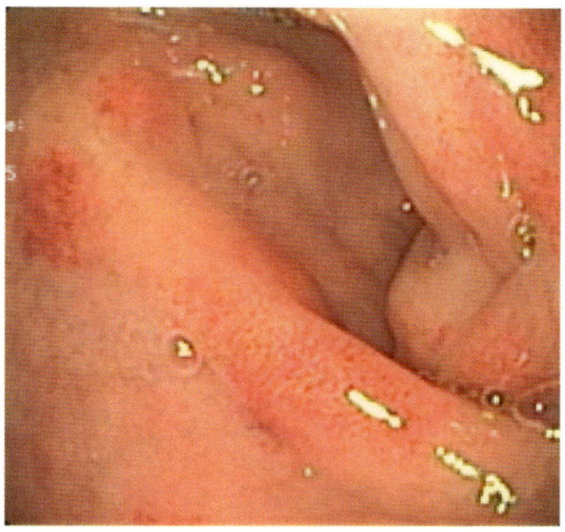

Fig. 5 Eosinophilic colitis

hypersensitivity process. Anyway, allergen-specific in vitro or in vivo tests are indicated in these patients, because, if positive, elimination of causative foods is effective on symptoms [74].

Therapy

Treatment of EGE includes dietetic and pharmacological approach. Surgery or other kind of therapy (i.e. paracentesis) may be needed in case of complications.

Dietetic therapy

Following the benefits obtained in patients with EoE, a dietetic approach was tested also in EGE subjects. Nowadays, data about efficacy of dietetic treatment are based on case reports or on small series of patients. Chehade demonstrated the effectiveness of elemental diet in six pediatric patients [75], while SFED diet was tested in one child with benefit [76]. Data available about IgE-targeted diet are discordant [63].

Pharmacological therapy

Corticosteroids therapy represents the main therapy for EGE and is effective in about 80% of patients [38]. There are not randomized trials for EGE therapy. In literature the most common first approach is systemic corticosteroid therapy with 20–40 mg/daily of prednisone for 2–6 weeks. In some cases this treatment was then continued with topic budesonide with benefit [77–79].

Other therapeutic approaches (mast cell stabilizers, omalizumab, mepolizumab, reslizumab, infliximab, leukotriene inhibitors, antihistaminic drugs, Th-2 inhibitors, such as suplatast and CRTH2) have been investigated, but their efficacy is not yet well defined, even because of the small number of patients involved.

Abbreviations

BANCR: BRAF-activated non-coding RNA; CAPN14: calpain 14; DSG1: desmoglein 1; EoE: eosinophilic esophagitis; EGE: eosinophilic gastroenteritis; EGIDs: eosinophilic gastrointestinal diseases; EGPA: eosinophilic granulomatosis with polyangiitis; GERD: gastroesophageal reflux disease; GM-CSF: granulocyte-macrophage colony-stimulating factor; HPF: high power field; iNKT: invariant natural killer T; NGF: neurotropic tyrosine kinase; NTRK1: neurotropic tyrosine kinase receptor type 1; PPI: proton pump inhibitor; SFED: six food elimination diet; SNP: single nucleotide polymorphism; SPT: skin prick test; TGF- β: transforming growth factor-beta; TNF-α: tumor necrosis factor alpha; TSLP: thymic stromal lymphopoietin.

Authors' contributions

ER conceived the study, contributed to the writing and coordinated the draft of the manuscript. IM, VM, contributed to the draft of the manuscript and to the revision of the article. All authors read and approved the final manuscript.

References

1. Liacouras CA, Furuta GT, Hirano I, et al. Eosinophilic esophagitis: updated consensus recommendations for children and adults. J Allergy Clin Immunol. 2011;128:3–20.

2. Hruz P. Epidemiology of eosinophilic esophagitis. Dig Dis. 2014;32:40–7.
3. van Rhijn BD, Verheij J, et al. Rapidly increasing incidence of eosinophilic esophagitis in a large court. Neurogastroenterol Motil. 2013;25:47–52.
4. Spergel JM. New genetic links in eosinophilic esophagitis. Genome Med. 2010;2:60.
5. Guarino MPL, Cicala M, Behar J. Eosinophilic esophagitis: new insight in pathogenesis and therapy. World J Gastroinest Pharmacol Ther. 2016;7(1):66–77.
6. Alexander ES, Martin LJ, Collins MH, et al. Twin and family studies reveal strong environmental and weaker genetic cues explaining heritability of eosinophilic esophagitis. J Allergy Clin Immunol. 2014;134(5):1084–92.
7. Abonia JP, Wen T, Stucke EM, et al. High prevalence of eosinophilic esophagitis in patients with inherited connective tissue disorders. J Allergy Clin Immunol. 2013;132(2):378–86.
8. Davis BP, Epstein T, Kottyan L, et al. Association of eosinophilic esophagitis and hypertrophic cardiomyopathy. J Allergy Clin Immunol. 2016;137(3):934–6.
9. Blanchard C, Wang N, Stringer KF, et al. Eotaxin-3 and uniquely conserved gene-expression profile in eosinophilic esophagitis. J Clin Invest. 2006;116:536–47.
10. Sherill JD, Gao P, Stucke EM, et al. Variation of thymic stromal lymphopoietin and its receptor associate with eosinophilic esophagitis. J Allergy Clin Immunol. 2010;126:160–5.
11. Blanchard C, Stucke EM, Burwinkel K, et al. Co-ordinate interaction between Il-13 and epithelial differentiation cluster genes in eosinophilic esophagitis. J Immunol. 2010;184:4033–41.
12. Blanchard C. Molecular pathogenesis of eosinophilic esophagitis. Curr Opin Gastroenterol. 2015;31:321–7.
13. Chandramouleeswaran PM, Shen D, Lee AJ, et al. Preferential secretion of thymic stromal lymphopoietin (TSLP) by terminally differentiated esophageal epithelial cells: relevance to eosinophilic esophagitis (EoE). PLoS ONE. 2016;11(3):e0150968.
14. Sherrill JD, Kc K, Wu D, et al. Desmoglein-1 regulates esophageal epithelial barrier function and immune responses in eosinophilic esophagitis. Mucosal Immunol. 2014;7:718–29.
15. Singla MB, Moawad FJ. An overview of the diagnosis and management of eosinophilic esophagitis. Clin Transl Gastroenterol. 2016;7:e155.
16. Gupta SK, Fitzgeraald JF, Kondratyuk T, HogenEsh H. Cytokine expression in normal and inflamed esophageal mucosa: a study into the pathogenesis of allergic eosinophilic esophagitis. J Pediatr Gastroenterol Nutr. 2006;42:22–6.
17. Blanchard C, Mingler MK, Vicario M, et al. IL-13 involvement in eosinophilic esophagitis: transcriptome analysis and reversibility with glucocorticoids. J Allergy Clin Immunol. 2007;120:1292–300.
18. Davis BP, Stucke EM, Khorki ME, et al. Eosinophilic esophagitis-linked calpain 14 is an IL-13-induced protease that mediates esophageal epithelial barrier impairment. JCI Insight. 2016;1(4):e86355.
19. Sherill JD, Kiran KC, Blanchard C, et al. Analysis and expansion of the eosinophilic esophagitis transcriptome by RNA sequencing. Genes Immun. 2014;15:361–9.
20. Rochman M, Kartashov AV, Caldwell JM, et al. Neurotrophic tyrosine kinase receptor 1 is a direct transcriptional and epigenetic target of IL-13 involved in allergic inflammation. Mucosal Immunol. 2015;8(4):785–98.
21. Zhang S, Wu X, Yu S. Prostaglandin D2 receptor D-type prostanoid receptor 2 mediates eosinophil trafficking into the esophagus. Dis Esophagus. 2014;27(6):601–6.
22. Niranjan R, Mavi P, Rayapudi M, Dynda S, Mishra A. Pathogenic role of mast cells in experimental eosinophilic esophagitis. Am J Physiol Gastrointest Liver Physiol. 2013;304(12):G1087–94.
23. Rayapudi M, Rajavelu P, Zhu X, et al. Invariant natural killer T-cell neutralization is a possible novel therapy for human eosinophilic esophagitis. Clin Transl Immunol. 2014;3:e9.
24. Jyonouchi S, Smith CL, Saretta F, et al. Invariant natural killer T cells in children with eosinophilic esophagitis. Clin Exp Allergy. 2014;44:58–68.
25. Roy-Ghanta S, Larosa DF, Katzka DA. Atopic characteristics of adult patients with eosinophilic esophagitis. Clin Gastroenterol Hepatol. 2008;6:531–5.
26. Noel RJ, Putnam PE, Rothenberg ME. Eosinophilic esophagitis. N Engl J Med. 2004;351:940–1.
27. Ridolo E, De Angelis GL, Dall'aglio P. Eosinophilic esophagitis after specific oral tolerance induction for egg protein. Ann Allergy Asthma Immunol. 2011;106:73–4.
28. Sánchez-García S, Rodríguez Del Río P, Escudero C, et al. Possible eosinophilic esophagitis induced by milk oral immunotherapy. J Allergy Clin Immunol. 2012;129(4):1155–7.
29. Lucendo AJ, Arias A, Tenias JM. Relation between eosinophilic esophagitis and oral immunotherapy for food allergy: a systematic review with meta-analysis. Ann Allergy Asthma Immunol. 2014;113(6):624–9.
30. Clayton F, Fang JC, Gleich GJ, et al. Eosinophilic esophagitis in adults is associated with IgG4 and not mediated by IgE. Gastroenterology. 2014;147:602–9.
31. Yamazaki K, Murray JA, Arora AS, et al. Allergen-specific in vitro cytokine production in adult patients with eosinophilic esophagitis. Dig Dis Sci. 2006;51:1934–41.
32. Mishra A, Hogan SP, Brandt EB, Rothenberg ME. An etiological role for aeroallergens and eosinophils in experimental esophagitis. J Clin Invest. 2001;107:83–90.
33. Ridolo E, Montagni M, Olivieri E, et al. Eosinophilic esophagitis: which role for food and inhalant allergens? Asia Pac Allergy. 2012;2:237–41.
34. Van Rhijn BD, van Ree R, Versteeg SA, et al. Birch pollen sensitization with cross-reactivity to food allergens predominates in adults with eosinophilic esophagitis. Allergy. 2013;68:1475–81.
35. Ridolo E, Montagni M, Melli V, et al. A role for pathogenesis-related proteins in poy-sensitized allergic patients with eosinophilic esophagitis: clinical and endoscopic features. J Allergy Ther. 2014;5:6.
36. Miehlke S. Clinical features of eosinophilic esophagitis. Dig Dis. 2014;32:61–7.
37. Joo MK, Park JJ, Kim SH. Prevalence and endoscopic features of eosinophilic esophagitis in patients with esophageal or upper gastrointestinal symptoms. J Dig Dis. 2012;13(6):296–303.
38. DeBrosse CW, Case JW, Putnam PE, et al. Quantity and distribution of eosinophils in the gastrointestinal tract of children. Pediatr Dev Pathol. 2006;9:201–8.
39. Dellon ES, Gonsalves N, Hirano I, et al. ACG clinical guideline: evidenced based approach to the diagnosis and management of esophageal eosinophilia and eosinophilic esophagitis (EoE). Am J Gastroenterol. 2013;108(5):679–92.
40. Alhmoud T, Hanson JA, Parasher G. Eosinophilic gastroenteritis: an underdiagnosed condition. Dig Dis Sci. 2016. [Epub ahead of print].
41. Kim HP, Vance RB, Shaheen NJ, Dellon ES. The prevalence and diagnostic utility of endoscopic features of eosinophilic esophagitis: a meta-analysis. Clin Gastroenterol Hepatol. 2012;10(9):988–96.
42. Gonsalves N, Policarpio-Nicolas M, Zhang Q, et al. Histopathologic variability and endoscopic correlates in adults with eosinophilic esophagitis. Gastrointest Endosc. 2006;64(3):313–9.
43. Shah A, Kagalwalla AF, Gonsalves N, et al. Histopathologic variability in children with eosinophilic esophagitis. Am J Gastroenterol. 2009;104(3):716–21.
44. Dohil R, Newbury RO, Aceves S. Transient PPI responsive esophageal eosinophilia may be a clinical sub-phenotype of pediatric eosinophilic esophagitis. Dig Dis Sci. 2012;57(5):1413–9.
45. Park JY, Zhang X, Nguyen N, et al. Proton pump inhibitors decrease eotaxin-3 expression in the proximal esophagus of children with esophageal eosinophilia. PLoS ONE. 2014;9(7):e101391.
46. Cianferoni A, Spergel JM. Eosinophilic esophagitis and gastroenteritis. Curr Allergy Asthma Rep. 2015;15:58.
47. Ahmed M. Eosinophilic esophagitis in adults. World J Gastrointest Pharmacol Ther. 2016;7(2):207–13.
48. Lucendo AJ, Arias A, De Rezende LC, et al. Subepithelial collagen deposition, profibrogenic cytokine gene expression, and changes after prolonged fluticasone propionate treatment in adult eosinophilic esophagitis: a prospective study. J Allergy Clin Immunol. 2011;128:1037–46.
49. Netzer P, Gschossmann JM, Straumann A, et al. Corticosteroid-dependent eosinophilic oesophagitis: azathioprine and 6-mercaptopurine can induce and maintain long-term remission. Eur J Gastroenterol Hepatol. 2007;19(10):865–9.
50. Attwood SE, Lewis CJ, Bronder CS, et al. Eosinophilic esophagitis: a novel treatment using Montelukast. Gut. 2003;52:181–5.

51. Beglinger C, Smith DA, Patel J, et al. Antiinterleukin-5 antibody treatment (mepolizumab) in active eosinophilic oesophagitis: a randomised, placebo-controlled, double-blind trial. Gut. 2010;59:21–30.
52. Dohil R, Broide DH, Aceves SS. Anti-IL-5 therapy reduces mast cell and IL-9 cell numbers in pediatric patients with eosinophilic esophagitis. J Allergy Clin Immunol. 2013;131:1576–82.
53. Spergel JM, Rothenberg ME, Collins MH, et al. Reslizumab in children and adolescents with eosinophilic esophagitis: results of a double-blind, randomized, placebo-controlled trial. J Allergy Clin Immunol. 2012;129:456–63.
54. Rothenberg ME, Wen T, Greenberg A, et al. Intravenous anti-IL-13 mAb QAX576 for the treatment of eosinophilic esophagitis. J Allergy Clin Immunol. 2015;135:500–7.
55. Kelly KJ, Lazenby AJ, Rowe PC, et al. Eosinophilic esophagitis attributed to gastroesophageal reflux: improvement with an amino acid-based formula. Gastroenterology. 1995;109(5):1503–12.
56. Peterson KA, Byrne KR, Vinson LA, et al. Elemental diet induces histologic response in adult eosinophilic esophagitis. Am J Gastroenterol. 2013;108(5):759–66.
57. Arias A, González-Cervera J, Tenias JM, Lucendo AJ. Efficacy of dietary interventions for inducing histologic remission in patients with eosinophilic esophagitis: a systematic review and meta-analysis. Gastroenterology. 2014;146(7):1639–48.
58. Gonsalves N, Yang GY, Doerfler B, et al. Elimination diet effectively treats eosinophilic esophagitis in adults; food reintroduction identifies causative factors. Gastroenterology. 2012;142(7):1451–9.
59. Kagalwalla AF, Sentongo TA, Ritz S, et al. Effect of six-food elimination diet on clinical and histologic outcomes in eosinophilic esophagitis. Clin Gastroenterol Hepatol. 2006;4(9):1097–102.
60. Schoepfer AM, Safroneeva E, Bussmann C, et al. Delay in diagnosis of eosinophilic esophagitis increases risk for stricture formation in a time-dependent manner. Gastroenterology. 2013;145(6):1230–6.
61. Dellon ES, Kim HP, Sperry SL, et al. A phenotypic analysis shows that eosinophilic esophagitis is a progressive fibrostenotic disease. Gastrointest Endosc. 2014;79(4):577–85.
62. Spergel JM, Brown-Whitehorn TF, Beausoleil JL, et al. 14 years of eosinophilic esophagitis: clinical features and prognosis. J Pediatr Gastroenterol Nutr. 2009;48(1):30–6.
63. Uppal V, Kreiger P, Kutsch E. Eosinophilic gastroenteritis: a comprehensive review. Clin Rev Allergy Immunol. 2016;50:175–88.
64. Reed C, Woosley JT, Dellon ES. Clinical characteristics, treatment outcomes, and resource utilization in children and adults with eosinophilic gastroenteritis. Dig Liver Dis. 2015;47(3):197–201.
65. Khan S, Orenstein SR. Eosinophilic gastroenteritis: epidemiology, diagnosis and management. Paediatr Drugs. 2002;4(9):563–70.
66. Klein NC, Hargrove RL, Sleisenger MH, Jeffries GH. Eosinophilic gastroenteritis. Medicine. 1970;49:299–319.
67. Yun MY, Cho YU, Park IS, et al. Eosinophilic gastroenteritis presenting as small bowel obstruction: a case report and review of the literature. World J Gastroenterol. 2007;13:1758–60.
68. Box JC, Tucker J, Watne AL, Lucas G. Eosinophilic colitis presenting as a left-sided colocolonic intussusception with secondary large bowel obstruction: an uncommon entity with a rare presentation. Am Surg. 1997;63:741–3.
69. Pineton de Chambrun G, Gonzalez F, Canva JY, et al. Natural history of eosinophilic gastroenteritis. Clin Gastroenterol Hepatol. 2011;9:950–6.
70. Chen MJ, Chu CH, Lin SC, et al. Eosinophilic gastroenteritis: clinical experience with 15 patients. World J Gastroenterol. 2003;9:2813–6.
71. von Wattenwyl F, Zimmermann A, Netzer P. Synchronous first manifestation of an idiopathic eosinophilic gastroenteritis and bronchial asthma. Eur J Gastroenterol Hepatol. 2001;13:721–5.
72. Ko HM, Morotti RA, Yershov O, et al. Eosinophilic gastritis in children: clinicopathological correlation, disease course, and response to therapy. Am J Gastroenterol. 2014;109:1277–85.
73. Maloney J, Nowak-Wegrzyn A. Educational clinical case series for pediatric allergy and immunology: allergic proctocolitis, food protein-induced enterocolitis syndrome and allergic eosinophilic gastroenteritis with protein-losing gastroenteropathy as manifestations of non-IgE-mediated cow's milk allergy. Pediatr Allergy Immunol. 2007;18:360–7.
74. Ishimura N, Furuta K, Sato S, et al. Limited role of allergy testing in patients with eosinophilic gastrointestinal disorders. J Gastroenterol Hepatol. 2013;28:1306–13.
75. Chehade M, Sicherer SH, Magid MS, et al. Multiple exudative ulcers and pseudopolyps in allergic eosinophilic gastroenteritis that responded to dietary therapy. J Pediatr Gastroenterol Nutr. 2007;45:354–7.
76. Yamada Y, Kato M, Isoda Y, et al. Eosinophilic gastroenteritis treated with a multiple-food elimination diet. Allergol Int. 2014;63(Suppl 1):53–6.
77. Iborra M, Alvarez-Sotomayor D, Nos P. Long-term safety and efficacy of budesonide in the treatment of ulcerative colitis. Clin Exp Gastroenterol. 2014;7:39–46.
78. Siewert E, Lammert F, Koppitz P, et al. Eosinophilic gastroenteritis with severe protein-losing enteropathy: successful treatment with budesonide. Dig Liver Dis. 2006;38:55–9.
79. Tan AC, Kruimel JW, Naber TH. Eosinophilic gastroenteritis treated with non-enteric-coated budesonide tablets. Eur J Gastroenterol Hepatol. 2011;13:425–7.

14

Pilot study: assessing the clinical diagnosis of allergy in atopic children using a microarray assay in addition to skin prick testing and serum specific IgE

Ru-Xin Foong[1,2*], Graham Roberts[3], Adam Tobias Fox[1] and George du Toit[1]

Abstract

Background: Children with atopic dermatitis (AD) are at risk of developing allergy. Alongside clinical history, testing modalities include skin prick tests (SPT), specific immunoglobulin-E (sp-IgE) and recently, microarray assays. The aim of this pilot study was to assess current tests and the ISAC sIgE-112 system in the diagnosis of food and aeroallergen allergy.

Methods: Children aged 0–11 years with moderate to severe AD were included. An initial allergy assessment including clinical history, SPT and sp-IgE was performed to determine food and aeroallergen sensitization. A second independent clinical assessment using the same information given to the first assessor and ISAC test results for food and aeroallergen sensitization was also made for each participant. The results from both were compared.

Results: 30 children [mean age 3.91 years (SD 3.3)] were included; 53.3 and 46.7 % had moderate and severe AD, respectively. Sp-IgE tests had a higher percentage of positive results compared to SPT and ISAC tests for common allergens. There was a significant difference between the three tests in detecting aeroallergen sensitization ($p = 0.038$), especially between sp-IgE and ISAC tests, but no significant difference between the tests for food allergen sensitization. There was good agreement between the two assessors; 70 % of the children had a change in diagnosis, with 60 % having at least one diagnosis added and 40 % having at least one diagnosis removed.

Conclusions: There is a role for the use of ISAC testing in diagnosing sensitization and allergy in children with AD as it leads to a change in diagnosis for many patients. Further work is required to assess its clinical and cost effectiveness.

Keywords: Aeroallergens, Atopic dermatitis, Diagnostic investigations, Food allergy

Background

Atopic dermatitis (AD) is a common inflammatory skin disease affecting 15–20 % of children in developed countries [1]. It usually starts in the first few months of life and is frequently outgrown by 15 years of age although there is a large amount of variability between children [2].

It is well known that there are close links between food allergy and AD as it is a significant risk factor for the development of food sensitization and food allergy [2–4]. Patients with higher levels of total Immunoglobulin-E (IgE) in their blood, which is often the case in children with AD, are more likely to be sensitised to foods [1, 5]. Kumar et al. found that children with AD had an 8.4-fold higher risk of developing a food allergy [6]. de Benedictis et al. demonstrated that of infants with AD in various countries around the world, 55.5 % were sensitised to at least one allergen and 52.9 % had a raised serum total IgE [7].

Due to the increased likelihood of children with AD being sensitised to various food allergens, it can be difficult to establish whether these children have true food

*Correspondence: ruxinfoong@gmail.com
[1] Division of Asthma, Allergy and Lung Biology, Guy's and St. Thomas' NHS Foundation Trust, London SE1 7EH, UK
Full list of author information is available at the end of the article

allergy. The European Academy of Allergy and Clinical Immunology (EAACI) guidelines recommend the use of clinical history, skin prick tests (SPT) and serum specific IgE (sp-IgE) tests in the investigation of food allergy but the gold standard for diagnosis remains the oral food challenge [8]. AD is often associated with aeroallergen sensitization and in the context of a high level of total IgE, there are often low levels of sp-IgE to numerous aeroallergens [1]. These are of unclear clinical significance.

Immunocap® ISAC-112 (Thermo Fisher/Phadia AB, Uppsala, Sweden) is an in vitro assay for the measurement of allergen sp-IgE antibodies in human plasma [9]. It is intended to aid in the diagnosis of IgE-mediated allergic disorders. There is currently no advice on the use of ISAC testing worldwide [8, 10]. The National Institute of Allergy and Infectious Diseases (NIAID) guidelines do not recommend the combined use of SPTs and sp-IgE tests for routine diagnosis of food allergy and instead recommend individual SPT and sp-IgE tests to help identify foods that might be provoking a reaction alongside clinical history [10]. Thus, the utilization of a broad screening test is controversial. Whilst it may facilitate a more accurate clinical allergy diagnosis for specific atopic conditions [11, 12], it has been suggested that identifying patterns of allergen responses for patients with AD is less reliable [12]. Spergel et al. [13] found that the predictive values of food-antigen sp-IgE were not clinically significant in predicting the development of food allergy in children with mild to moderate AD. However, this study performed sp-IgE only for common food allergens, potentially missing less common allergens [13].

The ISAC-112 has the potential as a single test modality, to identify food and aeroallergen sensitizations in at risk atopic children. Hatzler et al. [14] looked at the IgE response to grass pollen antigens and demonstrated that sensitization can occur years before the onset of clinical disease through a process called "molecular spreading". Therefore, the use of microarrays could be convenient in the setting where common food allergens have not yet been introduced thereby limiting the value of a detailed clinical history.

The aim of this pilot study was to assess the use of current diagnostic modalities (clinical consultation, SPT, sp-IgE) in a specialist allergy clinic in children with AD. We also assessed whether Immunocap® ISAC sIgE-112 testing could improve the diagnosis of food and aeroallergen allergy in these children.

Methods

Participants

We recruited children aged 0–11 years from the paediatric allergy clinic at St. Thomas' Hospital, London UK, an urban, tertiary referral centre. We identified children who had moderate to severe AD using any one of the LEAP study criteria [15]: parents or guardians' description of their child's AD severity as moderate or severe; use of topical creams and ointments containing corticosteroids or calcineurin inhibitors (defined as severe); or modified Scoring Atopic Dermatitis System (SCORAD) evaluation of at least 15 [16]. Written consent was obtained from the parents and child (if age relevant). Ethics approval was given by the NRES Committee London—Fulham (12/LO/1733).

Initial allergy assessment

The participants who fitted the criteria for moderate to severe AD underwent a detailed allergy clinical assessment (clinical history, SPT, sp-IgE tests) by a paediatric allergy consultant. A clinical diagnosis of food allergy and clinically significant aeroallergen sensitization was made based on these findings. The most common food and aeroallergens were tested for: peanut (Ara h1, Ara h2, Ara h3, Ara h8, Ara h9), egg (white or yolk), cow's milk, timothy grass pollen, birch tree pollen, *Dermatophagoides pteronyssinus* house dust mite, *Alternaria* mould, cat and dog. SPT were performed using Alyostal® Stallergenes allergen extracts by trained paediatric allergy nurses in the department. Sensitization to food and aeroallergens to the same allergens was measured by specific-IgE (Thermo Fisher, Uppsala, Sweden). Food allergy was defined by a history of IgE-mediated symptoms (e.g. rash, urticaria, wheeze, vomiting, hypotension, anaphylaxis) on exposure to a food antigen, in the presence of a positive SPT ($\geq$3 mm) or sp-IgE ($\geq$0.35 kU/l) [17]. Clinically significant aeroallergen sensitization was defined as positive SPT ($\geq$3 mm) or sp-IgE ($\mp$0.35 kU/l) in the presence of a history of worsening AD, allergic rhino-conjunctivitis or asthma symptoms when exposed to the relevant aeroallergen.

Second allergy assessment with ISAC

All participants then had an ISAC-112 (Thermo Fisher Scientific©) test performed of which blood was taken after the clinic appointment. Immunocap and ISAC-112 analysis were processed by the Viapath Analytics department at King's College Hospital, London UK. A positive ISAC was defined as $\geq$0.3 ISU-E for the same allergens tested for in the initial assessment. A second assessment was performed by a second paediatric allergy consultant who used the clinical history, SPT, sp-IgE and ISAC results to make an independent clinical assessment of the presence of food allergy and aeroallergen sensitizations.

Statistics

Statistical analysis was performed using (STATA, version 14, College Station, USA). Descriptive statistics were presented as means with standard deviation (SD) where appropriate and categorical variables presented as percentages. Kappa statistics were used to look at agreement between the tests results and allergic diagnoses. A Kappa of 0.01–0.4 is considered slight to fair agreement, 0.41–0.60 is moderate agreement and 0.61–0.99 is substantial to almost perfect agreement [18]. Chi square tests were used to compare the proportion sensitised to food allergens and aeroallergens based on the test performed. To compare the number of allergens that were positive for each participant for the difference tests and number of allergic diagnoses per participant, repeat measures ANOVA tests were used.

Results

A total of 30 participants were recruited for this study. The mean age of the children was 3.91 years (SD 3.3) and 60 % (n = 18) were male. Of the group, 53.3 % (n = 16) and 46.7 % (n = 14) had SCORAD scores suggestive of moderate and severe AD, respectively.

Comparison of SPT, sp-IgE and ISAC tests

We compared the percentage of children who had a positive test result on SPT, sp-IgE and ISAC for common food and aeroallergens (Fig. 1). Overall, apart from egg allergen, the sp-IgE tests had a higher percentage of positive results for each allergen compared to SPT and ISAC tests. When comparing SPT and ISAC tests a relatively similar percentage of positive results for allergens were noted. For example, for birch pollen, 36 % had a positive SPT and 36.7 % had a positive ISAC test.

We also looked at the agreement between the three different tests (Table 1). There was good agreement between the SPT and ISAC tests for sensitization to selected food and aeroallergens. There was relatively good agreement between sp-IgE and ISAC tests for house dust mite and *Alternaria* mould. There was also good agreement between SPT and sp-IgE for house dust mite. Other test and allergen comparisons showed low levels of agreement.

Comparison of positive sensitizations for each participant

The number of positive sensitizations for each participant for each test was compared. For aeroallergens, overall there was a significant difference between the results of the three tests (p = 0.038); subsequent pairwise comparisons found that the only significant difference was between the sp-IgE and ISAC tests results (Table 2). For food allergens, there was no overall significant difference found between the results from the different tests (p = 0.469). These results do require further consideration in the context of the specificity of the tests.

More specifically, we compared each participant's positive sensitizations based on the test performed. We found that 73.3 % of the participants had at least one positive aeroallergen based on their ISAC test compared to both their SPT or sp-IgE results, although the difference was not statistically significant (p = 0.35). For the food

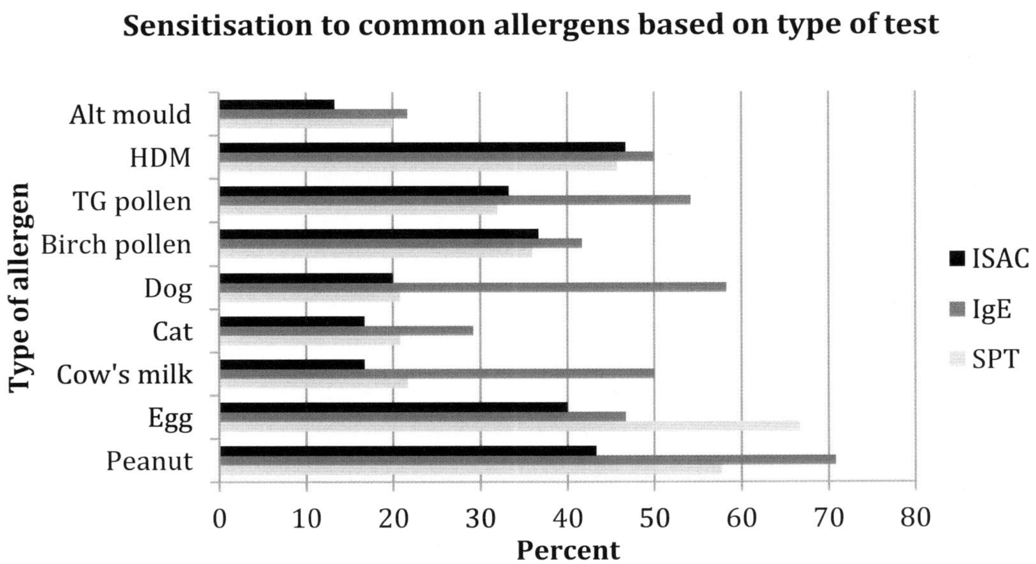

Fig. 1 Sensitization to common allergens based on the type of test performed. Figures are numerator/denominator (%) positive for each test for allergic sensitisation. Positive SPT was defined as ≥3 mm, positive specific IgE as ≥0.35 kU/l and positive ISAC as ≥0.3 ISU-E

Table 1 Agreement between the tests based on sensitization

Allergen	SPT and IgE	SPT and ISAC	IgE and ISAC
Peanut	0.42 (0.02)	0.54 (0.003)	0.36 (0.023)
Egg	0.29 (0.072)	0.43 (0.01)	0.19 (0.148)
Cow's milk	0.39 (0.010)	1.00 (<0.001)	0.38 (0.006)
Cat	0.53 (0.007)	0.86 (<0.001)	0.56 (0.003)
Dog	0.30 (0.029)	0.18 (0.192)	0.38 (0.008)
Birch pollen	0.20 (0.175)	0.65 (0.001)	0.55 (0.003)
Timothy grass pollen	0.28 (0.063)	0.73 (<0.001)	0.44 (0.005)
House dust mite	0.73 (<0.001)	0.58 (0.002)	0.92 (<0.001)
Alternaria mould	−0.25 (0.855)	0.06 (0.390)	0.70 (<0.001)

Figures are Kappa statistics (p values) where represent the level of agreement between allergen sensitization tests having taken into account any agreement that is expected by chance. Results of 0.61–0.99 signify excellent agreement, 0.41–0.60 signifies moderate agreement and 0.01–0.4 signifies only slight to fair agreement [18]

Table 2 Number of food and aeroallergen sensitizations by participant based on the type of test performed

Number of sensitizations	SPT (%)	Specific IgE (%)	ISAC (%)	P value
Aeroallergens				
0	13 (43.3)	9 (30.0)	8 (26.7)	0.038*
1	7 (23.3)	3 (10.0)	10 (33.3)	
2	3 (10.0)	6 (20.0)	1 (3.3)	
3	2 (6.7)	7 (23.3)	6 (20.0)	
4	2 (6.7)	1 (3.3)	5 (16.7)	
5	3 (10.0)	2 (6.7)	0 (0)	
6	0 (0)	2 (6.7)	0 (0)	
Food allergens				
0	7 (23.3)	8 (26.7)	11 (36.7)	0.469
1	13 (43.3)	8 (26.7)	11 (36.7)	
2	7 (23.3)	6 (20.0)	5 (16.7)	
3	3 (10.0)	8 (26.7)	3 (10.0)	

P values represent Chi square test. Given that this was significant for aeroallergens (*), pairwise comparisons were undertaken for aeroallergen sensitization: SPT vs. specific IgE ($p = 0.201$), specific IgE vs. ISAC ($p = 0.023$), SPT vs. ISAC ($p = 0.119$)

allergens, 76.7 and 73.3 % of participants were identified as sensitised by SPT or sp-IgE tests, respectively, compared to their ISAC test but the difference was not significant ($p = 0.50$).

Comparison of allergy diagnoses between the two assessors

We then compared allergy diagnoses outcomes between the two different assessors (Table 3). Overall, we found relatively good agreement between the two assessors. There was higher agreement for the food allergens

Table 3 Number (%) of food and aeroallergen diagnoses in 30 participants

Allergy diagnoses	Assessor 1	Assessor 2 (with ISAC results)	Chi square test
Aeroallergens			
0	11 (36.7 %)	9 (30.0 %)	0.588
1	4 (13.3 %)	3 (10.0 %)	
2	4 (13.3 %)	4 (13.3 %)	
3	4 (13.3 %)	3 (10.0 %)	
4	5 (16.7 %)	4 (13.3 %)	
5	2 (6.7 %)	2 (6.7 %)	
6	0 (0.0 %)	4 (13.3 %)	
7	0 (0.0 %)	1(3.3 %)	
Food allergens			
0	3 (10.0 %)	3 (10.0 %)	0.214
1	7 (23.3 %)	13 (43.3 %)	
2	11 (36.7 %)	4 (13.3 %)	
3	7 (23.3 %)	6 (20.0 %)	
4	2 (6.7 %)	4 (13.3 %)	

compared to the aeroallergens except for house dust mite and *Alternaria* mould allergy ($k = 0.92$ and $k = 0.70$, respectively). The mean number of allergies diagnosed by assessor 1 was 5.3 (SD 2.56) and was 5.9 (SD 2.98) by assessor 2, which were not significantly different ($p = 0.20$). The distribution of numbers of allergy diagnoses for the two assessors is presented in Table 3. There was no significant difference found between the number of allergy diagnoses for food allergens ($p = 0.214$) or aeroallergens ($p = 0.588$) between the two assessors.

As assessment 2 was made with the addition of the ISAC results, we were able to observe the effect the ISAC test had on allergy diagnoses (Table 4). When considering specific allergen diagnoses, a total of 20 diagnoses were removed based on the inclusion of ISAC results and 26 allergen diagnoses were added; 13 of those added were for food allergens not included in the SPT or sp-IgE screens. We found that 70 % (21/30) of the participants had a change in diagnosis between their two assessments with 60 % (18/30) having at least one allergic diagnosis added and 40 % (12/30) having at least one allergic diagnosis removed (Additional file 1: Table S1).

With regards to atopy, all the patients had a diagnosis of AD; therefore, there was 100 % agreement between the assessors ($k = 1.00$). For rhino-conjunctivitis, there were six diagnoses that were removed by assessor 2 and replaced by a diagnosis of non-allergic rhino-conjunctivitis. For asthma, there was no change with regards to diagnosis ($k = 0.42$) (Table 4).

Table 4 Allergy assessment by two assessors

Allergic diagnosis	Assessor 1	Assessor 2 (with ISAC results)	Diagnosis removed by assessor 2	Diagnosis added by assessor 2	Agreement between assessors
Atopic dermatitis	30 (100 %)	30 (100 %)	0 (0.0 %)	0 (0.0 %)	1.00
Rhino-conjunctivitis	14 (46.7 %)	8 (26.7 %)	6 (20.0 %)	0 (0.0 %)	0.59 (<0.001)
Asthma	4 (13.3 %)	4 (13.3 %)	0 (0.0 %)	0 (0.0 %)	0.42 (0.010)
Peanut	13 (43.3 %)	13 (43.3 %)	0 (0.0 %)	1 (3.3 %)	0.73 (<0.001)
Egg	15 (50.0 %)	18 (60.0 %)	3 (10.0 %)	1 (3.3 %)	0.67 (<0.001)
Cow's milk	9 (30.0 %)	7 (23.3 %)	1 (3.3 %)	1 (3.3 %)	0.66 (<0.001)
Other food allergy	21 (70.0 %)	19 (63.3 %)	1 (3.3 %)	13 (43.3 %)	0.85 (<0.001)
Cat	6 (20.0 %)	13 (43.3 %)	3 (10.0 %)	0 (0.0 %)	0.49 (0.001)
Dog	7 (23.3 %)	10 (33.3 %)	1 (3.3 %)	1 (3.3 %)	0.59 (<0.001)
House dust mite	11 (36.7 %)	17 (56.7 %)	2 (6.7 %)	2 (6.7 %)	0.49 (0.001)
Alternaria mould	6 (20.0 %)	10 (33.3 %)	1 (3.3 %)	2 (6.7 %)	0.67 (<0.001)
Birch pollen	10 (33.3 %)	13 (43.3 %)	1 (3.3 %)	2 (6.7 %)	0.79 (<0.001)
Timothy grass pollen	13 (43.3 %)	14 (46.7 %)	1 (3.3 %)	2 (6.7 %)	0.53 (0.002)
Horse	1 (3.3 %)	1 (3.3 %)	0 (0.0 %)	1 (3.3 %)	−0.03 (0.575)
Total			14 (46.7 %)	26 (86.7 %)	

Percentages represent the number (%) of participants given each diagnoses by each assessor. The number (%) of participants who had each specific allergy diagnosis removed or added by assessor 2 (impact of the ISAC test results) is also presented. Level of agreement between assessors is presented as Kappa statistics (p values)

Discussion

There is little published data on the use of ISAC testing in AD children. Prosperi et al. [12] found that ISAC testing had reasonable discrimination in detecting allergens associated with asthma, rhino-conjunctivitis, wheeze and airway hypersensitivity but it was not useful for detecting allergens associated with eczema in a paediatric cohort. Our study demonstrates that there is a high prevalence of food and aeroallergen sensitization in children with moderate to severe AD. Although the use of the ISAC-112 testing did not significantly change the number of allergic sensitizations or diagnoses compared to traditional test modalities of SPT and sp-IgE tests, the majority of participants had a change in specific allergy diagnoses when all of the ISAC-112 results were utilized.

Our results demonstrate that for the food allergens tested, sp-IgE testing yielded more positive results as compared to SPT and ISAC, despite the ISAC test covering a greater array of pre-set food allergen components. It has been suggested that the binding characteristics of the ISAC-112 are more specific as they bypass the high rates of sensitization that can occur in AD children who have a raised total IgE. However, the number of food and aeroallergen sensitizations was not lower using ISAC tests, which suggests that the ISAC test may not circumvent this issue.

In recent years, several studies have been performed which demonstrate strong correlation between the ISAC-112 test and other single-plex allergy tests (SPT, sp-IgE tests) [19, 20]. More specifically, studies have shown a good correlation between the testing methods for aeroallergens such as grass pollens [21] and house dust mite in allergic rhinitis patients [11]. In our cohort, the results available from the ISAC-112 test resulted in a change in diagnosis of allergic rhino-conjunctivitis to non-allergic rhino-conjunctivitis for six children. This supports the view that the ISAC test may be helpful at differentiating between allergic and non-allergic rhino-conjunctivitis compared to clinical history and single-plex tests. In fact, the WAO-ARIA-GA^{2}LEN consensus guidelines clarify the role that molecular allergy diagnostics such as ISAC-112 can have on resolving genuine versus cross-reactive sensitization in poly-sensitized patients, such as those with AD; hence facilitating a more accurate assessment of the severity of risks to allergens [22].

Another consideration that allergy diagnostic centres may have is the cost of running these diagnostic tests. In our study, SPT cost £15.95 per vial of allergen solution (Alyostal® Stallergenes), which is used for approximately 60 SPT (£0.27 per allergen per test). Skin prick testing requires a trained health care practitioner, safe medical facilities and time to perform and interpret the tests. Sp-IgE tests cost £14.30 per allergen compared to the ISAC test, which costs £250 for 112 allergen components. Both of these tests require phlebotomy services, laboratory staff and the necessary laboratory equipment. For the patients with a clinical history that identifies likely target allergens, confirmation by SPT and sp-IgE testing may prove sufficient and more cost-effective. However, in the poly-sensitised allergic patient with no identifiable causative allergens, based on costing in our tertiary centre, the ISAC test would prove to be more cost effective if the clinician wanted to test for more than 18 allergens or allergen components. Although this seems like a considerable number of allergens to test for, it is not an uncommon practice in investigating AD children. It is in the children with equivocal histories or poly-allergenicity that the ISAC test may provide clinicians with a more comprehensive overview of sensitization to common food and aeroallergens.

Limitations

The limitations of this study include small sample size recruited in a tertiary allergy clinic, which makes it difficult to extrapolate results to the general population. In smaller hospitals, ISAC testing may not be available which make these results less applicable to general clinical practice. However, our study focused on children with AD, which is an extremely common childhood atopic phenomena, of which allergic diagnoses can be challenging to diagnose. Although we tested for only a small number of allergens, these represent the most common food and aeroallergens in the UK. We assessed the additional diagnostic value of the ISAC-112 as opposed to the diagnostic performance of each of the modalities in isolation against a gold standard diagnostic provocation test. We also acknowledge that it would be beneficial to compare the different test modality outcomes for allergic diagnoses between AD children and a control population (i.e. children without AD) in future work. Also, the fact that the clinical examiners in this study were experienced specialist paediatric allergists can be seen as both an advantage and limitation of the study; this provides greater validity to the clinical diagnoses made, but different allergy tests may be interpreted differently in less experienced hands.

Conclusions

This pilot study demonstrates that there is a defined role for the use of ISAC testing in diagnosing sensitization and allergy in children with AD, which compares favourably with existing modalities of testing (i.e. SPT, sp-IgE tests). Depending on the clinical setting and the patient population (i.e. those with AD), the ISAC test may be useful in leading to a change in diagnosis and be more cost effective. Further investigation in a larger population, testing each test in isolation as well as against the gold standard (i.e. OFC), is needed.

Abbreviations

AD: atopic dermatitis; SPT: skin prick tests; Sp-IgE: specific immunoglobulin E; EAACI: European Academy of Allergy and Clinical Immunology; NIAID: National Institute of Allergy and Infectious Diseases; SCORAD: scoring atopic dermatitis system; SD: standard deviation.

Authors' contributions

RXF and GdT were both involved in the study design, application for ethics approval, data collection, data analysis and drafting of the manuscript. GR was involved in the study design, statistical analysis of the data and drafting of the manuscript. ATF was one of the main consultants involved in the data collection of the study. All authors read and approved the final manuscript.

Author details

[1] Division of Asthma, Allergy and Lung Biology, Guy's and St. Thomas' NHS Foundation Trust, London SE1 7EH, UK. [2] Institute of Child Health, University College of London, London, UK. [3] University of Southampton and National Institute for Health Research Respiratory Biomedical Research Unit, Southampton and David Hide Centre, Southampton, UK.

Acknowledgements

We would like to thank Rosemary Ebling and her laboratory staff in the Viapath Analytics department at King's College Hospital, London UK for their help in running the ISAC-112 tests.

Competing interests

Dr. Ru-Xin Foong has received funding from Thermofisher Scientific to cover conference fees for continued professional development. Dr. Graham Roberts has received research funding from ALK-Abello and Thermofisher Scientific and has his department has received consultancy fees from Novatitis, ALK-Abello and Danone. Dr. Adam Fox has received research funding from ALK-Abello and Danone and consultancy fees from Mead Johnson and Danone. Dr. George Du Toit has received research support from the ITN/NIAID for his involvement as part of the ITN LEAP Study Team. The National Peanut Board sponsored previous research, and currently part sponsors running costs of the KCL Clinical Trials Unit at St Thomas' Hospital. George is a voluntary scientific advisor for the Anaphylaxis Campaign; he has received lecture fees from the following commercial companies; Meda, Nestle-Nutrition, and Stallergenes.

Funding

Thermo Fisher Scientific© with the donation and analysis of ISAC 112 microarray chips; no input into the design or outcome of the study.

References

1. de Bruin Weller MS, Knulst AC, Meijer Y, Bruijnzeel-Koomen CA, Pasmans SG. Evaluation of the child with atopic dermatitis. Clin Exp Allergy. 2012;42(3):352–62.
2. Weidinger SNN. Atopic dermatitis (Seminar). Lancet. 2015;387(10023):1109–22.
3. Alduraywish SA, Lodge CJ, Vicendese D, Lowe AJ, Erbas B, Matheson MC, et al. Sensitization to milk, egg and peanut from birth to 18 years: a longitudinal study of a cohort at risk of allergic disease. Pediatr Allergy Immunol. 2015;27:83–91.
4. Gustafsson D, Sjoberg O, Foucard T. Development of allergies and asthma in infants and young children with atopic dermatitis–a prospective follow-up to 7 years of age. Allergy. 2000;55(3):240–5.
5. Wolkerstorfer A, Wahn U, Kjellman NI, Diepgen TL, De Longueville M, Oranje AP. Natural course of sensitization to cow's milk and hen's egg

in childhood atopic dermatitis: ETAC study group. Clin Exp Allergy. 2002;32(1):70–3.

6. Kumar R, Caruso DM, Arguelles L, Kim JS, Schroeder A, Rowland B, et al. Early life eczema, food introduction, and risk of food allergy in children. Pediatr Allergy Immunol Pulmonol. 2010;23(3):175–82.
7. de Benedictis FM, Franceschini F, Hill D, Naspitz C, Simons FE, Wahn U, et al. The allergic sensitization in infants with atopic eczema from different countries. Allergy. 2009;64(2):295–303.
8. Muraro A, Werfel T, Hoffmann-Sommergruber K, Roberts G, Beyer K, Bindslev-Jensen C, et al. EAACI food allergy and anaphylaxis guidelines: diagnosis and management of food allergy. Allergy. 2014;69(8):1008–25.
9. Thermoscientific. Phadia: allergy and autoimmunity—product catalog. 2013. http://www.phadia.com/Global/A%20Document%20Library/Product%20Catalogues/Product_Catalog_ID.pdf. Accessed July 2014.
10. Boyce JA, Assa'ad A, Burks AW, Jones SM, Sampson HA, Wood RA, et al. Guidelines for the diagnosis and management of food allergy in the United States: summary of the NIAID-sponsored expert panel report. Nutr Res. 2011;31(1):61–75.
11. Jung JH, Kang IG, Kim ST. Comparison of component-resolved diagnosis by using allergen microarray with the conventional tests in allergic rhinitis patients: the first using in Korea. Clin Exp Otorhinolaryngol. 2015;8(4):385–9.
12. Prosperi MC, Belgrave D, Buchan I, Simpson A, Custovic A. Challenges in interpreting allergen microarrays in relation to clinical symptoms: a machine learning approach. Pediatr Allergy Immunol. 2014;25(1):71–9.
13. Spergel JM, Boguniewicz M, Schneider L, Hanifin JM, Paller AS, Eichenfield LF. Food allergy in infants with atopic dermatitis: limitations of food-specific IgE measurements. Pediatrics. 2015;136(6):e1530–8.
14. Hatzler L, Panetta V, Lau S, Wagner P, Bergmann RL, Illi S, et al. Molecular spreading and predictive value of preclinical IgE response to Phleum pratense in children with hay fever. J Allergy Clin Immunol. 2012;130(4):894–901 **(e5)**.
15. Du Toit G, Roberts G, Sayre PH, Plaut M, Bahnson HT, Mitchell H, et al. Identifying infants at high risk of peanut allergy: the learning early about peanut allergy (LEAP) screening study. J Allergy Clin Immunol. 2013;131(1):135–43 **(e1–12)**.
16. Schmitt J, Langan S, Deckert S, Svensson A, von Kobyletzki L, Thomas K, et al. Assessment of clinical signs of atopic dermatitis: a systematic review and recommendation. J Allergy Clin Immunol. 2013;132(6):1337–47.
17. Muraro A, Dubois AE, DunnGalvin A, Hourihane JO, de Jong NW, Meyer R, et al. EAACI food allergy and anaphylaxis guidelines. food allergy health-related quality of life measures. Allergy. 2014;69(7):845–53.
18. Viera AJ, Garrett JM. Understanding interobserver agreement: the kappa statistic. Fam Med. 2005;37(5):360–3.
19. Huss-Marp J, Gutermuth J, Schaffner I, Darsow U, Pfab F, Brockow K, et al. Comparison of molecular and extract-based allergy diagnostics with multiplex and singleplex analysis. Allergo J Int. 2015;24:46–53.
20. Williams P, Onell A, Baldracchini F, Hui V, Jolles S, El-Shanawany T. Evaluation of a novel automated allergy microarray platform compared with three other allergy test methods. Clin Exp Immunol. 2016;184(1):1–10.
21. Ahlgrim C, Gutermuth J, Onell A, Borres MP, Schaffner I, Darsow U, et al. Comparison of molecular multiplex and singleplex analysis of IgE to grass pollen allergens in untreated German grass pollen-allergic patients. J Investig Allergol Clin Immunol. 2015;25(3):190–5.
22. Canonica GW, Ansotegui IJ, Pawankar R, Schmid-Grendelmeier P, van Hage M, Baena-Cagnani CE, et al. A WAO—ARIA—GA^{2}LEN consensus document on molecular-based allergy diagnostics. World Allergy Organ J. 2013;6(1):17.

15

The soft computing-based approach to investigate allergic diseases

Gennaro Tartarisco[1], Alessandro Tonacci[2], Paola Lucia Minciullo[3], Lucia Billeci[2], Giovanni Pioggia[1], Cristoforo Incorvaia[4*] and Sebastiano Gangemi[3]

Abstract

Background: Early recognition of inflammatory markers and their relation to asthma, adverse drug reactions, allergic rhinitis, atopic dermatitis and other allergic diseases is an important goal in allergy. The vast majority of studies in the literature are based on classic statistical methods; however, developments in computational techniques such as soft computing-based approaches hold new promise in this field.

Objective: The aim of this manuscript is to systematically review the main soft computing-based techniques such as artificial neural networks, support vector machines, bayesian networks and fuzzy logic to investigate their performances in the field of allergic diseases.

Methods: The review was conducted following PRISMA guidelines and the protocol was registered within PROSPERO database (CRD42016038894). The research was performed on PubMed and ScienceDirect, covering the period starting from September 1, 1990 through April 19, 2016.

Results: The review included 27 studies related to allergic diseases and soft computing performances. We observed promising results with an overall accuracy of 86.5%, mainly focused on asthmatic disease. The review reveals that soft computing-based approaches are suitable for big data analysis and can be very powerful, especially when dealing with uncertainty and poorly characterized parameters. Furthermore, they can provide valuable support in case of lack of data and entangled cause–effect relationships, which make it difficult to assess the evolution of disease.

Conclusions: Although most works deal with asthma, we believe the soft computing approach could be a real breakthrough and foster new insights into other allergic diseases as well.

Keywords: Allergy, Artificial intelligence, Artificial neural networks, Asthma, Fuzzy logic

Background

Recent advances in healthcare innovation have challenged us to think about the pioneering potential of big data coming from the digital world to invade the medical field. Big data introduces the exciting technological ability to digitize human beings in order to achieve a real personalization of medicine. Soft computing (SC) methods possess the extraordinary ability to exploit meaningful relationships of digital big data, making them suitable for the diagnosis, treatment and prediction of the outcome in many clinical scenarios. In the field of allergy these methods may be extremely useful to obtain important data and information on the characteristics and the management of many allergic diseases. Existing literature on the relationship between SC models and allergic diseases will be presented and discussed in this paper, highlighting the novel perspectives of this pioneering approach.

*Correspondence: cristoforo.incorvaia@gmail.com
[4] Cardiac/Pulmonary Rehabilitation, ASST PINI/CTO, Via Bignami 1, Milan, Italy
Full list of author information is available at the end of the article

Soft computing methods

SC is a branch of computer science introduced in the early 1990s [1]. It includes a collection of techniques that resemble biological processes more closely than

Table 1 Main soft computing uses in medicine

Main applications
Classification and prediction of disease categories
Diagnosis and prognosis
Medical decision-making processes
Physiological signal analysis
Epidemiological studies
Genetic association studies
Pharmacokinetics
Imaging
Geo-spatial distribution of diseases

traditional methodologies. SC deals with approximate reasoning, imprecision and uncertainty in order to achieve robustness and low-cost solutions for complex data analysis. This approach could excel in modern medicine, where the analysis and application of a large amount of knowledge are necessary to solve complex clinical problems, which in most cases are not deterministic. Table 1 lists the most important fields of application of SC methodologies in medicine.

SC models encompass automatic computing procedures, without human intervention, and are able to learn a task from a series of training examples. Moreover, they aim to generate sufficient output simple enough to be easily understood by the humans. Differently, classic statistical approaches are generally characterized by having an explicit model of probability, with the assumption that in most cases they require the intervention of an expert with regard to variable selection, transformation and overall structuring of the problem [2]. The general approach of SC modeling data analysis typically consists of four stages as shown in Fig. 1: (i) collection and encoding of clinical data in an electronic form suitable for further processing; (ii) data processing with techniques of feature extraction and dimension reduction (i.e., principal component analysis), selecting the most predictive parameters; (iii) pattern modeling selecting an SC model; (iv) extraction of knowledge by evaluating accuracy, sensitivity and specificity.

In the third step of Fig. 1, the most common SC models considered in this systematic review are shown: artificial neural networks (ANN), support vector machines (SVM), bayesian networks (BN), and fuzzy logic (FL).

Artificial Neural Networks

The ANN is a flexible non-linear model inspired by the brain's interconnections. ANNs possess an adaptable knowledge that is distributed over many neurons and synaptic connections. They are generally based on interconnected nodes (neurons), processing units able to compute input, activation and output functions. Each

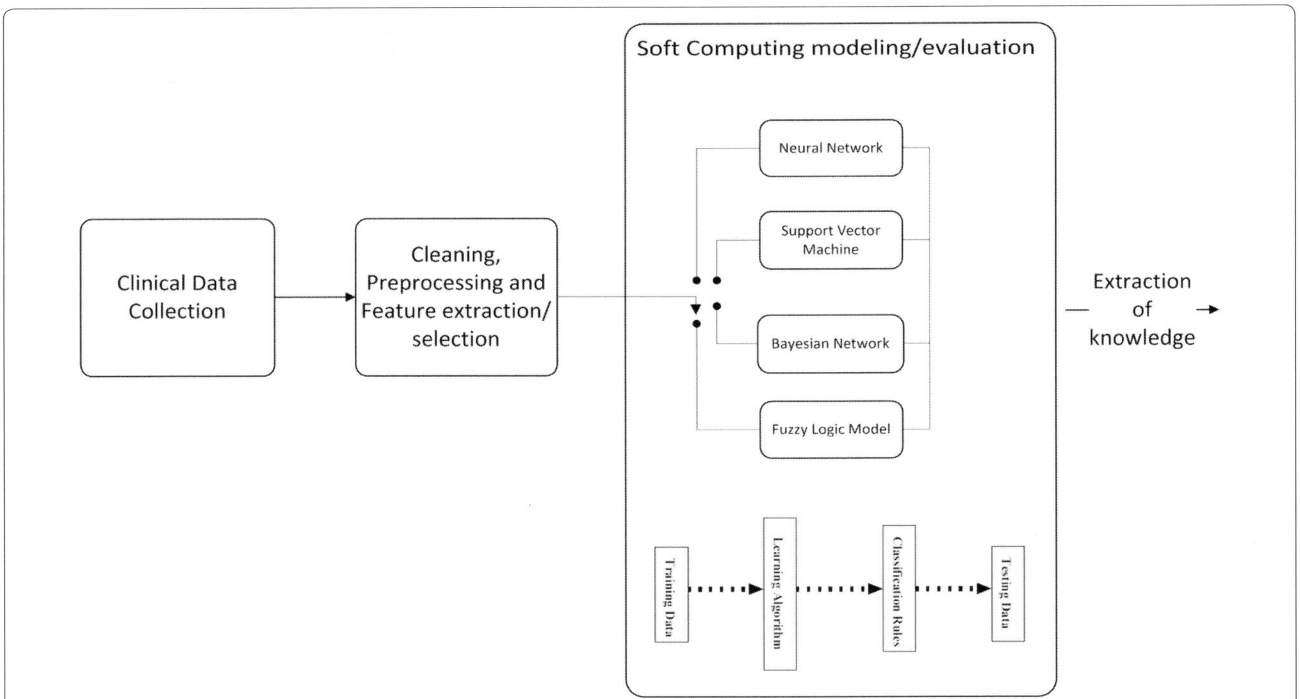

Fig. 1 Overview of soft computing-based data analysis process

connection (synapse strength) is provided by a weight adapted during the learning phase. The most common example of ANN is the multi-layer perceptron (MLP) [3]. The topology of the network is composed by interconnected nodes arranged in multiple layers. In the first layer each node corresponds to each input variable. The layers in the middle (hidden layers) represent the core of the non-linear model while the number of hidden nodes represents the complexity of the network. The relationships among variables are built using a sufficient number of training data and represented as functions using methods such as maximum likelihood estimation, maximum a posteriori or back propagation. The utility of ANN models lies in the fact that they can be used to infer a function from observations (training data). This is particularly useful in applications where the complexity of the data or tasks makes designing such a function by hand impractical. An interesting example of MLP, as shown in Fig. 2, was proposed by Hirsch et al. in 2001 to analyze an enormous amount of surveys to screen a population for asthma [4]. The trained neural network received as input 6825 screening questionnaires and was able to predict a final diagnosis of asthma with an accuracy of 74%.

The support vector machine

The SVM [5] is one of the most common machine learning models able to map the N input variables with a kernel function in an N-dimensional space (N-hyperplanes). The model is based on an algorithm able to find the best separating hyperplanes (maximum-margin hyperplane). Typically, SVM models are used for classification and regression analysis.

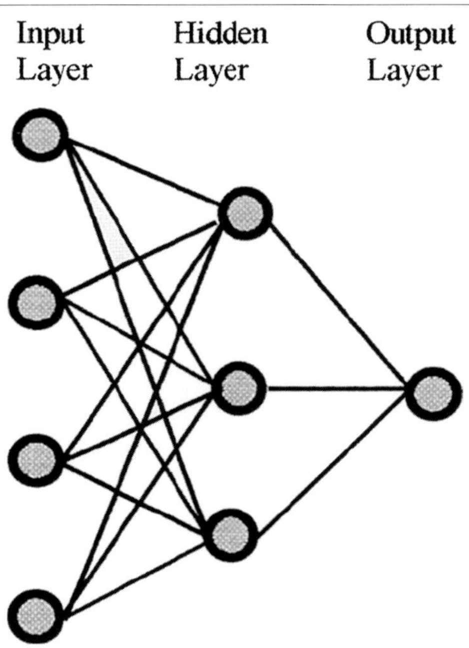

Fig. 2 The topology of multi-layer perceptron neural network to screen a population according to individual likelihood of asthma [4]. It is composed by interconnected nodes structured in three main layers. The input nodes represents questionnaire responses and the single output node represents probability of asthma

The Bayesian networks

The BN are suitable for providing a graphical representation of variables and their complex relationships. BN have the advantage of creating predictive models directly from data. The topology is an acyclic graph in which a set of nodes represents the variables, while the edges between nodes represent the probabilistic relationships between variables. More specifically, a node with an incoming arrow is conditioned by the node from which the arrow originates. Despite traditional regression approaches, BN are more flexible and accurate in small samples if we incorporate correct prior information and advantageous in handling missing data, which is prevalent in the clinical field. Moreover, they are not limited to representing the dependencies of a single outcome variable on predictor variables. Figure 3 reports an example of a BN model for studying asthma severity of Prosperi et al. [6]. The model reported in a tree topology was able to explain the main dependencies between severity and variables such as body mass index (BMI), forced expiratory flow (FEF), inhaled corti-costeroids (ICS), long-acting β_2-agonists (LABA) after a stepwise search in the whole original variable space.

The fuzzy logic model

While ANN, SVM and BN are important examples of SC models based on mathematical structures underlying learning, the FL approach [7] is based on integration of structured human knowledge into workable algorithms. Input and output of FL model are defined, converted to linguistic parameters (fuzzification) and the relationship among variables is generated through a set of rules (inference rules) defined by the experts. Finally, the output is represented by the aggregation of obtained results of input modules, converted into a numerical value (defuzzification) and classified. The FL approach is an alternative to the classic statistical methods where every proposition must either be "true" or "false". Instead, fuzzy logic asserts that things can be simultaneously "true" and "not true", with a certain membership degree to each class. FL techniques are used to deal with uncertainty and can be very powerful when there are poorly characterized parameters. In Fig. 4 an example of FL model provided by Zolnoori et al. to predict the level of asthma controls is reported [8]. The system is composed of 14 variables organized in five modules related to respiratory symptoms severity

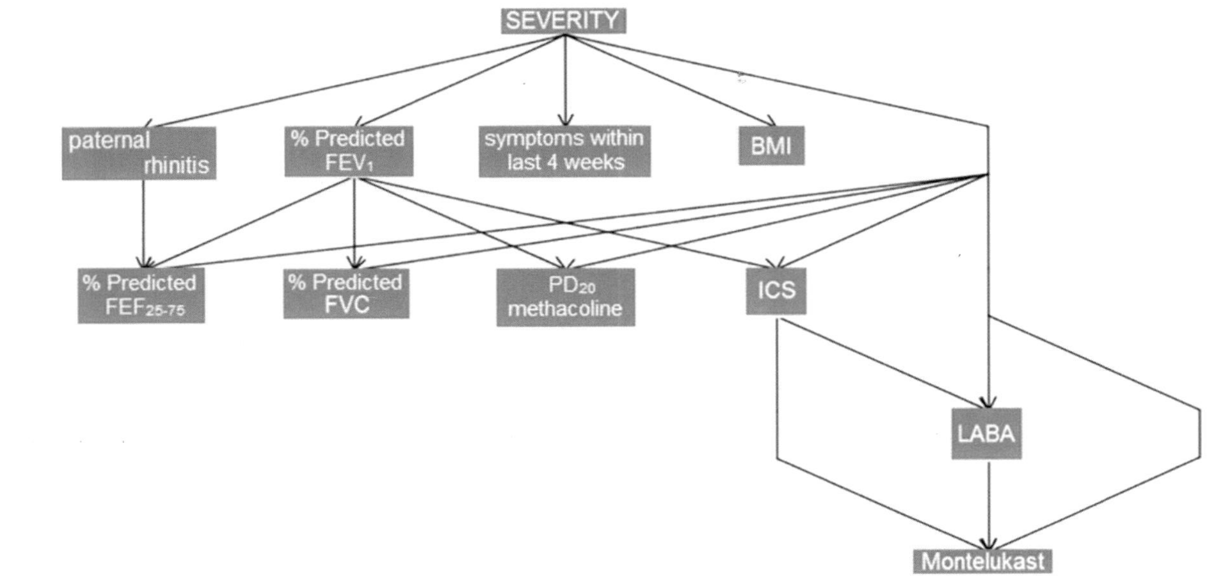

Fig. 3 Bayesian networks model evidences conditional dependencies between severity as diagnosed by the physician and the variable space selected by a stepwise search [6]. *BMI* body mass index, *FEF* forced expiratory flow, *ICS* inhaled corti-costeroids, *LABA* long-acting β_2-agonists

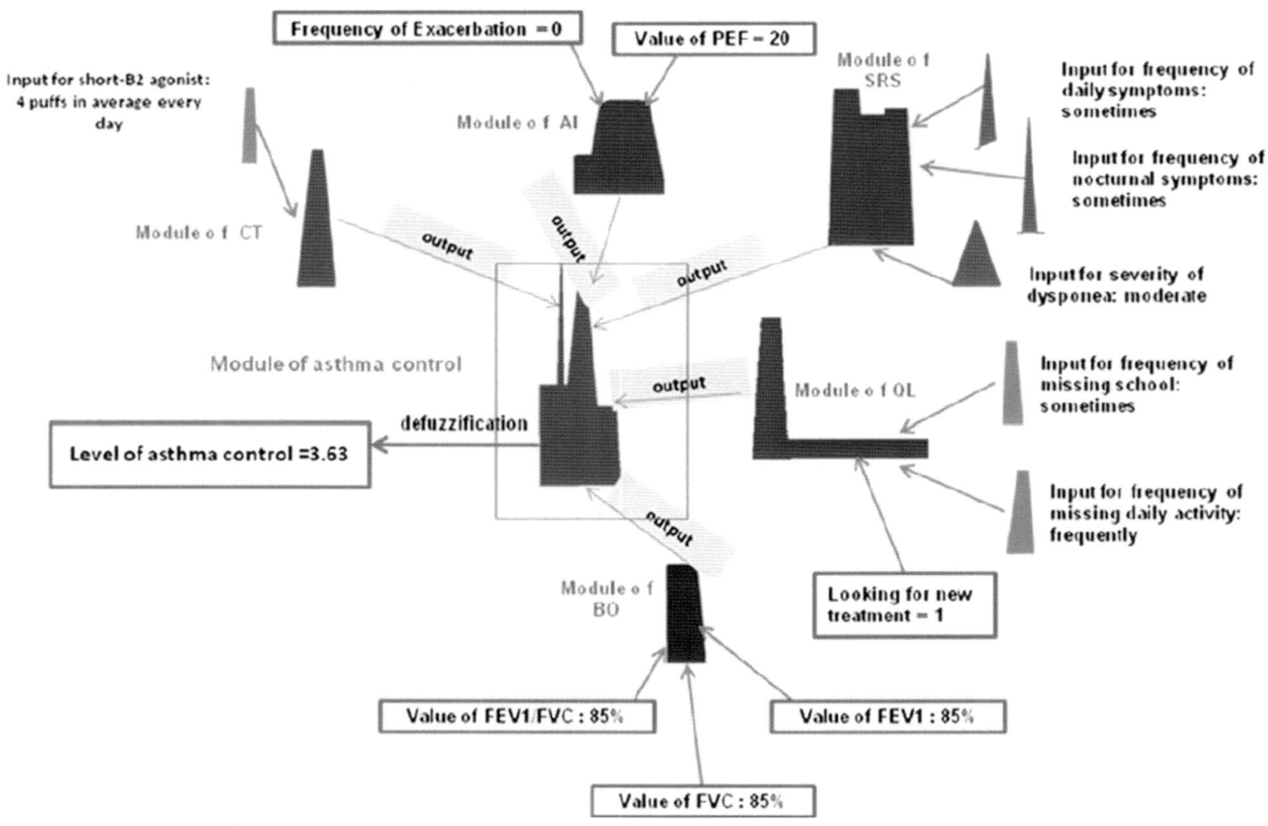

Fig. 4 Schematic view of fuzzy logic model able to combine input variables related to severity of respiratory symptoms (SRS), quality of life (QL), current medical treatment (CT), instability of asthma (AI), bronchial obstruction (BO) to infer the level of asthma control (AC) [8]

(SRS), bronchial obstruction (BO), asthma instability (AI), current treatment (CT), and quality of life (QL). All these variables are represented with fuzzy rules defined by experts and then aggregated in a fuzzy network. The output of the system is given by the degree of asthma control classified in five categories: excellent (0–1), good (1–3), fair (3–5), poor (5–7), and very poor (7–10).

Methods

Literature search

The research was performed on PubMed and ScienceDirect, covering the period starting from September 1, 1990 through April 19, 2016. We explored studies dealing with the most frequently adopted SC models (ANN, SVM, BN, FL) and allergic diseases. Research in PubMed was performed using medical subject headings (MeSH®) to report the most common SC methodologies employed to study the most frequent allergic diseases included under the Mesh term "hypersensitivity". The keywords used to search were based on the following logical linguistic pattern: ("Hypersensitivity"[Mesh]) AND ("Neural Networks [Computer]"[Mesh]) OR ("Support Vector Machines"[Mesh]) OR ("Bayes Theorem"[Mesh]) OR ("Fuzzy Logic"[Mesh]). Instead, the electronic search strategy on ScienceDirect was performed with the following queries: ("asthma" or "adverse drug reactions" or "allergic rhinitis" or "atopic dermatitis" or "allergic conjunctivitis") and ("artificial neural networks" or "support vector machine" or "Bayesian network" or "fuzzy logic").

Inclusion and exclusion criteria

The research was limited to clinical cross-sectional studies and case–control studies of articles published in peer-reviewed journals. Case–study reports, genetic association studies, cost-effectiveness healthcare studies, pollen/climate changes and classification of respiratory sounds were discarded from the review.

Study selection

The research was conducted independently by two authors, who evaluated whether the information of each reference was relevant or not. Each disagreement between the two reviewers was resolved by discussion until a consensus was reached. If the abstract did not include enough information to evaluate inclusion or exclusion, the full text of publication was reviewed if available. Otherwise, the paper was excluded. The selected papers were sorted by relevance and grouped for each allergic disease (Table 3). In this report, we first review recent findings for SC model-related allergic diseases (summarized in Table 2), evaluating the accuracy, sensitivity and specificity of SC models. We then critically discuss the potential strength and future implications for research in this field.

Results

We identified 10,643 references from citation database queries, respectively 10,486 from ScienceDirect and 157 from PubMed. The systematic review, whose details are shown in Fig. 5, revealed 27 papers dealing with clinical trials related to allergic diseases and SC models in the above-mentioned period.

In the present systematic review, the selected papers were grouped according to the specific type of allergy (Table 3): 18 works on asthma detection and diagnosis, six on adverse drug reactions (ADR), one on allergic rhinitis, one on allergic conjunctivitis and one on atopic dermatitis.

Studies on asthma

Findings from clinical studies about asthma suggest that SC models are mainly suitable for classification of exacerbations, severity, recognition of asthmatic patients vs. controls and for asthma level control. Predicting the correct category of exacerbation severity is challenging in order to assess the appropriate hospitalization of the patient [9]. Sanders et al. [10] first proposed an SC model to detect asthma exacerbation in patients from the pediatric emergency department. They employed a BN model analyzing variables related to past diagnoses, allergies, family history, medications, social history and vital signs (temperature, respiratory rate, and oxygen saturation). The output of the network was the probability of a patient being admitted to the emergency department with asthma exacerbation and being eligible for treatment using asthma-care guidelines (GINA). The implemented model was able to identify guideline-eligible patients with an accuracy of 96%. Dexheimer et al. [11], using the same database as Sanders et al. [10], compared BN and other SC methodologies such as ANN and Gaussian processes, for identifying asthma exacerbations. Here, the accuracies achieved were 96, 95.6 and 94%, respectively, with no significant differences. In a recent prospective study, Farion et al. [12] compared different SC models using tenfold cross-validation and BN achieved the best performances. In a second phase of work they compared BN results with predictions derived by the pediatric respiratory assessment measure (PRAM) score [10] and with those made by physicians, obtaining high comparable results. In another study, Finkelstein et al. [13] integrated the SC methodologies in a decision support home telemonitoring platform to predict asthma exacerbations. The study dataset was based on daily self-reports administered on 26 adult asthmatic patients at home. All the collected data were analyzed with a BN classifier and an SVM able to predict asthma exacerbation with an accuracy of 80%. Zolnoori et al. [14] developed an intelligent clinical decision support system

Table 2 Studies dealing with SC models and allergic diseases

Authors	Application	Subjects	Description	Input features	SC model	Findings
Prosperi et al. [6]	To predict asthma severity	383 children with asthma (age 6–18 years)	Use of unsupervised statistical learning techniques, such as exploratory factor analysis (EFA), hierarchical clustering (HC) to identify asthma phenotypes	Lung function, inflammatory and allergy markers, family history, environmental exposures, body mass index, age of asthma onset and medications	BN	Significant recognition of asthma severity
Farion et al. [12]	To predict asthma exacerbation	322 Phase 1: 240 children (age 1–17 years) Phase 2: 82 children (age 1–17 years)	Phase 1: selection of the most accurate machine learning model with WEKA tool Phase 2: comparison of performance of BN with PRAM score and Physicians	42 attributes corresponding to the patient's history, current asthma exacerbation, primary assessment and a selected secondary assessment	BN	Phase 1: Accuracy = 68% Phase 2: Accuracy = 70.7%
Finkelstein et al. [13]	To predict asthma exacerbation	26 adult asthmatic patients	Use of a modern telemonitoring system at home	Daily self-reports	SVM	Accuracy = 80% Sensitivity = 84% Specificity = 80%
Sanders et al. [10]	To predict asthma exacerbation	4023 patients (age 2–18 years)	Use of a SC model to identify patients eligible for asthma care guidelines	Past diagnoses, allergies, family history, medications, social history and vital signs (temperature, respiratory rate, and oxygen saturation)	BN	Accuracy = 96% Sensitivity = 90% Specificity = 88.3%
Dexheimer et al. [11]	Same of Sanders et al. [10]	4023 patients (age 2–18 years)	Comparison of machine learning models to best identify patients eligible for an asthma care guideline	Same of Sanders et al. [10]	ANN,BN, Gaussian processes (GP)	BN accuracy = 96% GP accuracy = 95.6% ANN accuracy = 94%
Pifferi et al. [20]	To classify asthma control levels	77 patients (age 7.5–17 years)	Assessment of spirometry and fractional exhaled nitric oxide (FeNO) measurements to classify asthma control according to GINA guidelines	1st model: values of spirometry; 2nd model: values of FeNO; 3rd model: values of spirometry and FeNO	ANN	3rd model achieved best performances of classification Accuracy = 86.4%
Pifferi et al. [17]	To classify asthmatic vs control	123 90 asthmatic children (age 9–16 years) and 33 controls (age 12–13 years),	Pattern recognition analysis of the exhaled breath temperature curve	The rate of temperature increase and the mean plateau value	ANN	Accuracy = 5% Sensitivity = 77.2% Specificity = 99%
Jaing et al. [21]	To classify how children manage their asthma	305 children (age 5–14 years)	Each participant was given 10 asthma-based problems and asked to manage them	Each management decision and its order	ANN	Significant classification of five major classes representing different approaches to solving an acute asthma case

Table 2 continued

Authors	Application	Subjects	Description	Input features	SC model	Findings
Kharroubi et al. [24]	To classify health state of patient with asthma	307 subjects	Estimation of a preference-based index for asthma (five-dimensional asthma quality of life utility index)	99 features about health statuscs	BN	BN model is more appropriate than conventionally used parametric random-effects model
Hirsch et al. [4]	To classify asthmatic vs control	6825 adults (age $\geq$ 16)	Respiratory questionnaires were analyzed by experts and compared with results provided by neural network	12 answers provided by the respiratory questionnaire (wheezing, chest tightness, shortness of breath, night cough), family history of asthma and associated conditions of hay fever or eczema	ANN	Accuracy = 74%
Chatzimichail et al. [19]	To classify asthmatic vs control	112 children (age 7–14 years)	Three step analysis:1-feature selection with Principal Component Analysis, 2-pattern classification, 3-performance evaluation	46 prognostic factors including data on asthma, allergic diseases, and lifestyle factors	SVM	Accuracy = 95.54% Sensitivity = 95.45% Specificity = 95.59%
Goulart et al. [32]	To classify allergic conjunctivitis vs control	102 48 with allergic conjunctivitis and 54 controls (age 3–14 years)	Allergic conjunctivitis questionnaires were analyzed by experts and compared with results provided by neural network	7 items selected from a questionnaire of 15 answers	ANN	Accuracy = 100%
Takahashi et al. [33]	To classify atopic dermatitis vs control	4610 answers, 2714 infants (12 months old) and 1896 children (2 years old)	To analyze the predictive accuracy of the predictive model for effect of atopic dermatitis in infancy, from the data of the epidemiological survey	Family history (father, mother, siblings, grand-father, grand-mother), food restriction, food allergy, age, food restriction of mother, egg introduced time, cow's milk introduced time	ANN	Accuracy = 96.4% Sensitivity = 88.6% Specificity = 99.5%
Christopher et al. [31]	To classify allergic rhinitis vs control	872 patients of all age groups	Allergic rhinitis reports of intradermal skin tests were analyzed by experts and compared with results provided by neural network	Patient's history and 40 clinically relevant allergens	ANN	Accuracy = 88.31% Sensitivity = 88.3% Specificity = 88.2%
De Matas et al. [23]	To predict the clinical effect of salbutamol	23 12 healthy volunteers and 11 mild asthmatics	In vivo and in vitro data of human subjects were analyzed using SC modeling	Demographic data and urinary levels of salbutamol and metabolite	ANN	Accuracy = 83.5%

Table 2 continued

Authors	Application	Subjects	Description	Input features	SC model	Findings
De Matas et al. [22]	To predict the clinical effect of salbutamol	18 mild-moderate asthmatic patients	SC modeling to predict the bronchodilator response at 10 (T10) and 20 (T20) min after receiving each of the 4 doses for each of the 3 different particle sizes	Aerodynamic particle size (APS), body surface area (BSA), age, pre-treatment forced expiratory volume in one-second (FEV1), forced vital capacity, cumulative emitted drug dose and bronchodilator reversibility	ANN	Accuracy = 88%
Gandhi et al. [25]	To predict hypersensitivity reaction	2458 reports concerning thrombotic events selected from AERS (adverse event reporting system) database	Retrospective analysis focused on thrombotic events associated with C1 esterase inhibitor products	Adverse events; demographic and administrative information; drug/biologic information; report sources; patient outcomes; drug therapy start and end dates; indications for use/diagnosis	BN	Potential signals of C1 esterase inhibitor product—associated thrombotic events among patients with hereditary angioedema were identified
Naranjo et al. [28]	To predict the posterior probability of a drug (BARDI tool)	51 patients	BARDI tool, calculates the posterior probability of a drug being the cause based on epidemiologic and case data	Reactions after receiving aromatic anticonvulsants	BN	Accuracy = 93% Sensitivity = 94% Specificity = 50%
Lanctot et al. [29]	To predict the posterior probability of a drug (BARDI tool)	27 cases of skin reactions	BARDI, combined with the LTA, a biochemical test that determines the percent of cell death because of toxic metabolites of a drug	Skin reactions associated with sulfonamide therapy	BN	Accuracy = 96% Sensitivity = 79% Specificity = 38%
Lanctot et al. [30]	To predict the posterior probability of a drug (BARDI tool)	106 challenging cases	BARDI, compared with the Adverse Drug Reaction Probability Scale (APS)	Drug- and nondrug-induced adverse events	BN	BN model discriminate better than ADR drug from nondrug-induced cases.
Kadoyama et al. [26]	To predict hypersensitivity reaction caused by anticancer agents	1,644,220 reported cases from 2004 to 2009 (AERS database)	SC model to detect important pattern related to anticancer agents-associated adverse events	Adverse events; demographic and administrative information; drug/biologic information; report sources; patient outcomes; drug therapy start and end dates; indications for use/diagnosis	BN	Potential signals were detected for paclitaxel-associated mild, severe, and lethal hypersensitivity reactions, and docetaxel-associated lethal reactions
Sakaeda et al. [27]	To predict hypersensitivity reactions caused by platinum agents	1,644,220 reported cases from 2004 to 2009 (AERS database)	The BN analysis aims to search for previously unknown patterns and automatically detect important signals, i.e., platinum agent-associat d adverse events, from such a large database	Adverse events; demographic and administrative information; drug/biologic information; report sources; patient outcomes; drug therapy start and end dates	BN	Significant association between the platinum agent-and mild, severe, and lethal hypersensitivity reactions

Table 2 continued

Authors	Application	Subjects	Description	Input features	SC model	Findings
Lurie et al. [16]	To classify asthma severity	113 patients (age 42.9 ± 16.3 years)	Implementation of a fuzzy model able to combine patients' and doctors' asthma perceptions	Doctor assessment, variables self-assessed by patients (dyspnea, perceived treatment efficacy, asthma-related quality of life questionnaire (AQLQ)), patients' sociodemographic characteristics, and asthma characteristics	FL	Accuracy = 73%
Zolnoori et al. [8]	To classify asthma control level	42 asthmatic patients	Implementation of a fuzzy model able to estimate the level of asthma control and help physicians to manage their patients more effectively	Respiratory symptom severity, bronchial obstruction, asthma instability, current treatment and quality of life	FL	Accuracy = 100%
Zolnoori et al. [14]	To classify asthma exacerbation	25 patients	Implementation of a fuzzy model able to estimate the level of asthma exacerbation and help physicians to manage their patients more effectively	Status of breathless, status of wheeze, status of alertness, status of respiratory rate, status of talk, status of pulse/min heart rate, value of PEF after initial bronchodilator, value of $paCO_2$, value of SaO_2%	FL	Accuracy = 100%
Zolnoori et al. [15]	To classify asthma severity	28 patients	Implementation of a fuzzy model able to estimate the four categories of asthma severity and help physicians to manage their patients more effectively	Bronchial obstruction, response to drug, skin prick test, severity of respiratory symptoms, instability of asthma, IgE value, quality of life	FL	Accuracy = 100%
Zolnoori et al. [18]	To classify asthmatic vs control	278 139 asthmatic patients and 139 non-asthmatic patients (age range 6–18)	Implementation of a fuzzy model to help physicians to manage their patients more effectively	Medical history, environmental factors, allergic rhinitis, genetic factors, consequences of asthma on lung tissues, response to laboratory tests and response to short-term medicine	FL	Sensitivity = 88% Specificity = 100%

SC soft computing, *ANN* artificial neural networks, *SVM* support vector machines, *BN* Bayesian networks, *FL* Fuzzy logic, *PRAM* pediatric respiratory assessment measure. *GINA* global initiative for asthma

(CDSS) based on the FL model to assess the level of asthma exacerbation. Input variables included the status of breathlessness, status of wheeze, status of alertness, status of respiratory rate, status of talk, status of pulse/min heart rate, value of PEF after initial bronchodilator, value of $paCO_2$, value of SaO_2%. The model was able to classify patients in four categories of asthma exacerbation including mild, moderate, severe and respiratory arrest imminent (RAI), achieving an accuracy of 100% (Cohen's coefficient $k = 1$). The studies analyzed so far suggested the high accuracy of an SC method to detect the correct level of asthma exacerbation. Within this review we also examined the role of SC methodologies in classifying the severity of asthma. Zolnoori et al. [15], in a second study, evaluated asthma severity by implementing a fuzzy rule expert system composed by seven input modules. Analyzed variables included bronchial obstruction, response to drugs, skin prick test, severity of respiratory symptoms, instability of asthma, IgE antibodies value and quality of life. This work evidenced a complete correspondence between model's and physician's evaluation (mild intermittent, mild persistent, moderate persistent, severe persistent) with and accuracy of 100% (Cohen's coefficient $k = 1$). In another study, Laure et al. [16] proposed the fuzzy approach to model the patient's perception of asthma severity. The model included variables self-assessed by patients (dyspnea, perceived treatment efficacy, asthma-related quality of life questionnaire (AQLQ), patients' socio-demographic characteristics, and asthma characteristics. The output of the model was compared with doctor assessment of asthma severity according to (GINA) guidelines. The study highlighted a clear tendency of the patient to underestimate asthma severity compared to the doctor assessment. This finding suggest that assessment of asthma severity should consider both patients' and doctors' perceptions of the disease and should include an AQLQ measure. Prosperi et al. [6] adopted BN to analyze non-linear relationships among variables and identified prognostic factors of asthma severity. Input variables included lung function, inflammatory and allergy markers, family history, environmental exposures, body mass index, age of asthma onset and medications. SC methodologies were found to help investigators to identify complex patterns and structures in the data, despite needing a thoughtful selection of input features and an appropriate data labeling in the case of identification of real asthma subgroups. Other studies examined the capabilities of SC methodologies to distinguish asthmatic patients from controls. Pifferi et al. [17] tested an ANN by extracting input features from the exhaled breath temperature curve (i.e., the rate of temperature increase and the mean plateau value). The model was tested in 90 asthmatic children and 33 healthy age-matched controls. ANN was able to recognize asthmatic children and controls with an accuracy of 99.3 and 70.3% respectively. In another study, an FL model was developed, and a sensitivity of 88% and specificity of 100% was obtained for a cutoff value of 0.7 of ROC curve [18].

These studies show the utility of an intelligent patient-based SC system to support asthma diagnosis, especially in developing countries, because of limitations on access to medical specialists and laboratory facilities. This review revealed that the use of SC methodologies could also have an important impact on analyzing huge amounts of screening questionnaires and to predict allergic diseases. In 2001 Hirsch et al. [4], proposed the use of ANN to screen a population for asthma, using the responses to a respiratory questionnaire. A random sample of 180 from 6825 respondents to a community survey underwent clinical review. Each survey was labeled according to likelihood of asthma, combining three independent expert opinions. The ANN was trained using the 12 questionnaire responses as input and the probability labels as outputs. Using the known probability labels from the training set, it was possible to derive the expected proportion of true asthmatic patients. In 2013 Chatzimichail et al. [19] proposed an intelligent approach based on SVM for asthma prediction in symptomatic preschool children based on questionnaire analysis. In this study 112 patients ranging from 7 to 14 years of age were analyzed. The performances of the SVM were evaluated by using the tenfold cross-validation approach and achieved an accuracy of 95.54%. Some studies emphasized the use of SC methodologies to objectivize the categorization of asthma control levels. Pifferi et al. [20] developed three ANNs (multi-layer perceptron) able to classify children with allergies according to three classes provided by GINA assessment (controlled, partially controlled and uncontrolled asthma) using only the input value of two simple measurements, namely spirometry and fractional exhaled nitric oxide (FeNO). Among the three tested models, only the input combination of values of spirometry and FeNO was able to provide high accuracy. More specifically, the model was able to recognize 100% of children with uncontrolled asthma, 74% with partially controlled asthma and 99% with totally controlled asthma. The same work presented a cross-sectional study of 77 children with allergic asthma. In this case the selected ANN model prospectively identified correctly 100% of uncontrolled, 79.5% of partially controlled and 79.6% of the controlled children. In another work, based on an FL model to predict the asthma control level, the clinical features of spirometry were combined with another four input classes of variables provided by the patients: respiratory symptom severity, asthma instability, current

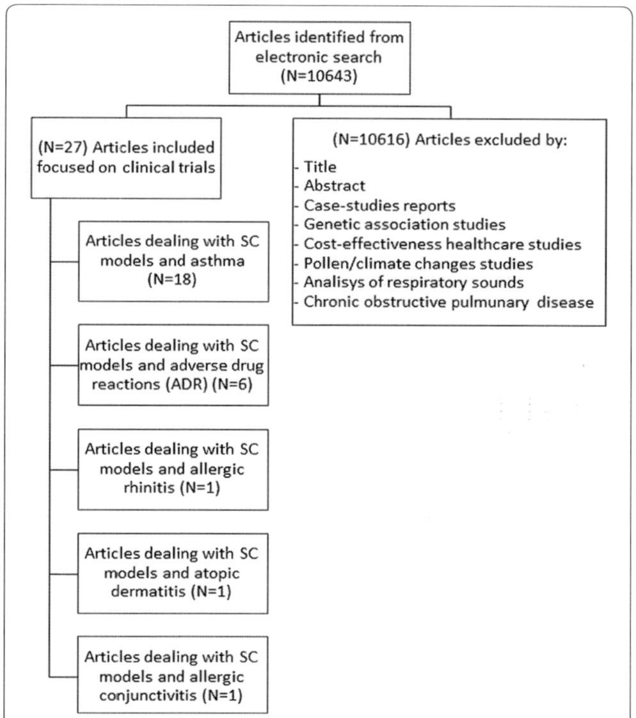

Fig. 5 Search strategy used to select articles included into this review

treatment and quality of life. The model was able to discriminate five categories of asthma control level: very poor, poor, fair, good, and excellent, achieving an accuracy of 100% (Cohen's coefficient k = 1) [8]. These findings suggest that the combination of clinical features (i.e., spirometry) and the subjective information provided by asthmatic patients can improve the performance of classification of SC models and help physicians to manage their patients more effectively. Another study demonstrates how SC models, through a training and pattern-recognition approach, can solve classification problems even when the specific category is not well-defined. In this regard, in a pilot study Jaing et al. [21] proposed the use of ANN to identify children's behavior categories representing different approaches of asthma management. This review also revealed that SC models are potentially useful for estimating pharmacokinetics performances. In two clinical trials, De Matas et al. [22, 23] used the ANN to model in vitro and in vivo data to predict the clinical effects of dry powder inhaler formulations containing salbutamol sulfate in individual subjects. In the first study, on healthy subjects the trained ANN was able to predict 83% of cumulative urinary excretion of salbutamol and metabolite 0–24 h post-inhalation. The correct prediction of ANN for mild asthmatic patients was 84%. In the second study, the ANN model was used to forecast the bronchodilator response defined as ΔFEV1 (%) measured at both 10 (T10) and 20 (T20) minutes after receiving each of the four doses of salbutamol sulfate puffs for each of the three different particle sizes (1.5, 3 and 6 μm).The average error between predicted and observed ΔFEV1(%) for individual subjects was <4% across the cumulative dosing regimen. These findings provide further evidence that ANNs supply a suitable approach for modeling complex biological data sets and have the potential to generate predictable models that can provide reliable estimations of clinical response to inhaled drug products in humans. The last clinical study about SC models and asthma disease was proposed by Kharroubi et al. [24], who explored the use of a non-parametric Bayesian method to classify the health state of people with asthma. The work presents the results of the non-parametric

Table 3 Overview of clinical studies related to SC models and allergic diseases

Type of allergy	No. of studies	Overall accuracy (%)	Application	ANN	SVM	BN	FL
Asthma	18	82.44 ± 23.71	To classify exacerbations [10–14]	1	1	2	1
			To classify severity [6, 15, 16]	–	–	1	2
			To classify pathologic vs control [4, 17–19]	2	1	–	1
			To classify asthma control level [8, 20]	1	–	–	1
			To classify how manage their pathology [21]	1	–	–	–
			To predict the clinical effect of salbutamol [22, 23]	2	–	–	–
			To classify health state[24]	–	–	1	–
ADR	6	94.5 ± 2.12	To predict the posterior probability of a drug (BARDI tool) [28–30]	–	–	3	–
			To predict hypersensitivity reaction (AERS database) [25–27]	–	–	3	–
Allergic rhinitis	1	88.31	To classify pathologic vs control [31]	1	–	–	–
Allergic conjunctivitis	1	100	To classify pathologic vs control [32]	1	–	–	–
Atopic dermatitis	1	96.4	To classify pathologic vs control [33]	1	–	–	–

model compared to the original model estimated using a conventional parametric random-effects model. This work evidenced that the non-parametric Bayesian models are theoretically more appropriate than previously used parametric models and provide better estimates of asthma quality of life.

Studies on adverse drug reactions

This review examined results about the use of SC models and adverse drug reactions (ADRs). Three studies evaluated the ADRs from the public version of the food and drug administration (FDA) adverse event reporting system (AERS). A large dataset of 1,644,220 case reports from 2004 to 2009 was analyzed through the use of a BN. In particular, Gandhi et al. [25] identified 10 combination cases of thrombotic events associated with the use of one C1 esterase inhibitor product (Cinryze) in patients with hereditary angioedema. Kadoyama et al. [26] evaluated the susceptibility to hypersensitivity reactions to anticancer agents using parameters based on a Bayesian confidence propagation neural network, and the empirical Bayes geometric mean. These indexes of pharmacovigilance provided signals of mild, severe and lethal hypersensitivity reactions associated with paclitaxel and docetaxel agents. In another study [27], the same group demonstrated with the same approach that carboplatin and oxaliplatin caused mild, severe, and lethal hypersensitivity reactions, whereas cisplatin did not. The use of dexamethasone affected oxaliplatin-induced mild hypersensitivity reactions, but had lesser effects on severe and lethal reactions. These findings highlight the significant potential of SC models to analyze huge amounts of data and the ability to discover patterns deeply hidden within the data. Another three studies highlighted the importance of a diagnostic tool for assessment of adverse drug events (BARDI). This computer program is based on BN and is able to perform a differential diagnosis on cutaneous reactions suspected of being drug-induced [28–30].

Studies on other allergic diseases

Finally, the review revealed that few studies about SC models and other allergic diseases are present in literature. In 2015 Christopher et al. [31]. presented a CDSS based on ANN to assist junior clinicians to diagnoses the presence or absence of allergic rhinitis analyzing reports of intradermal skin tests. The trained neural network achieved an accuracy of 88, 31%. In another work Goulart et al. [32] proposed the ANN to study an allergic conjunctivitis screening questionnaire. In this work the ANN predicted allergic diagnosis in 100% of cases using 7 of the 15 existent items. A study conducted in Japan by Takahashi et al. [33], proposed the use of ANN to predict the effects of atopic dermatitis in infancy from an epidemiological survey. A total of 4610 answered surveys were received: 2714 from mothers of infants (12 months old) and 1896 from mothers of children (2 years old). The sensitivity, specificity and predictive accuracy of the ANN model were respectively 88.6, 99.5 and 96.4%.

Discussion

Main findings

This systematic literature review explored the main SC methodologies to investigate allergic diseases. Results were obtained after an exhaustive literature research and examination of hundreds of papers focused on clinical trials. Several studies provided results about SC systems focused on early diagnosis of allergic diseases and the classification of illness categories (i.e., exacerbation, severity) obtaining a mean accuracy of 86.5%. More specifically, this review revealed that the SC approach could have an important impact on the analysis of an enormous amount of screening questionnaires and in the prediction of allergic diseases, discovering patterns deeply hidden within the still-unexplored data [32, 33]. This is possible because the SC models are flexible and able to generalize and predict on an individual basis the probability of diagnosis related to the specific disease of questionnaire respondents. In this specific case, the ANN and BN models are particularly suitable. Another important issue that the use of SC models can resolve concerns missing data in clinical trials. Frequently patients do not complete their follow-up according to a protocol for a variety of reasons, making data analysis more difficult. The BN is a good example of models naturally suitable for handling missing data, as suggested by Carpenter et al. [34, 35]. Another important result emerging from our review is that the SC models could have an important role in CDSS. Indeed, they provide an opportunity to assess the overall information of the main phenomena coming from patients (i.e., identifying information, family history, environmental exposure, perceived treatment efficacy, disease-related quality of life questionnaire) and clinicians (i.e., laboratory tests, values of spirometry), underlying critical features of the disease, treatment planning and the provision of warnings by adding new evidence through associative recall from historical data. In this regard, studies on clinical emergence coupling CDSS-human interaction with the clinician's knowledge and the suggestions of feedback signals are undertaken in order to generate patient-specific advice and to assist clinicians at the point of care [14, 31, 36]. SC models are also suitable for analyzing data when the likelihood is not defined and statistical tests are not appropriate. More specifically, the choice of an FL approach in substitution of other SC models can provide valuable support, since it starts from the context of a lack of experience data and entangled cause-and-effect relationships, which make it difficult to assess or diagnosis allergic diseases at an early stage [8, 16]. FL is extremely flexible, allowing the decision maker to use a broad range of linguistic variables and modifiers for finer discrimination. It is also a useful system in the case of the presence of a series of sub-decisions where available data is based on vagueness, uncertainty and opinion, such as questionnaires.

Strengths and limitations

Strengths of this review are related to an exhaustive literature search in PubMed and ScienceDirect databases. The research was performed following PRISMA guidelines and using recommended search queries with consensus finding. Moreover the protocol of this review was registered within the PROSPERO database, with the code CRD42016038894. We found most of SC works deal with asthma, six studies about ADR, and few studies about other allergic diseases. In this regard, in some cases their accuracy although high was quantitatively synthesized on few works. This result reveals how the SC approach is widely used to diagnose asthma, but it is still largely unexplored for other hypersensitivity diseases. Moreover, there are also limitations with the studies themselves. To date, a comparative analysis of SC performances with classic statistical methods was not possible due to the lack of studies comparing these models against a benchmark. This is due to the fact that in most cases the use of these advanced techniques needs to overcome obstacles including the need to establish multidisciplinary teams [37], the resistance to change in working practice especially from older clinicians [38] and the lack of appropriate gold standard clinical assessment procedures [39].

Conclusions

This systematic review, analyzing clinical trials employing SC methodologies, shows as these methodologies have been used in allergy field for several purposes such as for detecting patients with asthma exacerbations, to prompt clinicians to identify guideline-eligible patients, to evaluate putative ADR, to discriminate drug from nondrug-induced reactions, to improve the diagnostic accuracy and to enhance the management of patients with hypersensitivity reactions. The review also identify promising trends, especially in the diagnosis, prognosis and treatment of some allergic diseases, but also the need for a more extensive application as occurs in genetic association studies [40–43].

Such methods enable a new concept for modeling allergic diseases that combines the collection and mining of multimodal clinical evidence, with dynamic modeling of causal factors. We believe that the introduction of SC models can ease the exploration of big clinical data sets to enable better understanding of allergic disease subgroups, their pathophysiology and optimization of existing treatments. Clinicians should improve evidence by undertaking more randomized controlled trials to prove the efficacy of SC methodologies. In this regard, they should be trained to be more confident with the new perspective provided by these advanced techniques going over their standard methods of choice in interpreting medical data. The review provides evidence that SC methodologies can play a key role in predicting the onset, diagnosing, evaluating pathogenesis and prognosis and managing most of allergic diseases. Moreover, these methods can discover new patterns and evidence about early recognition of inflammatory markers and their relation to allergic diseases [44]. Nowadays most studies deal with asthma, however it is to be hoped that in the near future SC methodologies could be used to investigate all allergic diseases, with a particular attention to those pathologies with a huge burden on health for their impact on quality of life and their severity, such as urticaria and anaphylaxis.

Authors' contributions

GT, AT, LB and GP made substantial contribution to conception and design of the review. SG, PLM and CI participated in critical revision and drafting of the manuscript. LB, GP and SG participated in literature search and manuscript writing. All authors read and approved the final manuscript.

Author details

[1] Messina Unit, National Research Council of Italy (CNR)-Institute of Applied Science and Intelligent System (ISASI), Messina, Italy. [2] Pisa Unit, National Research Council of Italy (CNR)-Institute of Clinical Physiology (IFC), Pisa, Italy. [3] School and Division of Allergy and Clinical Immunology, Department of Clinical and Experimental Medicine, University Hospital "G. Martino", Messina, Italy. [4] Cardiac/Pulmonary Rehabilitation, ASST PINI/CTO, Via Bignami 1, Milan, Italy.

Acknowledgements

None.

References

1. Zadeh LA. Fuzzy logic, neural networks, and soft computing. Commun ACM. 1994;37:77–84.
2. Michie D, Spiegelhalter DJ, Taylor CC. Machine learning, neural and statistical classification. Ellis Horwood Limited; 1994.
3. Rosenblatt F. Principles of neurodynamics. Perceptrons and the theory of brain mechanisms. Cornell Aeronautical Laboratory, Report no. VG-1196-G-8; 1961.

4. Hirsch S, Shapiro JL, Turega MA, Frank TL, Niven RM, Frank PI. Using a neural network to screen a population for asthma. Ann Epidemiol. 2001;11:369–76.
5. Cortes C, Vapnik V. Support-vector networks. Mach Learn. 1995;20:273–97.
6. Prosperi MC, Sahiner UM, Belgrave D, Sackesen C, Buchan IE, Simpson A, et al. Challenges in identifying asthma subgroups using unsupervised statistical learning techniques. Am J Respir Crit Care Med. 2013;188:1303–12.
7. Zadeh LA. A note on prototype theory and fuzzy sets. Cognition. 1962;12:291–7.
8. Zolnoori M, Fazel Zarandi MH, Moin M, Taherian M. Fuzzy rule-based expert system for evaluating level of asthma control. J Med Syst. 2012;36:2947–58.
9. Dexheimer JW, Abramo TJ, Arnold DH, Johnson KB, Shyr Y, Ye F, et al. An asthma management system in a pediatric emergency department. Int J Med Inform. 2013;82:230–8.
10. Sanders DL, Aronsky D. Detecting asthma exacerbations in a pediatric emergency department using a Bayesian network. Am Med Inform Assoc Annu Symp Proc. 2006;2006:684–8.
11. Dexheimer JW, Brown LE, Leegon J, Aronsky D. Comparing decision support methodologies for identifying asthma exacerbations. In: Proceedings of the 12th World Congress on Health (Medical) Informatics; Building Sustainable Health Systems 880. IOS Press; 2007.
12. Farion KJ, Wilk S, Michalowski W, O'Sullivan D, Sayyad-Shirabad J. Comparing predictions made by a prediction model, clinical score, and physicians: pediatric asthma exacerbations in the emergency department. Appl Clin Inform. 2013;4:376–91.
13. Finkelstein J, Wood J. Predicting asthma exacerbations using artificial intelligence. ICIMTH. 2013;190:56–8.
14. Zolnoori M, Zarandi MH, Moin M. Application of intelligent systems in asthma disease: designing a fuzzy rule-based system for evaluating level of asthma exacerbation. J Med Syst. 2012;36:2071–83.
15. Zolnoori M, Zarandi MH, Moin M, Teimorian S. Fuzzy rule-based expert system for assessment severity of asthma. J Med Syst. 2012;36:1707–17.
16. Lurie A, Marsala C, Hartley S, Bouchon-Meunier B, Dusser D. Patients' perception of asthma severity. Respir Med. 2007;101:2145–52.
17. Pifferi M, Ragazzo V, Previti A, Pioggia G, Ferro M, Macchia P, et al. Exhaled air temperature in asthmatic children: a mathematical evaluation. Pediatr Allergy Immunol. 2009;20:164–71.
18. Zolnoori M, Fazel Zarandi MH, Moin M, Heidarnezhad H, Kazemnejad A. Computer-aided intelligent system for diagnosing pediatric asthma. J Med Syst. 2012;36:809–22.
19. Chatzimichail E, Paraskakis E, Sitzimi M, Rigas A. An intelligent system approach for asthma prediction in symptomatic preschool children. Comput Math Methods Med. 2013;2013:240182.
20. Pifferi M, Bush A, Pioggia G, Di Cicco M, Chinellato I, Bodini A, et al. Monitoring asthma control in children with allergies by soft computing of lung function and exhaled nitric oxide. Chest. 2011;139:319–27.
21. Jaing JT, Sepulveda JA, Casillas AM. Novel computer-based assessment of asthma strategies in inner-city children. Ann Allergy Asthma Immunol. 2001;87:230–7.
22. De Matas M, Shao Q, Silkstone VL, Chrystyn H. Evaluation of an in vitro in vivo correlation for nebulizer delivery using artificial neural networks. J Pharm Sci. 2007;96:3293–303.
23. De Matas M, Shao Q, Biddiscombe MF, Meah S, Chrystyn H, Usmani OS. Predicting the clinical effect of a short acting bronchodilator in individual patients using artificial neural networks. Eur J Pharm Sci. 2010;41:707–15.
24. Kharroubi SA, Brazier JE, Yang Y. Modeling a preference-based index for two condition-specific measures (asthma and overactive bladder) using a nonparametric Bayesian method. Value Health. 2014;17:406–15.
25. Gandhi PK, Gentry WM, Bottorff MB. Thrombotic events associated with C1 esterase inhibitor products in patients with hereditary angioedema: investigation from the United States Food and Drug Administration adverse event reporting system database. Pharmacotherapy. 2012;32:902–9.
26. Kadoyama K, Kuwahara A, Yamamori M, Brown JB, Sakaeda T, Okuno Y. Hypersensitivity reactions to anticancer agents: data mining of the public version of the FDA adverse event reporting system. Advers Event Report Syst J Exp Clin Cancer Res. 2011;30:93.
27. Sakaeda T, Kadoyama K, Yabuuchi H, Niijima S, Seki K, Shiraishi Y, et al. Platinum agent-induced hypersensitivity reactions: data mining of the public version of the FDA adverse event reporting system. Advers Event Report Syst Int J Med Sci. 2011;8:332–8.
28. Naranjo CA, Kwok MC, Lanctôt KL, Zhao HP, Spielberg SP, Shear NH. Enhanced differential diagnosis of anticonvulsant hypersensitivity reactions by an integrated Bayesian and biochemical approach. Clin Pharmacol Ther. 1994;56:564–75.
29. Lanctôt KL, Ghajar BM, Shear NH, Naranjo CA. Improving the diagnosis of hypersensitivity reactions associated with sulfonamides. J Clin Pharmacol. 1994;34:1228–33.
30. Lanctôt KL, Naranjo CA. Comparison of the Bayesian approach and a simple algorithm for assessment of adverse drug events. Clin Pharmacol Ther. 1995;58:692–8.
31. Christopher J, Jabez H, Khanna N, Kannan A. A clinical decision support system for diagnosis of allergic rhinitis based on intradermal skin tests. Comput Biol Med. 2015;65:76–84.
32. Goulart DA, Tacla MA, Marback PMF, Solé D, Paranhos Junior A, Perez HB, et al. Artificial neural networks applied to study allergic conjunctivitis screening questionnaire. Arq Bras Oftalmol. 2006;69:707–13.
33. Takahashi K, Hayasawa H, Tomita M. A predictive model for affect of atopic dermatitis in infancy by neural network and multiple logistic regression. Arerugi. 1999;48:1222–9.
34. Carpenter JR, Pocock S, Lamm CJ. Coping with missing data in clinical trials: a model-based approach applied to asthma trials. Stat Med. 2002;21(8):1043–66.
35. Carpenter JR, Roger JH, Kenward MG. Analysis of longitudinal trials with protocol deviation: a framework for relevant, accessible assumptions, and inference via multiple imputation. J Biopharm Stat. 2012;23:1352–71.
36. Dexheimer JW, Abramo TJ, Arnold DH, Johnson K, Shyr Y, Ye F, et al. Implementation and evaluation of an integrated computerized asthma management system in a pediatric emergency department: a randomized clinical trial. Int J Med Inform. 2014;83:805–13.
37. Dayhoff JE, De Leo JM. Artificial neural networks: opening the black box. Cancer. 2001;91:1615–35.
38. Anagnostou T, Remzi M, Lykourinas M, Djavan B. Artificial neural networks for decision-making in urologic oncology. Eur Urol. 2003;43:596–603.
39. Zhang XS, Huang JW, Roy RJ. Modeling for neuromonitoring depth of anesthesia. Crit Rev Biomed Eng. 2002;30:131–73.
40. Baurley JW, Conti DV. A scalable, knowledge-based analysis framework for genetic association studies. BMC Bioinformatics. 2013;14:312.
41. Li R, Conti DV, Diaz-Sanchez D, Gilliland F, Thomas DC. Joint analysis for integrating two related studies of different data types and different study designs using hierarchical modeling approaches. Hum Hered. 2013;74:83–96.
42. Pillai RR, Divekar R, Brasier A, Bhavnani S, Calhoun WJ. Strategies for molecular classification of asthma using bipartite network analysis of cytokine expression. Curr Allergy Asthma Rep. 2012;12:388–95.
43. Bunyavanich S, Schadt EE. Systems biology of asthma and allergic diseases: a multiscale approach. J Allergy Clin Immunol. 2015;135:31–42.
44. Hinks TS, Zhou X, Staples KJ, Dimitrov BD, Manta A, Petrossian T, et al. Innate and adaptive T cells in asthmatic patients: relationship to severity and disease mechanisms. J Allergy Clin Immunol. 2015;136:323–33.

16

How pregnancy can affect autoimmune diseases progression?

Marie-Pierre Piccinni[1,2*], Letizia Lombardelli[1,2], Federica Logiodice[1,2], Ornela Kullolli[1,2], Paola Parronchi[1,2] and Sergio Romagnani[1,2]

Abstract

Autoimmune disorders are characterized by tissue damage, caused by self-reactivity of different effectors mechanisms of the immune system, namely antibodies and T cells. Their occurrence may be associated with genetic and/or environmental predisposition and to some extent, have implications for fertility and obstetrics. The relationship between autoimmunity and reproduction is bidirectional. This review only addresses the impact of pregnancy on autoimmune diseases and not the influence of autoimmunity on pregnancy development. Th17/Th1-type cells are aggressive and pathogenic in many autoimmune disorders and inflammatory diseases. The immunology of pregnancy underlies the role of Th2-type cytokines to maintain the tolerance of the mother towards the fetal semi-allograft. Non-specific factors, including hormonal changes, favor a switch to Th2-type cytokine profile. In pregnancy Th2, Th17/Th2 and Treg cells accumulate in the decidua but may also be present in the mother's circulation and can regulate autoimmune responses influencing the progression of autoimmune diseases.

Keywords: Autoimmunity, T helper cells, Th1, Th2, Th17, Th22, Tfh pregnancy, Abortion, Allograft

Background

Autoimmune diseases include approximately 80 different disorders. Although, individually, each autoimmune disease affects a small number of individuals, as a whole, it is estimated that its prevalence is between 7.6 and 9.4 % [1]. It is well accepted that a disease can be classified as autoimmune if one shows that an immune response to a self-antigen causes the disease pathology. Indeed, autoimmune disorders are characterized by tissue damage, caused by self-reactivity of different effectors mechanisms of the immune system, namely antibodies and T cells. Their occurrence may be associated with genetic and/or environmental predisposition [2, 3] and to some extent, have implications for fertility and obstetrics.

The relationship between autoimmunity and reproduction seems to be bidirectional. Accordingly, autoimmune diseases may selectively affect women in their reproductive years and conversely pregnancy may affect the expression of autoimmune diseases. Thus, autoimmunity may have an influence on pregnancy outcomes. As the matter of fact, Gleicher et al. [4], performed PubMed, Google Scholar and Medline searches for the years 2000–2010 under various key words and phrases, referring to effects of autoimmunity/autoimmune diseases on pregnancy/pregnancy outcomes/pregnancy rates/reproduction/reproductive outcomes/fertility/infertility/fertility treatments/infertility treatments, and similar terms, toward significant impacts of autoimmunity on female reproductive success. They reported that autoimmunity not only increases miscarriage risks but also reduces female fecundity and infertility treatment success. However, pregnancy may have an influence on autoimmune diseases improvement or worsening. During pregnancy many autoimmune diseases go into remission, only to flare again in the early post-partum period. For example, Graves disease is an autoimmune thyroid disease which ameliorates during pregnancy, only to relapse post partum.

This review only addresses the impact of pregnancy on autoimmune diseases and not the influence of autoimmunity on pregnancy development.

*Correspondence: mppiccinni@hotmail.com
[2] Department of Experimental and Clinical Medicine, University of Florence, Largo Brambilla 3, 50134 Florence, Italy
Full list of author information is available at the end of the article

Pregnancy is related to T cell mediated-responses towards conceptus

The fact that women can successfully carry a conceptus, which is liken to an allograft, to full term without rejection is one of the most remarkable aspects of pregnancy.

Although conceptus/trophoblast does not express HLA class II molecules, it exhibits HLA class I molecules, the polymorphic HLA-C molecules, together with the non-polymorphic HLA-G and HLA-E. For the presence of paternal class I HLA-C molecules on the fetal-derived trophoblast cells, that invade the maternal *decidua basalis*, the conceptus has been considered to be a semi-allograft. After presentation of paternal alloantigens by maternal antigen presenting cells (APCs), the maternal T cells specific for these alloantigens, [5] could proliferate and secrete cytokines, promoting the activation of allograft rejection or tolerance mechanisms, respectively responsible for pregnancy failure or fetal survival.

In fact, on the basis of the profile of cytokines produced, T helper cells are classified in T helper (Th)1, Th2 and Th17 cells [6, 7]. CD4+ Th1 cells produce interleukin (IL)-2, tumor necrosis factor (TNF)-β and interferon (IFN)-γ and are the main effectors of phagocyte-mediated host defense, which are highly protective against infections sustained by intracellular pathogens. On the other hand, CD4+ Th2 cells, which are mainly responsible for phagocyte-independent host defense against extracellular pathogens, including nematodes, produce IL-4 (which together with IL-10 inhibit several macrophage functions and together with IL-13 produced by Th2 cells, stimulates IgE antibody production) and IL-5 (which promotes growth, differentiation and activation of eosinophils) [6]. An additional subset of CD4+ T helper cells named Th17, which produce IL-17A, IL-17F, IL-21, IL-26 and IL-22 [7], is protective against extracellular bacteria and may also play a role in inflammation [8]. A part of human IL-17A-producing cells were found to also produce interferon (IFN)-γ (they are named Th17/Th1) and both Th17 and Th17/Th1 exhibit plasticity towards Th1 cells in response to IL-12 produced by APCs [8]. Another part of the Th17 cells could also produce IL-4 (they are named Th17/Th2) in response to IL-4 present in the microenvironment of these cells or HLA-G5 produced by trophoblast cells and embryo at feto maternal interface [9, 10].

These three types of effector T helper cells play a central role in acute allograft rejection and tolerance. IFN-γ and IL-17 has been detected in rejecting allografts [11–13], indicating that some Th1- and Th17-dependent effector mechanisms play a central role in acute allograft rejection of transplanted tissues [14]. The production of the Th2-type cytokine IL-4 and IL-10, appears to be central for the induction and the maintenance of allograft tolerance [11, 15]. These findings indicate that Th1-type and Th17-type cytokines, that promote allograft rejection, may compromise pregnancy, whereas the Th2-type cytokines inhibiting in particular the Th1 responses, promote allograft tolerance and therefore may improve pregnancy success. Moreover, T reg cells, which dampen all the T helper responses has also been reported to be responsible for fetal alloantigens tolerance [16] and could induce fetoallograft tolerance through the production of IL-10 and TGF-β [17]. However recent studies in mice suggest that T reg cells play an important role in response to semen independently of placental antigen exposure, in preparing endometrium for implantation dampening uterine inflammation [18].

In mice many evidence confirmed the role of Th1- and Th2-type cytokines present at fetomaternal interface on the development of pregnancy [19–22]. Studies performed on unexplained recurrent abortion (URA), which is characterized by the loss of three or more consecutive pregnancies in the first trimester of pregnancy (with normal karyotype of the conceptus) has been chosen as model to study the first trimester of human pregnancy. Though multiple causes of URA are known (including structural, hormonal, infectious, autoimmune and thrombophilic causes), after evaluation, roughly half of all cases remain unexplained. The URA cases remained unexplained shed a light on the potential role of decidual effector CD4+ T helper on the maintenance of pregnancy.

Indeed, we reported a defect of IL-4 production by both CD4+ and CD8+ T cell clones and a defect of IL-10 by CD4+ T cell clones generated from the decidua of women suffering from URA undergoing a spontaneous abortion in comparison with women with successful pregnancy [23]. Thus, we found in URA a defective production of Th2-type cytokines which are essential for the fetal alloantigen tolerance in successful pregnancy. More recently, we reported that the purified human decidual CD4+ T cells obtained from successful pregnancy, which have not been activated in vitro, produce spontaneously IL-4, whereas they do never produce IFN-γ spontaneously, but only after stimulation with immobilized anti-CD3 monoclonal antibodies [24]. We also demonstrated that the purified CD4+ T cells were previously activated by the trophoblast cells in situ and expressed without any additional in vitro stimulation high levels of activation markers (CD25, CD69 and HLA-DR) [24]. These results confirm the prevalence of Th2 cells activated by trophoblast antigens at the feto-maternal interface [23, 25, 26]. Progesterone, which, at concentrations comparable to those present at the feto-maternal interface during pregnancy, is a potent inducer of production of IL-4 [27] could be at least in part responsible for a Th2 switch at feto-maternal interface.

Excessive Th17 activity has also been described to promote spontaneous abortion. Accordingly, Th17 cells has been reported to increase in decidua of patients with URA compared to healthy pregnant women [28, 29]. However, this significant increase seems to occur only in inevitable abortion with genital bleeding [29] and was suggested to be the consequence rather than the cause of miscarriage.

Very recently, we reported that an associated production of IL-4 and IL-17 is exhibited by a large number of decidual CD4+ T cells (named Th17/Th2 cells) in successful pregnancy and at embryo implantation site whereas pathogenic decidual Th17/Th1 cells are prevalent in URA and far from the embryo implantation site [10]. The differentiation of Th17 cells into Th17/Th2 cells is due to soluble HLA-G5, the soluble isoform of HLA-G, a non polymorphic Class I molecule produced by embryo and trophoblast cells in normal human pregnancy [10]. Thus, it seems that Th17 cells do not show a pathogenic role for pregnancy, but a beneficial role, when they also produce IL-4 whereas Th17/Th1 are pathogenic for pregnancy. In the intrauterine environment (both fetal and amniotic compartments) infection-related immunity seems to be preferentially directed towards combating extracellular microbial pathogens (responsible for a five fold increase of fetal resorption) with Th17-mediated immune responses [30] suggesting that Th17/Th2 cells could be essential for the success of pregnancy, because they may promote an adequate response to protect the mother against dangerous extracellular pathogens and induce fetoallograft tolerance together with Th2 cells and T reg cells.

Thus, T cells functions exacerbated during pregnancy characterized by a tolerogenic Th2-type profile, could have an influence on autoimmune disease improvement or worsening.

Autoimmunity is related to T cell mediated-responses

CD4+ T helper cells are critical for proper immune cell homeostasis and host defense, but are also major contributors to pathology of autoimmune and inflammatory diseases. Since the discovery of the Th1/Th2 dichotomy, many additional Th subsets were discovered, each with a unique cytokine profile, functional properties, and presumed role in autoimmune tissue pathology. This includes principally Th1, Th2, Th17 and Treg cells which are characterized by specific cytokine profiles described above. Cytokines, which are often categorized into pro-inflammatory and anti-inflammatory produced by these T helper subsets play a critical role in directing the effector response. The different T helper subsets in terms of cytokine profiles influence and shape the immune response, and could promote autoimmune and inflammatory diseases [31]. Therefore, autoimmune diseases develop as a result of abnormalities in immune response mediated by activated T cells-derived cytokines. Accordingly, IFN-γ produced by Th1 cells, has long been associated with pathology of several autoimmune diseases including autoimmune type 1 diabetes, multiple sclerosis (MS) and rheumatoid arthritis (RA). The association IFN-γ and autoimmune disorders is not surprising because IFN-γ is a potent proinflammatory cytokine which has a number of important roles including, increasing major histocompatibility gene complex (MHC) class I (MHC-I) and class II (MHC-II) antigen presentation, increasing the expression of toll-like receptors (TLR) by innate immune cells, promoting immunoglobulin G class switching, promoting the induction of chemokine secretion, macrophage activation and increased phagocytosis. Even before the discovery of Th1 cells, evidence for IFN-γ having detrimental effects on autoimmune diseases was provided by the observation that administration of IFN-γ to MS patients was deleterious and resulted in exacerbation of the disease [32].

However, there is some debate whether Th1 cells only play a pathogenic role in autoimmune diseases, or whether they also contribute to protective/anti-inflammatory immune responses. Experimental allergic encephalomyelitis (EAE) is an animal model of inflammatory demyelinating disease of the central nervous system. It is widely studied as an animal model of the human central nervous system demyelinating diseases, including MS. Experiments testing the impact of genetic deletion of IFN-γ on EAE showed that animals lacking IFN-γ developed disease with increased severity compared with IFN-γ sufficient controls [33]. Several hypotheses have been proposed to account for the apparent anti-inflammatory properties of IFN-γ including the downregulation of lymphocyte trafficking into the draining lymph-nodes [34], the control of T cell clonal expansion via induction of apoptosis [35] and the induction of indoleamine 2,3-dioxygenase (IDO), which exerts anti-inflammatory effects in lymph nodes and tissues [36].

Another T helper subset characterized by the production of IL-4, IL-5 and IL-13, the Th2 subset can promote pathology of several different autoimmune diseases, particularly those which are associated with humoral immune responses. Indeed, studies have demonstrated that aberrant and continued IL-4 expression in vivo can rescue autoreactive B cells from apoptosis, enhance their survival, and induce activation of autoreactive B cells and thereby promote autoimmune diseases [37]. Additionally, even in Th1 mediated immunopathology, Th2 cells may induce the generation of autoantibodies and enhance pathology. In contrast, Th2-type cytokines can mediate protection either by directly suppressing Th1/Th17 development via IL-4/IL-13 respectively, or by counteracting Th1-mediated inflammation. IL-4 is known to strongly suppress the development of Th1 cells even in an environment with high levels of IFN-γ, thereby antagonizing Th1 cell functions [38]. Anti-inflammatory properties of IL-4 include the inhibition of Th1-activated macrophages and suppression of the secretion of several potent pro-inflammatory mediators including IL-1, TNF and reactive oxygen species (ROS).

Even prior to the discovery of Th17 cells, which produce IL-17A, IL-17F and IL-22, IL-17 was noted to be overexpressed in a number of inflammatory/autoimmune conditions including MS [39], RA [40, 41], systemic lupus erythematosus (SLE) [42, 43] and airway inflammatory diseases [44] and thus has been implicated in their pathogenesis. Models of autoimmune diseases have substantiated Th17 cells as important contributors to tissue pathology and to the promotion of antibody responses. Much of the pathogenic functions of Th17 cells have been attributed to the secretion of IL-17, including the induction of the release of proinflammatory cytokines including TNF-α and IL-1β, the enhancing B cell functions, the recruitment of neutrophils and the activation of innate immune cells. Moreover, IL-17 induces the secretion of chemokines and other inflammatory mediators, the expression of adhesion molecule (ICAM-1), prostaglandin E2, as well as promoting tissue damage through the induction of matrix metalloproteinases and antimicrobial-peptides. In fact, increased IL-17 production sustains a pro-inflammatory environment and can cause excessive tissue damage [45]. Recently, it has been suggested that Th17 cells that have shifted towards Th1-phenotype seem to be more aggressive and more pathogenic than Th17 unshifted cells particularly in inflammatory diseases as MS, RA, psoriasis or inflammatory bowel diseases. Nonetheless, IL-17 could be dispensable for the development of organ-specific autoimmunity, as in EAE [46]. Although IL-17 could be dispensable, IL-23, which promotes the stability of Th17 cells, and T-bet, key transcription factor of Th1 cells, which regulates the expression of IL-23 receptor, are essential for autoimmune disorders.

Very recently, the newly identified T helper cell 22 (Th22) has been involved in autoimmune diseases pathogenesis. Th22 is a subset of CD4+ T helper cells obviously discrete from Th17 and Th1 subsets by production of interleukin (IL)-22 but not IL-17 or IFN-γ, and also with distinguished expression of aryl hydrocarbon receptor (AHR) as the key transcription factor. This T helper subset, by producing pro-inflammatory cytokines such as IL-22 and tumor necrosis factor-α (TNF-α), is implicated in the pathogenesis of autoimmune disease including RA, SLE, Behçet's disease, type 1 diabetes, immune thrombocytopenia [47], psoriasis and MS [48]. Thereby, Th22 cells and in particular IL-22 are implicated as a potential therapeutic target in autoimmune diseases.

Finally, not only Th1, Th2, Th17 and Th22 cells have been implicated in the pathogenesis of autoimmune disorders, the new subset follicular helper T cells (Tfh) seems to have a role in the pathogenesis of different autoimmune disorders [49]. Tfh has many features in common with Th17 cells, such as the ability to produce IL-21 and to express the IL-23 receptor (IL23R), the inducible co-stimulatory molecule ICOS, and the transcription factor c-Maf, all of them essential for expansion and establishment of the final pool of both Th17 and Th22 subsets. Tfh cells differ from Th17 by their ability to home to B cell areas in secondary lymphoid tissue through interactions mediated by the chemokine receptor CXCR5 that they express, and its ligand CXCL13. These CXCR5+ CD4+ T cells are considered an effector T cell type specialized in B cell help. The role of Tfh cells and its primary product, IL-21, on B cell activation and differentiation is essential for humoral immunity against infectious agents. However, when deregulated, Tfh cells seem to contribute to exacerbated humoral response and autoantibody production in autoimmune diseases. Accordingly, the presence of circulating Tfh cells as a potential biomarker of disease has been studied in various autoimmune conditions, including myasthenia gravis (MG), autoimmune thyroiditis, Sjögren's syndrome (SS), RA, MS, SLE, ulcerative colitis, Crohn's disease, ankylosing spondylitis, type 1 diabetes mellitus, autoimmune hepatitis, primary biliary cirrhosis and juvenile dermatomyositis. Alteration of Tfh cells have been reported in patients with various autoimmune diseases, such as RA, SLE and autoimmune thyroid diseases, where Tfh cells are present at increased frequency and show positive correlation with serum autoantibody titer. Therefore, a better understanding of the biology and the roles of Tfh cells is expected to contribute in clarifying the role of this subset in the pathogenesis of autoimmune disorders [49].

Some cytokines produced by non-T cells could stimulate the inappropriate activities of cells implicated in the pathogenesis of autoimmune diseases. Interleukin-27 (IL-27) is a member of the IL-12 family, is produced by activated antigen-presenting cells and plays an important role in the regulation of CD4+ T cell differentiation and immune response. IL-27 activates multiple signaling cascades, including the JAK-STAT and p38 MAPK pathways. Several studies have revealed that IL-27 promotes the differentiation of Th1 and Tr1, but inhibits Th2, Th17, and Treg cells. IL-27 displays both pro- and anti-inflammatory activities in different autoimmune diseases. The pro-/anti-inflammatory activity of IL-27 is influenced by the underlying immune effector pathways, the phase of the disease, the presence or absence of counter-regulatory cytokines/T cell subsets, and the tissue/cell type under study. Meka et al. [50] discussed the role of IL-27 in RA, MS, colitis, SLE, psoriasis, type 1 diabetes, and uveitis. Most of this information is derived from experimental models of these autoimmune diseases.

Despite a spectrum of outcomes in various autoimmune diseases, mostly anti-inflammatory and immunomodulatory effects of T cell cytokines have been observed in these disorders. Accordingly, T cell cytokines, but also inducers/inhibitors of some T cell-secreted cytokines represent a novel, promising target/agent for the treatment of autoimmune diseases.

T cell responses in autoimmune disorders are influenced by pregnancy

In the light of what described before, Th1 and Th17-type autoimmune disorders could be improved when there is a rise in Th2-type cytokines in pregnancy (e.g. RA, Graves disease and MS [51–54]) and Th2-type autoimmune disorders could get worse in pregnancy when Th2-type cytokines increased (e.g. SLE [55]). By contrast, in the post partum period, when the Th2-type cytokines decreases Th1 and Th17-type inflammatory and autoimmune disorders could get worse and Th2-type autoimmune disorders could improve. As the matter of fact, during pregnancy, SLE flares are associated with antiphospholipids (aPL) antibodies, synergic changes of pregnancy on Th1 and Th2 cytokines, that interact with hormones such as estrogen and prolactin that amplify the inflammatory effect. From the clinical point of view, SLE activity at pregnancy onset, thrombocytopenia, lupus nephritis, arterial hypertension, aPL syndromes, preeclampsia is associated with lupus flares and fetal complications. The SLE flares during pregnancy make the difference between an uncomplicated pregnancy and pregnancy with maternal and fetal complications [55]. Pregnancy and the postpartum period have a profound effect not only on SLE, but also on autoimmune thyroid disease. Graves disease ameliorates during pregnancy, only to relapse postpartum, whereas postpartum thyroiditis is caused by destructive thyroiditis during the first few months after delivery [51]. Similarly, pregnant women with MS typically have a greatly reduced relapse rate, whereas very soon after the delivery, the disease activity returns, often even at a higher level than seen in the pre-pregnancy year. The reasons for the increased postpartum activity are not entirely clear, but factors such as the abrupt decrease in estrogen levels immediately after the delivery and the loss of the immunosuppressive state of pregnancy are likely of importance [54]. There is compelling evidence that estrogen, progesterone, and testosterone control autoimmune disorders. In particular these hormones control MS by influencing immune responses and by contributing to repair mechanisms in the nervous system. Similarly to many other autoimmune diseases, MS is more common among women than men, and its incidence among women is rising. There are also qualitative differences in the disease course between men and women, with male patients experiencing increased disease progression, brain atrophy and cognitive impairment.

Hormones, which seems to contribute to autoimmune disorders worsening or improvement by influencing T cell cytokine responses involved in the pathogenesis of these disorders, may offer important insights into autoimmune disease prevention and treatment (Table 1).

Hormone-controlled T cell cytokine profile influences progression of autoimmune and inflammatory diseases

Women mount more vigorous antibody- and cell-mediated immune responses following either infection or vaccination than men. A large number of autoimmune diseases are more prevalent in women. Thus, it seems that sex influences susceptibility to autoimmune diseases (e.g. RA, for which the female-to-male ratio is 3:1 has been reported [56]). Many ideas mainly based on hormonal and genetic factors that influence the autoimmune systems of females and males differently, have been proposed to explain this predominance. These hypotheses have gained credence mostly because many of these diseases appear or fluctuate when there are hormonal changes such as in late adolescence and pregnancy. Differences in X chromosome characteristics between men and women with an autoimmune disease have led researchers to think that the genetic background of this group of diseases also relates to the genetic determinants of gender. Thus, the hormonal changes as well as the genetic factors, could explain why women are more prone to develop autoimmune diseases [57].

Table 1 Pregnancy influences autoimmune diseases progression

Autoimmune disease	Influence on pregnancy
Rheumatoid arthritis (RA)	Improved
Systemic lupus erythematosus (SLE)	Worse
Multiple sclerosis (MS)	Improved
Graves' disease	Improved
Systemic sclerosis (SS)	Worse
Hashimoto thyroiditis	Improved

During pregnancy Th2-type autoimmune disease get worsen and Th1/Th17-type autoimmune disease improved

Female hormonal stimulation of immune responses could be responsible for the higher incidence of most autoimmune diseases in women than in men. Prior the discovery of Th17 cells, the first evidence of the role of hormonal changes on the autoimmune disorders progression derived from studies performed on Th1- and Th2- type cells. Indeed, it has been demonstrated that both androgens and estrogens are able to regulate the Th1/Th2 balance. Androgens were described as hormones which promote autoimmune diseases with a profile of Th1-type cytokines, such as RA, whereas estrogens were described as inducers of autoimmune diseases with a Th2-type cytokine profile, like SLE. Thus, Th1-type autoimmune diseases could be improved when decrease Th1-type cytokines, or when there is a rise in Th2-type cytokines (increased estrogens, as in pregnancy), whereas Th2-type autoimmune diseases could be improved when Th2-type cytokines are diminished (decreased estrogen, as in post-partum period) or when Th1-type response is stimulated [58].

This idea has gained credence because, in particular for RA, the peak incidence in women coincides with the time of menopause, when estrogen levels rapidly drop, connecting sex hormones to disease etiology [59]. In contrast, men have rather continuous levels of estrogen throughout their adult lives, and estrogen levels are lower in postmenopausal women than in men of corresponding age [60]. In a well-established experimental model of RA, the collagen-induced arthritis (CIA), it has repeatedly been shown that estrogen ameliorates disease development [61, 62]. In contrast to RA, estrogen aggravates systemic lupus erythematosus [63]. Estrogen is a potent immunomodulatory agent and can exert stimulatory as well as regulatory effects on the immune system, such as enhancing B cell antibody production, reducing B and T lymphopoiesis and inhibiting T cell-dependent inflammation [64, 65].

More recently with the discovery of Th17 cells, RA has been associated as MS, to Th17-mediated inflammatory diseases. Effects of estrogen on Th17 cells have mostly been studied in the context of the experimental MS, called EAE, where an estrogen is protective. Estrogen decreases production of IL-17 in EAE and inhibits Th17 differentiation and disease progression, dependent on estrogen receptor α (ERα) in T cells [66]. Furthermore, the regulatory role of estrogen has been demonstrated in CIA, where the estrogen metabolite 2-methoxyestradiol decreased IL-17 mRNA in arthritic joints [67], regulates the localization of Th17 cells, resulting in increased Th17 in lymph nodes but decreased Th17 in joints of CIA [56].

Progesterone is also able to decrease the Th17 cell activity [68] and could decrease the progression of IL-17-mediated autoimmune and inflammatory diseases. Progesterone is also a potent Th2-inducer [27] that could influence the progression of Th2 and Th1-mediated autoimmune disorders, by worsening Th2-type autoimmune disorders and improving Th1-mediated autoimmune and Th17/Th1-mediated inflammatory disorders. During pregnancy, the rise in Th2-type cytokines could be mostly due to progesterone, which is 10- to 50-fold higher at feto-maternal interface than in peripheral blood and which can inhibit the development and function of Th1 and macrophages cells [69], thus preventing the trophoblast alloantigen rejection.

Therefore, during pregnancy, hormonal changes which could play a critical role in determining the effector CD4+ T cell cytokine profile at fetomaternal interface, could explain why in some conditions pregnant women are more prone to develop Th2-type autoimmune diseases, whereas in pregnant women the Th1- and Th17-type autoimmune and inflammatory diseases are improved (Fig. 1).

Conclusion

The immunology of pregnancy underlies the role of CD4+ T cell cytokine profile. Indeed, the mother must maintain tolerance of the fetal semi-allograft while not suppressing her own immune system and exposing herself and the fetus to infection. Non-specific factors, including probably not only hormonal changes [26, 27, 70], but also trophoblast key immunomodulatory molecules (e.g. HLA-G5, [10]) favoring a switch to a predominantly Th2-type cytokine profile, may play some part in the maintenance of transient tolerance to paternal antigens in pregnancy [23, 25, 26]. The generation of specific Th2 and Th17/Th2 cells and T reg cells, is key to the maintenance of pregnancy. These cells preferentially accumulate in the decidua but may also be present

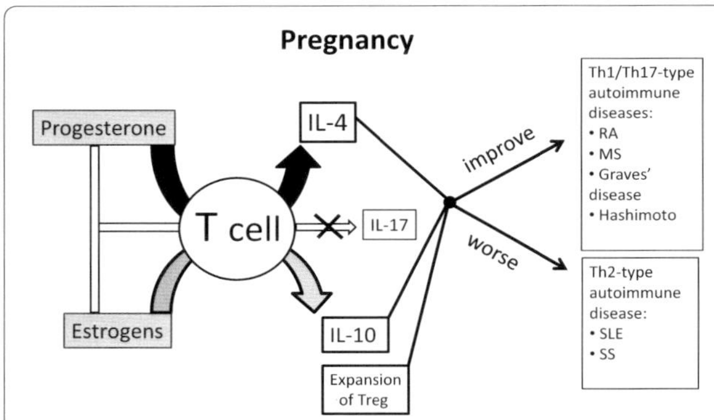

Fig. 1 Hormone-controlled T cell responses influence the progression of autoimmune diseases: progesterone and estrogens inducing Th2-type response and decreasing Th1/Th17 response influence the improvement and the worsening of Th1/Th17-type autoimmune diseases, and Th2-type autoimmune diseases, respectively

in the mother's circulation and are thus capable of regulating coincidental autoimmune responses to remission or worsening of the related Th1-/Th17- or Th2-autoimmune diseases, respectively [51]. The postpartum exacerbation of some Th1/Th17 autoimmune disorders may reflect an imbalance in Th2-type cells and T reg cells, which is caused by the rapid fall in the numbers of these cells after delivery.

Autoimmune disorder development could also be influenced by the transplacental transfer of cells between mother and fetus, which occurred during pregnancy even years before the onset of the disorder. The fetal microchimerism is acquired by the mother during pregnancy and this fetal cells are maintained in the mother for decades. Similarly, there is also a maternal microchimerism acquired by an infant during pregnancy. In mouse models it is possible to study the bi-directional transfer of cells in pregnancy using fluorescent tags. Years ago, we showed that systemic sclerosis (SSc), an immunologically mediated disorder of the connective tissue, is characterized by a predominant activation of IL-4-producing Th2 cells, which may account for the clinical and serological similarities of SSc to chronic graft versus host disease (cGVHD), in which T cells from involved tissues produce Th2-type cytokines. We showed that offspring CD4+ T cells present in the blood and skin of women with SSc are able react with maternal MHC antigen and exhibit a Th2-type profile, supporting the possibility that cGVHD reaction attributable to long-term microchimerism plays a pathogenic role of SSc [71, 72]. The fetal microchimerism has been described in many other autoimmune diseases [73]. More recently, it has been demonstrated that maternal microchimerism could play a role in type 1 diabetes of children [74].

Therefore, pregnancy is able to influence the onset and progression of autoimmune and inflammatory diseases by influencing the T cell cytokine-mediated responses during the gestation period, the post-partum period, but also decades after the pregnancy period.

Abbrevations

Th: T helper; APC: antigen presenting cell; IL: interleukin; HLA: human leukocyte antigen; TNF: tumor necrosis factor; IFN: interferon; URA: unexplained recurrent abortion; MS: multiple sclerosis; RA: rheumatoid arthritis; MHC: major histocompatibility complex; EAE: experimental allergic encephalomyelitis; TLR: toll like receptor; IDO: indoleamine 2,3-dioxygenase; ROS: reactive oxygen species; SLE: systemic lupus erythematosus; AHR: aryl hydrocarbon receptor; MG: myasthenia gravis; SS: Sjögren's syndrome; CIA: collagen-induced arthritis; Erα: estrogen receptor α; SSc: systemic sclerosis; cGVHD: chronic graft versus host disease.

Authors' contributions

MPP conceived, designed, and wrote the manuscript. LL, FL, OK, PP and SR have been involved in the submission and have given final approval of the version to be published. All authors read and approved the final manuscript.

Author details

[1] Center of Excellence for Research, Transfer and High Education DENOTHE of the University of Florence, Florence, Italy. [2] Department of Experimental and Clinical Medicine, University of Florence, Largo Brambilla 3, 50134 Florence, Italy.

Acknowledgements

MPP was supported by Intramural Scientific Research funds (ex-60 %) of the University of Florence. The work performed in MPP laboratory was supported by the European NoE EMBIC (LSHM-CT-2004-512040).

Funding

The work performed in MPP laboratory was supported by the European NoE EMBIC (LSHM-CT-2004-512040).

References

1. Cooper G, Bynum M, Somers E. Recent insights in the epidemiology of autoimmune diseases: improved prevalence estimates and understanding of clustering of diseases. J Autoimmun. 2009;33:197–207.
2. Rose NR, MacKay IR. The autoimmune diseases. 5th ed. London: Elsevier Academic Press; 2006.
3. Kochi Y. Genetics of autoimmune diseases: perspectives from genome-wide association studies. Int Immunol. 2016;28:155–61.
4. Gleicher N, Weghofer A, Barad DH. Cutting edge assessment of the impact of autoimmunity on female reproductive success. J Autoimmun. 2012;38:J74–80.
5. Tilburgs T, Scherjon SA, van der Mast BJ, Versteeg-VD Voort-Maarschalk M, et al. Fetal–maternal HLA-C mismatch is associated with decidual T cell activation and induction of functional T regulatory cells. J Reprod Immunol. 2009;82:148–57.
6. Romagnani S. T-cell responses in allergy and asthma. Curr Opin Allergy Clin Immunol. 2001;1:73–8.
7. Harrington LE, Hatton RD, Mangan PR, Turner H, Murphy TL, Murphy KM, Weaver CT. Interleukin 17-producing CD4+ effector T cells develop via a lineage distinct from the T helper type 1 and 2 lineages. Nat Immunol. 2005;6:1123–32.
8. Annunziato F, Cosmi L, Santarlasci V, Maggi L, Liotta F, Mazzinghi B, et al. Phenotypic and functional features of human Th17 cells. J Exp Med. 2007;204:1849–61.
9. Cosmi L, Maggi L, Santarlasci V, Capone M, Cardilicchia E, Frosali F, et al. Identification of a novel subset of human circulating memory CD4(+) T cells that produce both IL-17A and IL-4. J Allergy Clin Immunol. 2010;125:222–30.
10. Lombardelli L, Logiodice F, Aguerre-Girr M, Kullolli O, Haller H, Casart Y, et al. Interleukin-17-producing decidual CD4+ T cells are not deleterious for human pregnancy when they also produce interleukin-4. Clin Mol Allergy. 2016;14:1. doi:10.1186/s12948-016-0039-y.

11. Strom TB, Roy-Chaudury R, Manfro R, Zheng XX, Nickerson PW, Wood K, Bushell A. The Th1/Th2 paradigm and allograft response. Curr Opin Immunol. 1996;8:688–93.
12. Li XC, Zand MS, Li Y, Zheng XX, Strom TB. On histocompatibility barriers, Th1 to Th2 immune deviation, and the nature of the allograft responses. J Immunol. 1998;161:2241–7.
13. Chen H, Wang W, Xie H, Xu X, Wu J, Jiang Z, et al. A pathogenic role of IL- 17 at the early stage of corneal allograft rejection. Transpl Immunol. 2009;21:155–61.
14. Burns WR, Wang Y, Tang PC. Recruitment of CXCR3+ and CCR5+ T cells and production of interferon-gamma-inducible chemokines in rejecting human arteries. Am J Transplant. 2005;5:1226–36.
15. Wang C, Tay SS, Tran GT, Hodgkinson SJ, Allen RD, Hall BM, et al. Donor IL-4-treatment induces alternatively activated liver macrophages and IDO-expressing NK cells and promotes rat liver allograft acceptance. Transpl Immunol. 2010;22:172–8.
16. Graca L, Cobbolt SP, Waldmann H. Identification of regulatory T cells in tolerated allografts. J Exp Med. 2002;195:1641–6.
17. Zenclussen AC, Gerlof K, Zenclussen ML, Ritschel S. Zambon Bertoja A, Fest S, Hontsu S, Ueha S, Matsushima K, Leber J, Volk HD. Regulatory T cells induce a privileged tolerant microenvironment at the fetal-maternal interface. Eur J Immunol. 2006;36:82–94.
18. Robertson SA, Prins JR, Sharkey DJ, Moldenhauer LM. Seminal fluid and the generation of regulatory T cells for embryo implantation. Am J Reprod Immunol. 2013;69:315–30.
19. Lin H, Mosmann TR, Guilbert L, Tuntipopipat S, Wegmann TG. Synthesis of T helper 2-type cytokines at maternal-fetal interface. J. Immunol. 1993;151:4562–73.
20. Wegmann TG, Lin H, Guilbert L, Mossmann TR. Bidirectional cytokine interactions in the maternal-fetal relationship: is successful pregnancy a Th2 phenomenon? Immunol Today. 1993;14:353–6.
21. Chaouat G, Assal-Meliani A, Martal J, Raghupathy R, Elliott JF, Mosmann T, et al. IL-10 prevents naturally occuring fetal loss in the CBA X DBA/2 mating combination and local defect in IL-10 production in this abortion-prone combination is corrected by in vivo injection of IFN-γ. J Immunol. 1995;154:4261–8.
22. Krishnan L, Guilbert LJ, Russell AS, Wegmann TG, Mosmann TR, Belosevic M. Pregnancy impairs resistance of C57BL/6 mice to leishmania major infection and causes decreased antigen-specific IFN-gamma response and increased production of T helper 2 cytokines. J Immunol. 1996;156:644–52.
23. Piccinni MP, Beloni L, Livi C, Maggi E, Scarselli G, Romagnani S. Defective production of both leukemia inhibitory factor and type 2 T-helper cytokines by decidual T cells in unexplained recurrent abortions. Nat Med. 1998;4:1020–4.
24. Lombardelli L, Aguerre-Girr M, Logiodice F, Kullolli O, Casart Y, Polgar B, et al. HLA-G5 induces IL-4 secretion critical for successful pregnancy through differential expression of ILT2 receptor on decidual CD4+ T cells and macrophages. J Immunol. 2013;191:3651–62.
25. Piccinni MP, Scaletti C, Vultaggio A, Maggi E, Romagnani S. Defective production of LIF, M-CSF and Th2-type cytokines by T cells at fetomaternal interface is associated with pregnancy loss. J Reprod Immunol. 2001;52:35–43.
26. Piccinni MP, Lombardelli L, Logiodice F, Kullolli O, Romagnani S, Le Bouteiller P. T helper cell mediated-tolerance towards fetal allograft in successful pregnancy. Clin Mol Allergy. 2015;13:9. doi:10.1186/s12948-015-0015-y.
27. Piccinni MP, Giudizi MG, Biagiotti R, Beloni L, Giannarini L, Sampognaro S, et al. Progesterone favors the development of human T helper cells producing Th2-type cytokines and promotes both IL-4 production and membrane CD30 expression in established Th1 cells clones. J Immunol. 1995;155:128–33.
28. Wang WJ, Hao CF, Yi-Lin Yin GJ, Bao SH, Qiu LH, et al. Increased prevalence of T helper 17 (Th17) cells in peripheral blood and decidua in unexplained recurrent spontaneous abortion patients. J Reprod Immunol. 2010;84:164–70.
29. Nakashima A, Ito M, Shima T, Bac ND, Hidaka T, Saito S. Accumulation of IL-17-positive cells in decidua of inevitable abortion cases. Am J Reprod Immunol. 2010;64:4–11.
30. Witkin SS, Linhares IM, Bongiovanni AM, Herway C, Skupski D. Unique alterations in infection-induced immune activation during pregnancy. BJOG. 2011;118:145–53.
31. Raphael I, Nalawade S, Eagar TN, Forsthuber TG. T cell subsets and their signature cytokines in autoimmune and inflammatory diseases. Cytokine. 2015;74:5–17.
32. Panitch HS, Hirsch RL, Schindler J, Johnson KP. Treatment of multiple sclerosis with gamma interferon: exacerbations associated with activation of the immune system. Neurology. 1987;37:1097–102.
33. Ferber IA, Brocke S, Taylor-Edwards C, Ridgway W, Dinisco C, Steinman L, et al. Mice with a disrupted IFN-gamma gene are susceptible to the induction of experimental autoimmune encephalomyelitis (EAE). J Immunol. 1996;156:5–7.
34. Flaishon L, Topilski I, Shoseyov D, Hershkoviz R, Fireman E, Levo Y, Marmor S, et al. Cutting edge: anti-inflammatory properties of low levels of IFN-gamma. J Immunol. 2002;168:3707–11.
35. Refaeli Y, Van Parijs L, Alexander SI, Abbas AK. Interferon gamma is required for activation-induced death of T lymphocytes. J Exp Med. 2002;196:999–1005.
36. Mellor AL, Munn DH. IDO expression by dendritic cells: tolerance and tryptophan catabolism. Nat Rev Immunol. 2004;4:762–74.
37. Illera VA, Perandones CE, Stunz LL, Mower DA Jr, Ashman RF. Apoptosis in splenic B lymphocytes. Regulation by protein kinase C and IL-4. J Immunol. 1993;151:2965–73.
38. Swain SL, Weinberg AD, English M, Huston G. IL-4 directs the development of Th2-like helper effectors. J Immunol. 1990;145:3796–806.
39. Lock C, Hermans G, Pedotti R, Brendolan A, Schadt E, Garren H, et al. Gene-microarray analysis of multiple sclerosis lesions yields new targets validated in autoimmune encephalomyelitis. Nat Med. 2002;8:500–8.
40. Kotake S, Udagawa N, Takahashi N, Matsuzaki K, Itoh K, Ishiyama S, et al. IL-17 in synovial fluids from patients with rheumatoid arthritis is a potent stimulator of osteoclastogenesis. J Clin Invest. 1999;103:1345–52.
41. Hirota K, Yoshitomi H, Hashimoto M, Maeda S, Teradaira S, Sugimoto N, et al. Preferential recruitment of CCR6-expressing Th17 cells to inflamed joints via CCL20 in rheumatoid arthritis and its animal model. J Exp Med. 2007;204:2803–12.
42. Wong CK, Lit LC, Tam LS, Li EK, Wong PT, Lam CW, et al. Hyperproduction of IL-23 and IL-17 in patients with systemic lupus erythematosus: implications for Th17-mediated inflammation in auto-immunity. Clin Immunol. 2008;127:385–93.
43. Doreau A, Belot A, Bastid J, Riche B, Trescol-Biemont MC, Ranchin B, et al. Interleukin 17 acts in synergy with B cell-activating factor to influence B cell biology and the pathophysiology of systemic lupus erythematosus. Nat Immunol. 2009;10:778–85.
44. Linden A, Hoshino H, Laan M. Airway neutrophils and interleukin-17. Eur Respir J. 2000;15:973–7.
45. Zhu S, Qian Y. IL-17/IL-17 receptor system in autoimmune disease: mechanisms and therapeutic potential. Clin Sci. 2012;122:487–511.
46. Haak S, Croxford AL, Kreymborg K, Heppner FL, Pouly S, Becher B, et al. IL-17A and IL-17F do not contribute vitally to autoimmune neuro-inflammation in mice. J Clin Investig. 2009;119:61–9.
47. Azizi G, Yazdani R, Mirshafiey A. Th22 cells in autoimmunity: a review of current knowledge. Eur Ann Allergy Clin Immunol. 2015;47:108–17.
48. Tian T, Yu S, Ma D. Th22 and related cytokines in inflammatory and autoimmune diseases. Expert Opin Ther Targets. 2013;17:113–25.
49. Mesquita D Jr, Cruvinel WM, Resende LS, Mesquita FV, Silva NP, Câmara NO, et al. Follicular helper T cell in immunity and autoimmunity. Braz J Med Biol Res. 2016;49:e5209. doi:10.1590/1414-431X20165209.
50. Meka RR, Venkatesha SH, Dudics S, Acharya B, Moudgil KD. IL-27-induced modulation of autoimmunity and its therapeutic potential. Autoimmun Rev. 2015;14:1131–41.
51. Weetman AP. Immunity, thyroid function and pregnancy: molecular mechanisms. Nat Rev Endocrinol. 2010;6:311–8.
52. De Man YA, Dolhain RJ, Hazes JM. Disease activity or remission of rheumatoid arthritis before, during and following pregnancy. Curr Opin Rheumatol. 2014;26:329–33.
53. Pozzilli C, Pugliatti M. ParadigMS Group. An overview of pregnancy-related issues in patients with multiple sclerosis. Eur J Neurol. 2015;22(Suppl 2):34–9.
54. Airas L. Hormonal and gender-related immune changes in multiple sclerosis. Acta Neurol Scand. 2015;132:62–70.
55. Jara LJ, Medina G, Cruz-Dominguez P, Navarro C, Vera-Lastra O, Saavedra MA. Risk factors of systemic lupus erythematosus flares during pregnancy. Immunol Res. 2014;60:184–92.

56. Andersson A, Stubelius A, Karlsson MN, Engdahl C, Erlandsson M, Grahnemo L, et al. Estrogen regulates T helper 17 phenotype and localization in experimental autoimmune arthritis. Arthritis Res Ther. 2015;17:32. doi:10.1186/s13075-015-0548-y.
57. Quintero OL, Amador-Patarroyo MJ, Montoya-Ortiz G, Rojas-Villarraga A, Anaya JM. Autoimmune disease and gender: plausible mechanisms for the female predominance of autoimmunity. J Autoimmun. 2012;38:J109–19.
58. González DA, Díaz BB. Rodríguez Pérez Mdel C, Hernández AG, Chico BN, de León AC. Sex hormones and autoimmunity. Immunol Lett. 2010;133:6–13.
59. Khosla S, Melton LJ 3rd, Atkinson EJ, O'Fallon WM. Relationship of serum sex steroid levels to longitudinal changes in bone density in young versus elderly men. J Clin Endocrinol Metab. 2001;86:3555–61.
60. Ostensen M. Sex hormones and pregnancy in rheumatoid arthritis and systemic lupus erythematosus. Ann N Y Acad Sci. 1999;876:131–43.
61. Engdahl C, Jochems C, Windahl SH, Börjesson AE, Ohlsson C, Carlsten H, et al. Amelioration of collagen-induced arthritis and immune-associated bone loss through signaling via estrogen receptor α, and not estrogen receptor β or G protein-coupled receptor 30. Arthritis Rheum. 2010;62:524–33.
62. D'Elia HF, Larsen A, Mattsson LA, Waltbrand E, Kvist G, Mellström D, et al. Influence of hormone replacement therapy on disease progression and bone mineral density in rheumatoid arthritis. J Rheumatol. 2003;30:1456–63.
63. Rijhsinghani AG, Thompson K, Bhatia SK, Waldschmidt TJ. Estrogen blocks early T cell development in the thymus. Am J Reprod Immunol. 1996;36:269–77.
64. Straub RH. The complex role of estrogens in inflammation. Endocr Rev. 2007;28:521–74.
65. Leipe J, Grunke M, Dechant C, Reindl C, Kerzendorf U, Schulze-Koops H, et al. Role of Th17 cells in human autoimmune arthritis. Arthritis Rheum. 2010;62:2876–85.
66. Lélu K, Laffont S, Delpy L, Paulet PE, Périnat T, Tschanz SA, et al. Estrogen receptor α signaling in T lymphocytes is required for estradiol-mediated inhibition of Th1 and Th17 cell differentiation and protection against experimental autoimmune encephalomyelitis. J Immunol. 2011;187:2386–93.
67. Plum SM, Park EJ, Strawn SJ, Moore EG, Sidor CF, Fogler WE. Disease modifying and antiangiogenic activity of 2-methoxyestradiol in a murine model of rheumatoid arthritis. BMC Musculoskelet Disord. 2009;10:46.
68. Xu L, Dong B, Wang H, Zeng Z, Liu W, Chen N, et al. Progesterone suppresses Th17 cell responses, and enhances the development of regulatory T cells, through thymic stromal lymphopoietin-dependent mechanisms in experimental gonococcal genital tract infection. Microbes Infect. 2013;15:796–805.
69. Bashyam H. Th1/Th2 cross-regulation and discovery of IL-10. J Exp Med. 2007;204:237.
70. Piccinni MP, Bani D, Beloni L, Manuelli C, Mavilia C, Vocioni F, et al. Relaxin favors the development of activated human T cells into Th1-like effectors. Eur J Immunol. 1999;29:2241–7.
71. Scaletti C, Vultaggio A, Maggi E, Romagnani S, Piccinni MP. Microchimerism and systemic sclerosis. Int Arch Allergy Immunol. 2001;125:196–202.
72. Scaletti C, Vultaggio A, Bonifacio S, Emmi L, Torricelli F, Maggi E, et al. Th2-oriented profile of male offspring T cells present in women with systemic sclerosis and reactive with maternal major histocompatibility complex antigens. Arthritis Rheum. 2002;46:445–50.
73. Adams Waldorf KM. Nelson JL. Autoimmune disease during pregnancy and the microchimerism legacy of pregnancy. Immunol Invest. 2008;37:631–44. doi:10.1080/08820130802205886.
74. Ye J, Vives-Pi M, Gillespie KM. Maternal microchimerism: friend or foe in type 1 diabetes? Chimerism. 2014;5:21–3.

17

Allergic sensitization to common pets (cats/dogs) according to different possible modalities of exposure

G. Liccardi[1,2*], L. Calzetta[2,3], G. Baldi[4], A. Berra[5], L. Billeri[6], M. Caminati[7], P. Capano[8], E. Carpentieri[9], A. Ciccarelli[10], M. A. Crivellaro[11], M. Cutajar[12], M. D'Amato[13], I. Folletti[14], F. Gani[15], D. Gargano[16], D. Giannattasio[17], M. Giovannini[18], C. Lombardi[19], M. Lo Schiavo[20], F. Madonna[21], M. Maniscalco[22], A. Meriggi[23], C. Micucci[24], M. Milanese[25], C. Montera[20], G. Paolocci[14], R. Parente[26], A. Pedicini[27], R. Pio[20], F. Puggioni[28], M. Russo[1], A. Salzillo[1], P. Scavalli[29], N. Scichilone[30], B. Sposato[31], A. Stanziola[13], G. Steinhilber[32], A. Vatrella[33], P. Rogliani[2,3], G. Passalacqua[34] and On behalf of Italian Allergic Respiratory Diseases Task Force

Abstract

Background: The query "are there animals at home?" is usually administered for collecting information on anamnesis. This modality to consider exposure to pet allergens constitutes a potential bias in epidemiological studies and in clinical practice. The aim of our study was to evaluate/quantify different modalities of exposure to cat/dog in inducing allergic sensitization.

Methods: Thirty Italian Allergy units participated in this study. Each centre was required to collect the data of at least 20 consecutive outpatients sensitized to cat/dog allergens. A standardized form reported all demographic data and a particular attention was paid in relieving possible modalities of exposure to cat/dog.

Results: A total 723 patients sensitized to cat/dog were recorded, 359 (49.65%) reported direct pet contact, 213 patients (29.46%) were pet owners, and 146 subjects (20.19%) were exposed to pets in other settings. Other patients were sensitized by previous pet ownership (150–20.75%) or indirect contact (103–14.25%), in 111 subjects (15.35%) any contact was reported.

Conclusions: Only 213 patients (29.46%) would be classified as "exposed to animals" and 510 (70.54%) as "not exposed" according to usual query. Our classification has shown that many "not-exposed" subjects (399–55.19%) were "really exposed". The magnitude of exposure to pet allergens at home is not related exclusively to pet ownership. These considerations should be taken into account during the planning of epidemiological studies and in clinical practice for the management of pet allergic individuals.

Keywords: Allergic rhinitis, Allergic sensitization, Bronchial asthma, Cat, Dog, Pets exposure, Hypersensitivity, Pets

*Correspondence: gennaro.liccardi@tin.it
[2] Postgraduate School of Respiratory Medicine. Department of Experimental Medicine and Surgery, University of Rome "Tor Vergata", Rome, Italy
Full list of author information is available at the end of the article

Background

Exposure to animal allergens constitutes a relevant risk factor for the development of allergic sensitization and respiratory allergic diseases, such as asthma and rhino-conjunctivitis in susceptible individuals [1]. In all developed countries cats and dogs are the most common pets living in indoor environments and the frequency of their ownership is highly variable, according to cultural differences and environmental factors [2, 3]. Cat and dog allergens should be considered ubiquitous because they are found not only in indoor environments, where these animals are kept, but also in other indoor private or public places where cats/dogs have been never kept [4]. Although the presence of a pet at home is considered usually the main risk factor for allergic sensitization, dynamic distribution of the main pet allergens indoors is complex and depends by production, aero-dispersion, sedimentation and passive transport through clothes and other items [5–9]. These variables determine a diffuse presence of pet allergens (indirect exposure) also in indoor environments without pets and in environments where pets are no longer present for a long time (e.g. voluntary removal or re-location, natural death etc.) [10–12]. The query "are there animals at home?" is common and usually administered by researchers, physicians and pulmonologists/allergologists to patients for collecting information on anamnesis [13]. This prevalent modality to consider exposure to pet allergens constitutes a potential bias in large epidemiological studies on the relationship between pet-exposure and allergic sensitization [14]. We believe that an accurate medical history on pet exposure is essential also in clinical practice for an objective evaluation of the risk and the clinical significance of the skin-prick-test (SPT) positivity to pet (cat/dog) allergens, as well as for the management of sensitized patients (pet-avoidance measures, allergen immunotherapy, pharmacological treatment of respiratory symptoms etc.) [14]. The aim of our study was to evaluate and quantify the role of different modalities of exposure to cat/dog in inducing allergic sensitization in a consistent population of cat and/or dog sensitized individuals living in Italy.

Methods

Thirty Allergy units, distributed over the whole national territory and belonging to the "Italian Allergic Respiratory Diseases Task Force" participated in this cross-sectional study. Each centre collected data of at least 20 consecutive outpatients, referred for actual asthma and/or rhinitis and sensitized to cat/dog allergens. Data were collected from January 1 to June 30 2013. All centres followed the same protocol, recorded the results in a previously agreed form and obtained an informed consent. Subjects with occupational exposure to cat/dog (farmers, stable-men, or veterinary doctors) were not considered to avoid possible inhibition of SPT responses as a consequence of exposure to higher amounts of pet allergens. Patients with chronic infectious diseases, malignancies or dysmetabolic diseases, severe cutaneous disorders, negative skin reaction to histamine, or treated with drugs interfering with the skin response were excluded from the study [15]. The standardized form reported: demographic data, type and duration of respiratory symptoms, results of the SPTs. Since the absence of a pet at home does not exclude a direct exposure to pet outside and the presence of a pet at home must not be considered the only criterion of pet contact, the assessment of further possible modalities of exposure to cat/dog was considered with specific regard (Fig. 1). The forms had to be filled by the allergist, who also verified the consistency of clinical history and SPT results. Then, the same doctor confirmed the diagnosis of respiratory allergy according to the International Guidelines [16, 17]. The commercial allergen extracts used for screening SPTs were provided by ALK Abello Group, Milan Italy. All centres used the same standard panel of allergens including: *Dermatophagoides pteronyssinus, Dermatophagoides farinae, Alternaria alternata, Cladosporium herbarum*, cat dander, dog dander, *Parietaria*, Grass mix, *Artemisia vulgaris, Olea europaea, Betula pendula, Cupressus sempervirens*, and *Corylus avellana*. These allergens covered the majority of allergens causing respiratory allergy in Italy. Positive (10 mg/ml histamine HCl) and negative (saline solution in glycerine-phenol solution) controls were used. SPTs were carried out and interpreted according to international guidelines [18]. The results were read after 15 min and expressed as the mean of the major wheal diameter plus its orthogonal. A skin reaction of 3 mm or greater was considered positive. SPTs were always performed by the same operator in each centre. The profiles of the wheals were outlined using a fine-point marking pen and transferred by adhesive tape onto patient's form.

Results

The participating centres were distributed over the Italian territory. A total of 723 patients sensitized to cat/dog as well as to other allergens were registered, and the main characteristics of these subjects are summarized in Table 1. No patients were mono-sensitized to the common pets, the low percentage of pet-mono-sensitized patients has been described also by other authors [19]. Since all cat/dog-sensitized patients showed multiple cutaneous positivity to other common allergens (mites, pollens and moulds), we could not quantify the role of cat/dog sensitization on the entire duration of allergic symptoms during the year. As shown in Table 2, 359 patients (49.65%) reported direct pet contact, 213

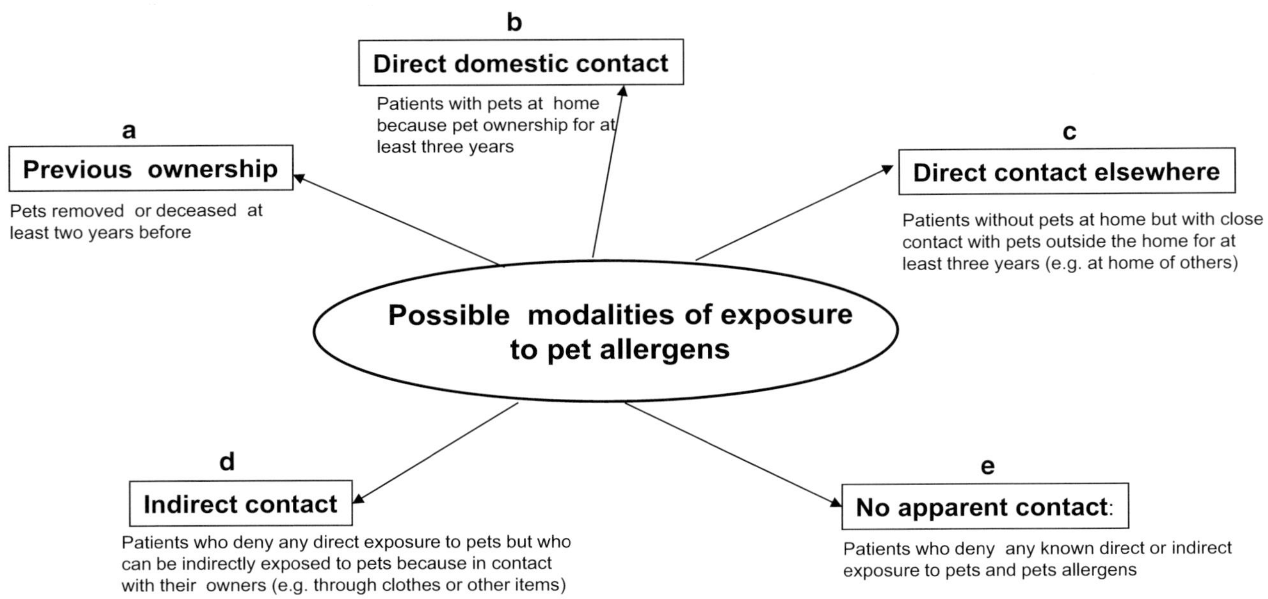

Fig. 1 An overview of modalities of exposure to pet allergens reported in our standardized form (Modified from [10])

patients (29.46%) were pet owners (pets at home), and 146 subjects (20.19%) were directly exposed to pets in other settings (for at least 3 years in both groups). The remaining patients were likely sensitized because previous pet ownership (150–20.75%) or indirect contact through pet-contaminated items (103–14.25%), in 111 individuals (15.35%) any apparent (direct/indirect) contact was reported. In Table 3 the number and % of patients reporting a worsening of respiratory symptoms after direct exposure to pets is shown. Three hundred seventy-five patients (51.8%) reported an evident aggravation of rhino-conjunctivitis/asthma following pet contact, while 10 patients (1.3%) denied any clinical effects. The cat allergy was more common than that to dog in inducing acute respiratory symptoms in susceptible individuals (259 vs. 56 subjects, respectively). Because monoclonal antibody-based methods to measure the amount of cat/dog allergens in the dust of indoor environments were not available in Italy, we have not information about the levels of indoor exposure to pet allergens.

Discussion and conclusions

Common pet ownership with a stable presence of the animal indoors is usually considered the main index of exposure to cat/dog, with the consequent risk of inducing allergic sensitization. "Are there animals at home?" is the common query administered by doctors to patients in order to collect information on anamnesis during epidemiological studies on the relationship between exposure to pets and development of allergic sensitization (e.g. during the first phase of life to evaluate a "protective effect" of early exposure to cat/dog). The same query is commonly used also in clinical practice to establish the clinical significance of a SPT positivity to cat/dog allergens and, thus, to manage the sensitized patients (pet-avoidance measures, allergen immunotherapy, pharmacological treatment of respiratory symptoms etc.). This commonly used question should not be considered the main factor of exposure to pet allergens and, consequently, the main risk factor for allergic sensitization either in clinical practice and large epidemiological studies [12, 20, 21]. In fact, Fig. 1 shows that only the condition b is reported usually in the questionnaires utilized for large epidemiological studies as well as in clinical practice for collecting data on anamnesis. In the conditions a, c and d the presence of a pet at home should be considered "formally negative" in the questionnaires or anamnestic report, but the level of direct/indirect exposure to pet allergens could be significant [4–7]. Only the condition e should be considered at the lower risk of pet allergen exposure after having excluded any direct/indirect contact with pets. Therefore, the simple answer "yes or no" on the question regarding the presence of pet at home can lead to misleading interpretation of the clinical significance of positive SPTs as well as the real risk of exposure to allergens of dog/cat in epidemiological studies. Consequently, we have previously suggested a new, more realistic, classification of modalities of exposure to pet allergens in "real life" based on the five possible conditions reported in Fig. 1. We have used this classification

Table 1 Characteristics of the patients sensitized to dog/cat allergens (total no. = 723)

	No (%)
Age range (years)	
0–20	202 (28.0)
21–40	318 (44.0)
41–60	159 (22.0)
> 60	44 (6.0)
Sex: male/female	384/339 (53.1/46.8)
Family history of atopy (yes/no)[a]	358/365 (49.5/50.4)
Intermittent/mild persistent asthma[b]	137 (17.2)
Moderate/severe persistent asthma[b]	80 (10.1)
Intermittent/mild persistent rhinitis[b]	274 (34.4)
Moderate/severe persistent rhinitis[b]	305 (38.3)
Allergic sensitization to common pets	
Dog	160 (22.1)
Cat	256 (35.4)
Dog/cat	307 (42.5)
Allergic sensitization only to cat/dog	0 (0)
Age of onset of respiratory symptoms (years)	
0–20	493 (68.2)
21–40	176 (24.3)
41–60	51 (7.1)
> 60	3 (0.4)
Smoking habit	
Never	479 (66.3)
Actual	105 (14.5)
Past	79 (10.9)
Passive smoke only	60 (8.3)
Previous immunotherapy	
No	622 (86.0)
Yes (none for pets)	101 (14.0)

[a] At least one parent with history of asthma/allergic rhinitis/atopic dermatitis/food allergy

[b] Diagnosis of asthma and/or rhinitis (the majority of patients have shown both symptoms)

of exposure either for common pets and large animal such as horse, for which we have provided some specific modifications [10, 21–27]. To the best of our knowledge, this is the first study on the application of these new queries on the modality of exposure to pet allergens. As shown by Table 2, only a limited amount of patients sensitized to pets should be classified as "exposed to animals", whereas the majority of patients should be classified as "not exposed" as a consequence of usual query "are there animals at home?. On the other hand and in agreement with our classification, a high percentage of formally "not-exposed" subjects were "really exposed" to pets. As a consequence of the present classification, only few patients were really "not-exposed" because no apparent direct/indirect exposure to pets or pet-derived materials. Another important finding of our study is that only half of our pet-sensitized individuals reported a clinically relevant symptoms worsening as a consequence of a close contact with pets, especially with cats. If we consider the modality of exposure, it is likely that these individuals belong to the groups directly exposed to pets at home or elsewhere [28]. These findings confirm that in already pet-sensitized patients a direct and prolonged exposure to animals may represent a relevant risk factor for exacerbations of respiratory symptoms [29]. It is important to note that 338 individuals (46.7%) failed to respond presumably because the symptoms were considered negligible, or not related with the contact of animals.

This is a possible limitation of this study. Other limitations are the lack of data on the presence of pet allergens at home for the reasons previously reported, and the lack of data on the general population regarding the exposure to pets in the first years of life.

In conclusion, this study suggests that our novel classification could be of particular importance to correctly evaluate the modality of pet exposure at home in the countries characterized by a high frequency of pet ownership. It is likely that, in these countries, the "average amount" of pet allergens indoors could be high (or very high in some particular conditions) also in the absence of a pet at home. The magnitude of exposure to pet allergens at home is not exclusively related to pet ownership/presence of a pet indoors, but can be also relevant without a pet living with the inhabitants. In addition, we have previously demonstrated, by using in vivo [30] and in vitro [31] methods, that allergic sensitization to common pets significantly increases the risk of developing sensitization to other furry animals, likely for cross-sensitization

Table 2 Possible modalities of exposure to pet allergens in 723 pet-sensitized patients (no and %)

Possible modalities of exposure to pets	No (%)	DOG, no (%)	CAT, no (%)	DOG/CAT, no (%)
Previous ownership	150 (20.75 %)	65 (8.9)	62 (8.5)	23 (3.2)
Direct domestic contact	213 (29.46 %)	104 (14.3)	88 (12.1)	21 (2.9)
Direct contact elsewhere	146 (20.19 %)	50 (6.9)	57 (7.9)	39 (5.4)
Indirect contact	103 (14.25 %)	23 (3.2)	46 (6.3)	34 (4.7)
No apparent contact	111 (15.35 %)	12 (1.7)	16 (2.2)	83 (11.5)

Table 3 Triggering of respiratory symptoms after exposure to pet allergens in 723 pet-sensitized patients (no and %)

	Type of response	Total, no (%)	DOG, no (%)	CAT, no (%)	DOG/CAT, no (%)
Are allergic respiratory symptoms triggered by direct pet contact?	Positive	375 (51.8)	56 (7.8)	259 (35.8)	60 (8.3)
	Negative	10 (1.3)	5 (0.6)	3 (0.4)	2 (0.3)
	No response	338 (46.7)	(*) All pets		
		Patients no (%)			
		723 (100)			

(*) No response regards both pets without distinction

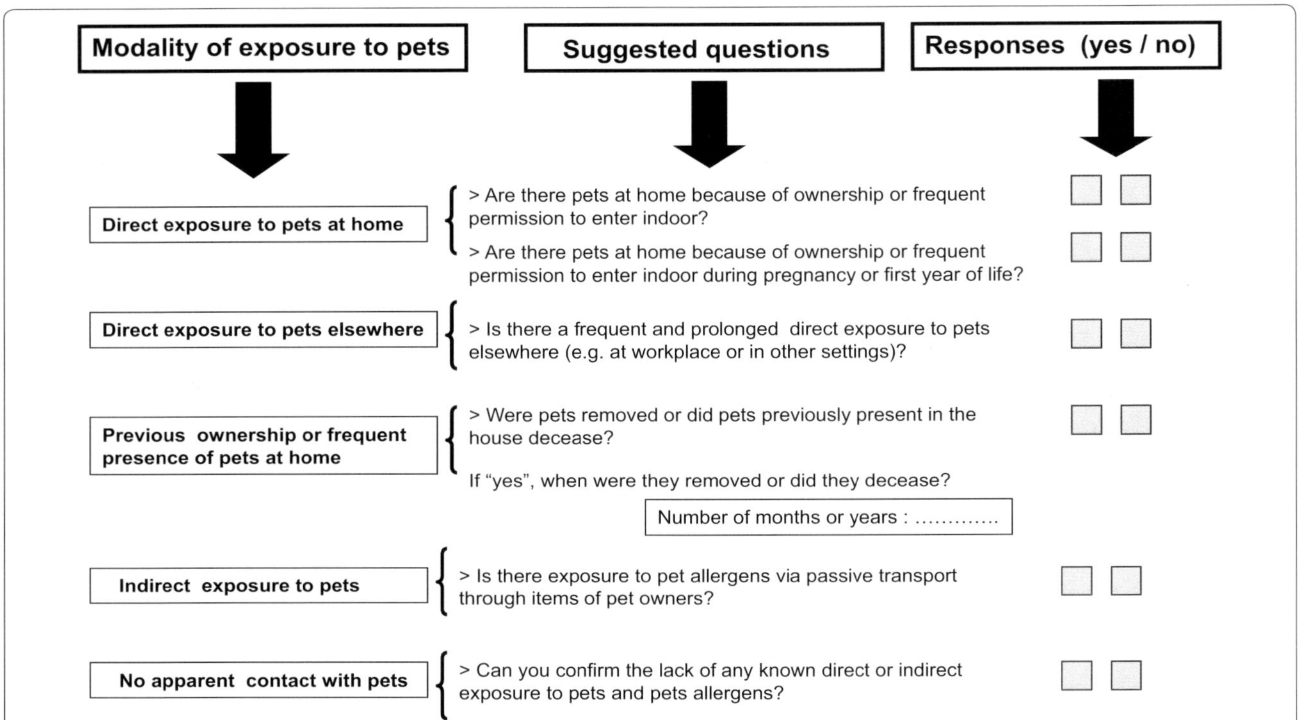

Fig. 2 Suggested items to assess exposure to pet allergens in epidemiological studies and in clinical practice (Modified from [14])

mechanism involving albumins and lipocalins. These considerations should be taken into account during the planning of epidemiological studies on the relationship between exposure to pet and development of allergic sensitization to pet allergens. In clinical practice, a real assessment of the risk and clinical significance of allergic sensitization to pet allergens is crucial for the management of patients (pet-avoidance measures, allergen immunotherapy, pharmacological treatment of respiratory symptoms etc.). In this context we have suggested few and well-defined questions to assess pet exposure in "real life" (Fig. 2) [14]. Finally, we believe that the topic of animal allergy is very important for both clinical and emotional implications in pet-owner patients, and especially in children. The love for animals in general and for pets in particular is increasing world-wide, so we wish to underline the necessity of an adequate assessment of risk factors for allergic sensitization, and possible prevention strategies by using a more realistic evaluation of possible modalities of exposure.

Authors' contributions

GL conceived the idea, designed this study and wrote manuscript first draft. BG, BA, CM, CP, CE, CA, CMA, CMAR, DAM, FI, GF, GD, GDOM, MC, MM, MC, PG, PR, PA, PR, PF, SA, SP, SN, SB, SA, SG and VA recruited pet-sensitized patients. CL, RP, PG, collected the data and RM performed the statistical analyses. All co-authors drafted the manuscript and gave input and agreed to the final submitted version. All authors read and approved the final manuscript.

Author details

[1] Department of Pulmonology, Haematology and Oncology. Division of Pneumology and Allergology, High Speciality "A. Cardarelli" Hospital, Naples, Italy. [2] Postgraduate School of Respiratory Medicine. Department of Experimental Medicine and Surgery, University of Rome "Tor Vergata", Rome, Italy. [3] Department of Experimental Medicine and Surgery, University of Rome Tor Vergata, Rome, Italy. [4] Respiratory Medicine Unit, ASL (District 66), Salerno, Italy.

[5] Respiratory Allergy Unit, G. Da Procida Hospital, Salerno, Italy. [6] Department of Laboratory Medicine, University Hospital Padova, Padua, Italy. [7] Asthma Center and Allergy Unit, Verona University and General Hospital, Verona, Italy. [8] Unit of Pulmonary Immunology and Respiratory Diseases Ospedale "Santa Maria Della Speranza", Battipaglia, Salerno, Italy. [9] Division of Pneumology, "Santa Maria Novella" Hospital, Galatina, Lecce, Italy. [10] Allergy Unit, Loreto Crispi Hospital, Naples, Italy. [11] Unit of Allergy and Occupational Medicine, University Hospital Padova, Padua, Italy. [12] Allergy Center, Division of Internal Medicine, Ospedali Riuniti Penisola Sorrentina, Sorrento, Naples, Italy. [13] Department of Respiratory Disease, "Federico II" University – AO "Dei Colli", Naples, Italy. [14] Department of Medicine, Section of Occupational Medicine, Respiratory Diseases and Toxicology, Terni Hospital, University of Perugia, Perugia, Italy. [15] Allergy Unit, S. Luigi Gonzaga Hospital, Orbassano, Turin, Italy. [16] Allergy Unit, High Speciality "San Giuseppe Moscati" Hospital, Avellino, Italy. [17] Respiratory Physiopathology and Allergy, High Speciality Center, "Mauro Scarlato" Hospital, Scafati, Salerno, Italy. [18] Pulmonary Diseases Department, Mirandola Hospital, Modena, Italy. [19] Departmental Unit of Allergy, Clinical Immunology and Respiratory Diseases, Fondazione Poliambulanza, Brescia, Italy. [20] Allergy and Clinical Immunology, "G. Fucito" Hospital, S. Giovanni di Dio e Ruggi D'Aragona University Hospital, Salerno, Italy. [21] Allergy Unit, ASL (Sanitary District n°12), Caserta, Italy. [22] Pulmonary Rehabilitation Unit, ICS Maugeri, Telese Terme, Benevento, Italy. [23] Allergy and Immunology Unit, Fondazione "Salvatore Maugeri", Institut of Research and Care, Scientific Institute of Pavia, Pavia, Italy. [24] Division of Pneumology and Allergology Hospital "Carlo Urbani", Jesi, Ancona, Italy. [25] Division of Pneumology, S. Corona Hospital, Pietra Ligure, Savona, Italy. [26] Division of Allergy and Clinical Immunology, University of Salerno, Salerno, Italy. [27] Division of Internal Medicine and Allergy, Fatebenefratelli Hospital, Benevento, Italy. [28] Respiratory Diseases Department-IRCCS Humanitas Research and Clinical Center, Rozzano, Milan, Italy. [29] Unit of Respiratory Physiopathology, Allergy and Occupational Medicine, ASL Viterbo, Viterbo, Italy. [30] Biomedical Department of Specialistic and Internal Medicine, University of Palermo, Palermo, Italy. [31] Pneumology Unit, Azienda Ospedaliera "Misericordia", Grosseto, Italy. [32] Division of Pneumology, Spedali Civili Brescia, Brescia, Italy. [33] Department of Medicine and Surgery, University of Salerno, Fisciano, Italy. [34] Allergy and Respiratory Diseases, Policlinico San Martino, University of Genoa, Genoa, Italy.

Acknowledgements
The authors would like to thank the veterinarian doctor Dr. Giovanni Menna as pet consultant and Mr. Gaetano Francesco Salzillo for technical assistance in the preparation of tables and figures.

Italian Allergic Respiratory Diseases Task Force (other components) Ilaria Baiardini, Caterina Bucca, Giorgio Walter Canonica, Maria Teresa Costantino, Stefano Del Giacco, Enrico Heffler, Stefania La Grutta, Vincenzo Patella, Erminia Ridolo, Giovanni Rolla, Oliviero Rossi, Eleonora Savi, Gianenrico Senna, Carlo Filippo Tesi, Giovanni Viegi.

References

1. Konradsen JR, Fujisawa T, van Hage M, Hedlin G, Hilger C, Kleine-tebbe J, Matsui EC, Roberts G, Ronmark E, Platts-Mills TAE. Allergy to furry animals: new insights, diagnostic approaches, and challenges. J Allergy Clin Immunol. 2015;135:616–25.
2. Eller E, Roll S, Chen CM, Herbarth O, Wichman HE, Berg A, Krämer U, Mommers M, Thijs C, Wijga A, Brunekreef B, Fantini MP, Bravi F, Forastiere F, Porta D, Sunyer J, Torrent M, Høst A, Halken S, Lødrup Carlsen KC, Carlsen KH, Wickman M, Kull I, Wahn U, Willich SN, Lau S, Keil T, Heinrich J. Meta-analysis of determinants for pet ownership in 12 European birth cohort on asthma and allergies: a GA2LEN initiative. Allergy. 2008;63:1491–8.
3. Sheikh SI, Pitts J, Ryan-Wenger NA, McCoy KS, Hayes D. Racial differences in pet ownership in families of children with asthma. World J Pediatr. 2016;12:343–6.
4. Liccardi G, D'Amato G, D'Amato L, Salzillo A, Piccolo A, De Napoli I, Dente B, Cazzola M. The effect of pet ownership on the risk of allergic sensitization and bronchial asthma. Respir Med. 2005;99:227–33.
5. Chan-Yeung M, McClean PA, Sandell PR, Slutsky AS, Zamel N. Sensitization to cat without direct cat exposure. Clin Exp Allergy. 1999;29:762–5.
6. Munir AKM, Einarsson R, Schou C, Dreborg SKG. Allergens in school dust.I. The amount of the major cat (*Fel d* 1) and dog (*Can f* 1) allergens in dust from Swedish schools is high enough to probably cause perennial symptoms in most children with asthma who are sensitized to cat and dog. J Allergy Clin Immunol. 1993;91:1067–74.
7. Liccardi G, D'Amato G, Russo M, Canonica GW, D'Amato L, Passalacqua G. Focus on cat allergen (Fel d 1): immunological and aerodynamic characteristics, modality of airway sensitization and avoidance strategies. Int Arch Allergy Immunol. 2003;132:1–12.
8. D'Amato G, Liccardi G, Russo M, Barber D, D'Amato M, Carreira J. Clothing is a carrier of cat allergens. J Allergy Clin Immunol. 1997;99:577–8.
9. Liccardi G, Barber D, Russo M, D'Amato M, D'Amato G. Human hair: an unexpected source of cat allergen exposure. Int Arch Allergy Immunol. 2005;137:141–4.
10. Liccardi G, Salzillo A, Calzetta L, Piccolo A, Menna G, Rogliani P. Can the presence of cat/dog at home be considered the only criterion of exposure to cat/dog allergens? A likely underestimated bias in clinical practice and in large epidemiological studies. Eur Ann Allergy Clin Immunol. 2016;48:61–4.
11. Liccardi G, Salzillo A, Calzetta L, Pignatti P, Rogliani P. Can pet keeping be considered the only criterion of exposure toc at/dog allergens in the first year of life ? Allergol Immunopathol (Madr). 2016;44:387–8.
12. Liccardi G, Salzillo A, Cecchi L, D'Amato M, D'Amato G. Is cat-keeping the main determinant of new-onset adulthood cat sensitization ? J Allergy Clin Immunol. 2012;129:1689–90.
13. Apfelbacher C, Frew E, Xiang A, Apfel A, Smith H. Assessment of pet exposure by self-report in epidemiological studies of allergy and asthma: a systematic review. J Asthma. 2016;53:363–73.
14. Liccardi G, Salzillo A, Calzetta L, Piccolo A, Rogliani P. Assessment of pet exposure by questionnaires in epidemiological studies (but also in clinical practice!): why the questions should be simplified? J Asthma. 2016;53:879–81.
15. Bousquet J, Michel FB. Precision of prick and puncture tests. J Allergy Clin Immunol. 1992;90:870–2.
16. Bousquet J, The ARIA, Workshop Group. Allergic rhinitis and its impact on asthma. J Allergy Clin Immunol. 2001;108:S147–336.
17. Global Initiative for Asthma. http://ginasthma.com.
18. Bousquet J, Heinzerling L, Bachert C, Papadopoulos NG, Bousquet PJ, Burney PG, Canonica GW, Carlsen KH, Cox L, Haahtela T, Lodrup Carlsen KC, Price D, Samolinski B, Simons FE, Wickman M, Annesi-Maesano I, Baena-Cagnani CE, Berg-mann KC, Bindslev-Jensen C, Casale TB, Chiriac A, Cruz AA, Dubakiene R, Durham SR, Fokkens WJ, Gerth-van-Wijk R, Ka-layci O, Kowalski ML, Mari A, Mullol J, Nazamova-Baranova L, O'Hehir RE, Ohta K, Panzner P, Passalacqua G, Ring J, Rogala B, Romano A, Ryan D, Schmid-Grendelmeier P, Todo-Bom A, Valenta R, Woehrl S, Yusuf OM, Zuberbier T, Demoly P. Global allergy and asthma european network; allergic rhinitis and its impact on asthma. Practical guide to skin prick tests in allergy to aeroallergens. Allergy. 2012;67:18–24.
19. Galvão CES, Graudenz GS, Kalil J, Castro FFM. Sensitization to cat allergen and its association with respiratory allergies: cross-sectional study. Sao Paulo Med J. 2017;135:488–90.
20. Liccardi G, Salzillo A, Calzetta L, Piccolo A, Rogliani P. Chronic cat allergen exposure and low sensitization: possible limitations in patients' selection? J Allergy Clin Immunol. 2016;137:1621–2.

21. Liccardi G, D'Amato G, Canonica GW, Dente B, Passalacqua G. Severe respiratory allergy induced by indirect exposure to rabbit dander: a case report. Allergy. 2004;59:1237–8.
22. Liccardi G, Piccolo A, Dente B, Salzillo A, Gilder JA, Russo M, D'Amato G. Rabbit allergens: a significant risk for allergic sensitization in subjects without occupational exposure. Respir Med. 2007;101:333–9.
23. Liccardi G, Passalacqua G, on behalf of the Allergy Study Group of the Italian Society of Respiratory Medicine (SIMeR). Sensitization to rabbit allergens in Italy—a multicentre study in atopic subjects without occupational exposure. Int Arch Allergy Immunol. 2006;141:295–9.
24. Liccardi G, Salzillo A, Dente B, Piccolo A, Lobefalo G, Russo M, Gilder JA, D'Amato G. Horse allergens: an underestimated risk for allergic sensitization in an urban atopic population without occupational exposure. Respir Med. 2009;103:414–20.
25. Liccardi G, Salzillo A, Sofia M, Piccolo A, Dente B, Russo M, D'Amato M, Stanziola A, D'Amato G. Sensitization to rodents (mouse/rat) in an urban atopic population without occupational exposure living in Naples. Italy. Eur Ann Allergy Clin Immunol. 2012;44:200–4.
26. Liccardi G, Salzillo A, Piccolo A, Russo M, D'Amato G. Sensitization to furry animals in an urban atopic population living in Naples, Italy. Allergy. 2011;66:1500–1.
27. Liccardi G, D'Amato G, Antonicelli L, Berra A, Billeri L, Canoni-ca GW, Casino G, Cecchi L, Folletti I, Gani F, Lombardi C, Lo Schiavo M, Meriggi A, Milanese M, Passalacqua G, Pio R, Rolla G, Russo M, Scaccianoce S, Senna GE, Scavalli P, Scichilone N, Sposato B, Siracusa A, Ventura MT, Allergy Study Group of the Italian Society of Respiratory Medicine (SIMeR). Sensitization to horse allergens in Italy: a multicentre study in urban atopic subjects without occupational exposure. Int Arch Allergy Immunol. 2011;155:1103–14.
28. Heinrich J, Bedada GB, Zock JP, Chinn S, Norbäck D, Olivieri M, Svanes C, Ponzio M, Verlato G, Villani S, Jarvis D, Luczynska C, Indoor Working Group of the European Community Respiratory Health Survey II. Cat allergen level: its determinants and relationship to specific IgE to cat across European centers. J Allergy Clin Immunol. 2006;118:674–81.
29. Zeidler MR, Goldin JG, Kleerup EC, Kim HJ, Truong DA, Gjertson DW, Kennedy NJ, Newman KB, Tashkin DP, Silverman JM, Corren J. Small airways response to naturalistic cat allergen exposure in subjects with asthma. J Allergy Clin Immunol. 2006;118:1075–81.
30. Liccardi G, Passalacqua G, Salzillo A, Piccolo A, Falagiani P, Russo M, Canonica GW, D'Amato G. Is sensitization to furry animals an independent allergic phenotype in non-occupationally exposed individuals ? J Investig Allergol Clin Immunol. 2011;21:137–41.
31. Liccardi G, Meriggi A, Russo M, Croce S, Salzillo A, Pignatti P. The risk of sensitization to furry animals in patients already sensitized to cat/dog: a in vitro evaluation using molecular-based allergy diagnostics. J Allergy Clin Immunol. 2015;135:1664–6.

18

Urban air pollution and climate change: "The Decalogue: Allergy Safe Tree" for allergic and respiratory diseases care

Vincenzo Patella[1,2,3*†], Giovanni Florio[1,2†], Diomira Magliacane[1†], Ada Giuliano[4†], Maria Angiola Crivellaro[3,5†], Daniela Di Bartolomeo[3,6†], Arturo Genovese[2,3†], Mario Palmieri[3,7†], Amedeo Postiglione[3,8†], Erminia Ridolo[3,9†], Cristina Scaletti[3,10†], Maria Teresa Ventura[3,11†], Anna Zollo[3,12†] and Air Pollution and Climate Change Task Force of the Italian Society of Allergology, Asthma and Clinical Immunology (SIAAIC)

Abstract

Background: According to the World Health Organization, air pollution is closely associated with climate change and, in particular, with global warming. In addition to melting of ice and snow, rising sea level, and flooding of coastal areas, global warming is leading to a tropicalization of temperate marine ecosystems. Moreover, the effects of air pollution on airway and lung diseases are well documented as reported by the World Allergy Organization.

Methods: Scientific literature was searched for studies investigating the effect of the interaction between air pollution and climate change on allergic and respiratory diseases.

Results: Since 1990s, a multitude of articles and reviews have been published on this topic, with many studies confirming that the warming of our planet is caused by the "greenhouse effect" as a result of increased emission of "greenhouse" gases. Air pollution is also closely linked to global warming: the emission of hydrocarbon combustion products leads to increased concentrations of biological allergens such as pollens, generating a mixture of these particles called particulate matter (PM). The concept is that global warming is linked to the emission of hydrocarbon combustion products, since both carbon dioxide and heat increase pollen emission into the atmosphere, and all these particles make up PM10. However, the understanding of the mechanisms by which PM affects human health is still limited. Therefore, several studies are trying to determine the causes of global warming. There is also evidence that increased concentrations of air pollutants and pollens can activate inflammatory mediators in the airways. Our Task Force has prepared a Decalogue of rules addressing public administrators, which aims to limit the amount of allergenic pollen in the air without sacrificing public green areas.

Conclusions: Several studies underscore the significant risks of global warming on human health due to increasing levels of air pollution. The impact of climate change on respiratory diseases appears well documented. The last decades have seen a rise in the concentrations of pollens and pollutants in the air. This rise parallels the increase in the number of people presenting with allergic symptoms (e.g., allergic rhinitis, conjunctivitis, and asthma), who often require emergency medical care. Our hope is that scientists from different disciplines will work together with institutions, pharmaceutical companies and lay organizations to limit the adverse health effects of air pollution and global warming.

*Correspondence: info@allergiasalerno3.it
†All authors contributed equally to this manuscript
[1] Division Allergy and Clinical Immunology, Department of Medicine ASL Salerno, "Santa Maria della Speranza" Hospital, Battipaglia, Salerno, Italy
Full list of author information is available at the end of the article

Background

Climate change is already underway and is expected to continue in the next decades: temperatures are increasing, global precipitation patterns are changing, ice and snow are melting, and global average sea level is rising. Moreover, the impact of global warming on human health has been documented by several reports from the World Health Organization (WHO) [1], which illustrate that a major concern about this phenomenon is the increase in air pollution levels. In this respect, the last report of the European Environment Agency (EEA) indicates that up to 96% of the urban population in the European Union are exposed to particulate and fine dust levels in excess of threshold values [2]. In addition to air pollution produced by hydrocarbon combustion emissions, there is another issue: the formation of particles related to global warming, and the presence of gases, such as ozone, with generation of a mixture of particles in the atmosphere, called particulate matter (PM) or particle pollution. Environmental PM is a heterogeneous mixture of particles produced by various processes, whose size ranges from 2.5 to 10 μm. The fine particulate fraction (PM2.5) (also known as "fine particles") consists of particles with a size of 2.5 microns (or smaller), while the ultrafine particulate fraction (also known as "ultrafine particles") consists of particles with a size smaller than 0.1 μm. The latter has a variable chemical composition, with the highest volatility, which is obviously due to its smaller size. It should also be noted that, although the ultrafine fraction represents less than 1% of the particulate mass, it is suspected of causing the greatest harm to the exposed population [3–6]. Importantly, this particulate fraction can reach the deepest parts of the bronchial tree, leading to major inflammatory and procarcinogenic effects on the bronchial mucosa [6]. Of note, PM is also involved in other diseases, including cardiovascular disorders such as coronary heart disease and heart failure. These conditions are mainly due to the oxidative stress generated by the inflammatory response, with both short- and long-term adverse effects on human health through a variety of mechanisms [7–11]. In addition, it has been demonstrated that exposure to ozone and PM2.5 induces adverse health effects, including various pulmonary diseases and lung cancer. Overall, air pollution-related global mortality has been associated with several emission sources; therefore, air pollution control can be an effective strategy to reduce mortality [12]. Both concentrations and chemical composition of PM show a large variability not only geographic, but also seasonal. PM concentrations are usually higher in urban areas than in rural areas. With regard to seasonal variability, PM levels increase significantly during the winter due to increased emissions from road traffic and residential heating, and decrease during spring and summer when pollen concentrations are typically highest [13].

Some particulates are naturally occurring and originate from volcanoes, dust storms, forest and grassland fires, living vegetation, and sea spray. Although most aerosols remain suspended in the atmosphere for short periods (typically between 4 days and a week), they can travel vast distances. Dust plumes from the Sahara often cross the Atlantic and reach the Caribbean. Winds sweep a mixture of Asian aerosols, including dust from the Gobi desert and pollution from China, to the east over Japan and toward the central Pacific Ocean. Smoke from wildfires in Siberia and Canada can go as far as the Arctic ice cap [11]. Sea spray from the Mediterranean Sea and mineral dust from Sahara in North Africa can contribute to the chemical composition of PM in Southern Europe [14, 15].

Human activities, including the combustion of fossil fuels in vehicles, power plants, and many industrial processes [10], can also generate significant amounts of particulates. Coal combustion in developing countries is the primary means to generate energy and heat homes. Although salt spray is the most common form of particulate in the atmosphere over the oceans, anthropogenic aerosols, i.e. those that are generated by human activities, currently account for about 10% of the total mass of aerosols in the atmosphere [11].

In recent years, air quality has improved in industrialized Western countries, while it has worsened in developing countries. In Asia, for example, anthropogenic emissions have increased in recent decades with the rapid development of urbanization and industrialization. On the contrary, aerosol emissions have declined in North America and Europe with the relocation of factories to developing countries and with the adoption of more stringent clean air regulations in Western countries. However, it may be difficult to define the amount of air pollution in different areas of the world, since most aerosols remain suspended in the atmosphere for short periods, typically between 4 days and a week. PM particles in the atmosphere can move at 5 m (16.4 ft) per second, and may travel thousands of kilometres in a week, making it difficult to accurately measure pollution levels; consequently, any predictions about the deterioration of air quality can be distorted by this initial bias, especially with regard to time.

Air pollution and climate change-related health impacts

Global warming is a major public health emergency. Global temperature has risen markedly over the last 50 years and is still rising, as demonstrated by warming of the oceans, rising sea levels, melting of glaciers, retreating of Arctic sea ice, and diminishing snow cover in the Northern Hemisphere. Climate change is also associated with extreme weather events such as heat waves, droughts, floods, and hurricanes. These changes are probably due to increased emissions of greenhouse gases (namely, carbon dioxide, methane and nitrous oxide), largely from anthropogenic sources. Projections of future greenhouse gas emissions indicate a worsening of the situation with further increase in average temperatures and temperature extremes by the end of the twenty-first century [16].

A large body of evidence suggests that climate change have significant health impacts, both direct and indirect. Direct health impacts include morbidity and mortality associated with direct exposure to hazardous weather conditions such as heat waves, floods, cyclones, etc. Indirect health impacts, which include the majority of climate change-related diseases, are mediated by environmental conditions which affect the spatial and temporal distribution of aeroallergens, the generation and dispersion of air pollutants, and the population of disease-transmitting vectors like mosquitoes and ticks.

Several epidemiological studies have demonstrated a close association between global warming, air pollution and respiratory allergic diseases, such as bronchial asthma and rhinitis. Climate changes affect the quantity, quality, timing and distribution of aeroallergens [17]. The increased atmospheric carbon dioxide concentrations due to fossil fuel burning stimulate the growth of plants, including allergenic species. On top of that, higher temperatures can lead to earlier and longer pollination seasons, leading to increased pollen sensitization rate and symptom duration. Individuals with asthma are at increased risk of developing obstructive airway attacks when exposed to gaseous and particulate components of air pollution [17]. In addition, air pollution can modify the allergenic potential of pollens, especially in the presence of favourable weather conditions. Air pollution—in particular PM, diesel exhaust particles (DEP), ozone, nitrogen dioxide, and sulfur dioxide—have been shown to have an inflammatory effect on the airways of susceptible subjects, causing increased mucosal permeability, facilitating the penetration and access of inhaled allergens to the cells of the immune system [18]. There are also data suggesting that air pollution can lead to the development of asthma. Therefore, climate change combined with air pollution may have severe impacts on respiratory health, especially in children.

Thunderstorms occurring during the pollen season have been shown to induce severe asthma attacks in pollinosis patients [18, 19]. The thunderstorm-related epidemics are limited to late spring and summer when there are high levels of pollen grains in the atmosphere. The main hypotheses for thunderstorm-related asthma claim that thunderstorms can concentrate pollen grains at ground level which rupture due to osmotic shock and release allergenic particles of respirable size into the atmosphere [19].

Rising temperatures, a higher concentration of carbon dioxide in the atmosphere, heavier rainfalls, and higher humidity induce faster proliferation of pollens, moulds, and fungi [20]. In addition, increases in humidity associated with higher temperatures may encourage the growth of cockroaches, house dust mites, and moulds, and, thus, allergen load [17]. Higher temperatures can also induce the migration of stinging and biting insects into new environments, as well as increasing the population of existing insect species [19]. Indeed, climate changes and globalization are altering the distribution and consistency of allergenic species including venomous insects. In particular, given the expansion of native species and the colonization of invasive ones, one can predict, despite the uncertainty of current models, that stinging Hymenoptera will pose new challenges in the future [21].

Many studies have reported the impact of climatic changes on the spatial and temporal distribution of infectious diseases such as vector-borne, rodent-borne, food-borne and water-borne diseases, including in particular malaria, tick-borne diseases, cholera and other diarrhoeal diseases. Importantly, several vector-borne diseases have emerged in Europe in recent years; these include vivax malaria, West Nile fever, dengue fever, Chikungunya fever, Leishmaniasis, Lyme disease, and tick-borne encephalitis [22, 23].

Chronic exposure to air pollution is also associated with pulmonary inflammation, chronic obstructive pulmonary disease (COPD), and lung cancer. Several studies suggest that chronic exposure to outdoor air pollution increases the prevalence and incidence of COPD [24]. Moreover, among individuals with COPD, air pollution is associated with increased respiratory symptoms, loss of lung function, COPD exacerbations and higher mortality [24]. Air pollution is also linked to lung cancer, and the International Agency for Research on Cancer (IARC) has classified the particulate matter in outdoor air pollution as carcinogenic to humans [25].

Studies from across the world have consistently demonstrated that exposure to particulate air pollution is associated with a host of cardiovascular diseases, including myocardial ischaemia and infarctions, heart failure, arrhythmias, strokes and increased cardiovascular mortality [26]. Acute exposure may contribute to plaque instability and trigger acute cardiovascular events, including myocardial ischaemia and infarction, stroke, heart failure, arrhythmias, and sudden death, particularly in high-risk subjects, while chronic exposure may favour the development and progression of atherosclerosis and possibly of hypertension in the long term [27].

Finally, a number of studies have reported an association between air pollution and higher risk of neuroinflammation and neurodegeneration [28, 29]. In particular, there is some evidence that chronic exposure to airborne pollutants in the early years of life may contribute to neurodegenerative disease processes including Alzheimer's disease and Parkinson's disease [30].

In summary, air pollution and climate change-related health impacts are enormous and are expected to increase during the next decades. As a result, also the social and economic costs of climate change are enormous and will increase in the future. Nevertheless, there is a relative scarcity of economic studies on the health impacts of climate change. Most studies have estimated the economic costs of extreme weather events or the impacts of climate change on respiratory diseases and infectious diseases (vector borne, water related, and food borne). However, these economic studies are heterogeneous in terms of objectives and methodology. To this end, a review has pointed out the need for climate change-specific health economic guidelines to provide a standardized approach and stimulate economic research [31]. A more recent review, conducted to evaluate the health costs resulting from human exposure to weather-related extreme events such as heat waves, droughts, floods, storms and hurricanes, has highlighted a lack of evidence about the potential cost-effectiveness of interventions that exploits the capacity of natural ecosystems to reduce exposure to extreme events, despite the observations that evidence that poor land management increases the vulnerability to these events [32]. However, all studies identified in this review indicate that the health costs associated with the impacts of extreme events are substantial. For example, six climate change-related events that struck the United States between 2000 and 2009, accounted for about $14 billion in lost lives and health costs [33].

Mechanisms responsible for allergic and respiratory diseases

The mechanisms by which PM affects human health are still debated [34]. The atmosphere is the medium of transit not only for pollutant gases and particles, but also for a wide variety of biogenic materials of plant and animal origin. Among biogenic materials, there is the bioaerosol, which consists of different kinds of airborne particles such as viruses, bacteria, moulds, plant fibres, and also pollen with variable sizes, ranging from tens of nanometers to a few hundreds of micrometers. These biological substances are involved in allergic and respiratory diseases, and act both directly and indirectly on airway epithelial cells. The increased concentration of pollen and air pollutants can activate different epithelial and immune cells in the airways, leading to the release of inflammatory mediators [35]. However, the specific components and the mechanisms responsible for oxidative stress following exposure to PM are not fully understood. Direct oxidant production by air pollution particles in epithelial cells of the respiratory mucosa has been reported. This effect has been attributed to both organic components and a number of heavy metals (e.g., arsenic, cadmium, chromium, mercury, nickel, lead, and thallium). These metals have a wide distribution in the environment as a result of their multiple industrial, domestic, agricultural, medical, and technological applications, which raises many concerns about their potential effects on human health and the environment. The main consequences of oxidative stress include the activation of specific cellular reactions (including activation of kinases and transcription factors), the release of inflammatory mediators, and eventually cell damage or apoptosis [36]. All this promotes bronchial hyperreactivity as well as a decline in pulmonary function, increasing the risk of allergic sensitisation, asthma, chronic obstructive pulmonary disease, and cancer. Recent epigenetic studies have shown that a number of genes controlling immune and inflammatory responses are sensitive to tropospheric ozone. Indeed, atmospheric pollutants like diesel exhaust particles [particulate] (DEPs) and ozone are directly involved in asthma pathogenesis [37]. Importantly, DEPs are a major component of traffic-related particulate air pollution in most urban areas. In addition, a number of evidence indicates that DEPs may facilitate entry of allergens into the airways eliciting immunopathological response, and can also bind pollen, dog, cat, and house dust mite allergens [38–40]. Due to their very fine size, DEPs can facilitate the penetration of these allergens into the lungs, thereby increasing the amount of allergens interacting with the airway epithelium. It has also been demonstrated that DEPs can disrupt pollen particles causing the release of allergenic sub-pollen particles. Interestingly, a detailed analysis of pollen taken from air-polluted areas showed an increased amount of allergenic proteins with higher allergenic potential. In another study, comparing recent and decade-old pollen extracts, the recent pollen extract showed higher allergenic potency. In addition, the recent pollen extract obtained from the urban area had a higher allergenic potency than the recent pollen extract from the suburban area [39]. More recently, the same authors of the above study demonstrated that a recent pollen extract from an urban area significantly exposed to pollution and climate change was more effective at inducing transepithelial permeability and ROS production in cultured airway epithelial cells [41]. This DEPs ability seems to be strongly dependent on a range of variables. However, the latest scientific findings indicate that DEPs are likely involved in exacerbations of already existing disease processes, and not in the development of new diseases. The latter hypothesis is based on the enhancement of Th2-dependent responses induced by DEPs [42]. Nonetheless, there are a variety of mechanisms involved in exposure to asthma triggers that do not depend on IgE-mediated responses. These observations have been partially confirmed by epigenetic studies. Epigenetics refers to changes in gene expression that are not caused by alterations in DNA sequences; these changes can be associated with environmental factors such road traffic and smoke pollution [43]. With regard to this issue, recent studies have been focused on mutation hotspots and DNA methylation, involving the so called CpG islands, which are located near the promoter region of many genes. In particular, one of these studies showed significant differences in methylation levels of CpG islands in eosinophils from asthmatic patients compared with non-asthmatic individuals, with the lowest levels of methylation in the subjects with asthma. This study also showed significant associations between IgE and low methylation at 36 loci concentrated in CpG islands [44]. In addition to the above, changes in histone acetyltransferase and deacetylase activity have been observed in cells from patients with lung disorders such as severe asthma and chronic obstructive pulmonary disease (COPD) [45]. Considering that the anti-inflammatory effects of glucocorticoids are dependent on histone deacetylase activity, this finding may be relevant for patients with severe asthma and COPD who are insensitive to glucocorticoid therapy. Indeed, it has been shown that glucocorticoid-insensitive asthmatics have an increased activation of p38 mitogen-activated protein kinase (MAPK), which can reduce the ligand-binding affinity of the glucocorticoid receptor (GR) leading to impaired corticosteroid sensitivity [46]. This can contribute to poor disease control in patients with chronic asthma and COPD. In this respect, it is worth mentioning that also disruption of circadian rhythms may impair asthma control. For example, the degree of asthma control has been shown to strongly correlate with sleep quality. In fact, individuals whose asthma is not well controlled take longer to fall asleep, awake more often, and spend more time awake during the night compared to those with well controlled asthma [47]. Interestingly, many other immunological and allergic diseases, including allergic rhinitis, atopic eczema, chronic urticaria, and rheumatoid arthritis, show a circadian rhythm in the intensity of symptoms and disease severity, which suggests the importance of chronotherapy as a strategy to achieve symptoms control [47].

Of note, not all studies support the hypothesis that air pollution has a greater deleterious effect on asthmatic patients compared to non-asthmatic individuals. However, experimental and clinical studies have demonstrated that asthmatic patients have an increased inflammatory response to air pollutants like PM2.5-10 [48] and especially ozone [49]. Several factors may contribute to the adverse effects of ozone in asthmatic patients by impairing innate immune responses [50].

Epidemiological studies indicate that older people are at higher risk of hospitalisation. In particular, increased exposure to air pollution has been linked to increased mortality, hospital admissions and emergency-room visits in the elderly [51]. These effects are mainly due to exacerbations of chronic diseases or to respiratory tract infections (e.g., pneumonia), and may be modulated by ambient temperature as demonstrated by several studies showing that the elderly are particularly vulnerable to heat waves. In general, it seems that elderly subjects are more vulnerable to PM than to other pollutants, with greater effects on cardiorespiratory mortality and acute hospital admissions [51]. The elderly are at greater risk than other age groups due to their enhanced susceptibility to air pollutants as a result of normal and pathological ageing and related processes. In fact, ageing has been associated with a decline in immune defences and respiratory function, resulting in a higher predisposition to respiratory infections. Moreover, among the chronic diseases that affect the elderly population, COPD and asthma can accelerate pulmonary function decline and increase the risk of mortality [52].

The relationship between short-term exposure to air pollution and cardiorespiratory morbidity and mortality in the elderly is well-documented. A systematic review and meta-analysis conducted by Bell et al. [53] found strong, consistent evidence of a higher risk of PM-associated hospitalisation and death in the elderly. The results of this meta-analysis showed that a 10 μg/m3 increase in PM10 exposure was associated with a higher risk of death of 0.64% (95% confidence interval (CI) 0.50, 0.78) for older populations compared with 0.34% (95% CI 0.25, 0.42) for younger populations. In another systematic review by Bell et al. [54], regarding sensitivity to mortality or hospital admission from short-term ozone exposure, mortality risk was also higher for older persons (1.27%; 95% CI 0.76–1.78) than for younger persons (0.60%; 95% CI 0.40–0.80).

Further evidence of an association between air pollution and mortality in the elderly was provided by another study, which showed that a 3–4% increase in daily deaths for all causes and for cardiovascular disease in the elderly was associated with an increase in fine particulate matter and sulfur dioxide from the 10th to the 90th percentile [55]. The increase in mortality was even higher (6%) for respiratory deaths. Cardiovascular deaths were also associated with levels of carbon monoxide (4% increase in daily deaths). On the contrary, the associations between air pollution and mortality were not statistically significant in children under 5 years. In summary, there was a significant trend of increased risk of death based on age, with effects more evident for individuals over 65 years old. The effect of air pollution was even larger in areas with higher socioeconomic level [55].

With regard to the effects of socioeconomic vulnerability on the risk of mortality in populations exposed to high PM concentrations, an Asian study showed that economic inactivity had the greatest influence on the risk of mortality (Table 1) [56]. People who were economically inactive had a 5.5% higher risk of all-cause mortality and a 5.6% higher risk of cardiorespiratory mortality from a 10 μg/m^3 increase in PM10–2.5 compared with those who were employed during a day with an extreme dust event. Also, the elderly and non-married people had higher risks of mortality during days with extreme dust events. People aged 65 years and older had a 4.4% higher risk of all-cause mortality and a 5.3% higher risk of cardiorespiratory mortality compared with those who were under the age of 65. People who were not married had a 4.1% higher risk of all-cause mortality and a 4.7% higher risk of cardiorespiratory mortality than those married [56].

Importantly, it has been observed that antioxidant metabolic pathways become increasingly compromised with ageing. Older people are also particularly sensitive to the short-term effects of ozone exposure [50]. It is becoming increasingly clear that ageing is strongly associated with senescence of the immune system [57–61]. To this regard, outdoor traffic pollution exposure is the most important predictive factor for asthma in the elderly [62–66]. Indeed, higher levels of outdoor and indoor exposures to DEPs, combined with obesity and atopic state, are associated with inadequate asthma control in the elderly [67]. There is also evidence that heat waves are associated with an increased risk of hospitalisation and higher mortality in the elderly [68]. In particular, two studies have shown that severe cardiovascular and respiratory diseases can be induced by the elevated air pollution associated with heat waves, especially in the elderly [69, 70].

Environmental pollution exposure significantly increases the risk of respiratory diseases, particularly asthma. Both adult and young patients, smokers or nonsmokers, are prone to acute asthma attacks as a result of greater exposure to air pollution. In particular, children from low-income backgrounds have been found to be more susceptible to acute asthma attacks due to air pollution. However, larger studies are required to confirm the relevance of these interactions, and to further explore the risk factors for asthma associated with long-term air pollution exposure in patients of different ages. Moreover, when differentiating between the effects of various risk factors, it is important to remember that asthma is not a single disease [71]. In addition, the risk of both allergic and non-allergic asthma seems to increase with increasing BMI as previously reported in children [72]. Finally, associations between early-life environmental exposures and asthma have been found in non atopic subjects [73, 74].

Recently, air pollution has also been associated with increased plasma viscosity and cardiac functions abnormalities, mainly due to cardiac arrhythmias [75–77]. Therefore, elderly patients are more susceptible than younger patients to the adverse effects of climate change due to their higher incidence of cardiovascular disease. Another important issue is the relationship between climate change and microbial infections. It has been suggested that the rapid and intense climate changes related to global warming can create conditions that promote the spread of epidemic diseases. For instance, heavy rainfalls increase the availability of breeding places for pests such as bugs and rats, which contaminate drinking water supplies. Moreover, parasitic and viral diseases transmitted by mosquitoes are very sensitive to climate changes [78–80].

Other mechanisms involved in climate change include air temperature increases in urban areas, a phenomenon called "heat island." This effect is particularly relevant for people living in these areas, especially those who are affected by cardiovascular and/or respiratory diseases. It also has a significant impact on the most fragile

Table 1 Effect modification of socioeconomic vulnerability for 10 mg/m^3 increase of PM10-2.5, with 95% confidence interval. Modified from Ho et al. [56]

Socioeconomic vulnerability (individual level)	OR at lag 0 (all cause mortality)	OR at lag 0 (cardiorespiratory mortality)
Age		
>65	*1.044 [1.029, 1.059]*	1.053 [1.029, 1.078]
<65	1.047 [0.994, 1.103]	1.045 [0.920, 1.186]
Gender		
Female	1.057 [1.014, 1.102]	1.062 [0.998, 1.131]
Male	1.033 [1.018, 1.049]	1.030 [1.009, 1.052]
Socioeconomic status		
Economically inactive	*1.055 [1.039, 1.070]*	*1.056 [1.030, 1.081]*
Economically active	1.024 [0.992, 1.057]	1.019 [0.974, 1.066]
Marital status		
Non-married	*1.041 [1.018, 1.065]*	*1.047 [1.004, 1.093]*
Married	1.034 [1.013, 1.056]	1.030 [1.003, 1.056]

Italic text indicates results with significant difference between vulnerable and non-vulnerable groups

population groups (e.g., elderly and poor people). In fact, these people have less access to air conditioning and tend to stay more outdoors (e.g., streets, squares) where they are more exposed to urban overheating. In addition, exposure to outdoor air pollution combined with exposure to allergenic pollen can trigger severe asthma attacks. A reduction in emergency hospital admissions after the implementation of prevention programs supports the view of a causal link between air pollution and exacerbations of chronic respiratory diseases [80].

The SIAAIC task force on air pollution and climate change: the decalogue "Allergy Safe Tree"

In April 2014, the Italian Society of Allergology, Asthma and Clinical Immunology (Società Italiana di Allergologia, Asma ed Immnunologia Clinica, SIAAIC) established the Task Force (TF) on "Air Pollution and Climate Change."

The SIAAIC TF launched a project divided into 3 successive steps. The first step involved the establishment of a multidisciplinary expert group, including high-profile academic, institutional and associative figures working in the field of "Air Pollution and Climate Change" at the legal, environmental and institutional levels. SIAAIC Allergists and Clinical Immunologists were clearly involved in this group. The second step of the project ("exploratory step") included the collection of national and European data on climate and environmental changes. The third step of the TF's work, still underway, focused on the preparation of a final document (Report or Guidelines) to raise awareness about "Air Pollution and Climate Change" and their impact on Immunological and Allergic Diseases. The TF also planned the production of a "synthetic" version of the document intended for the public, as well as the preparation of a Decalogue to be sent to local administrators with a set of rules aimed at protecting public health. Starting from this initial proposal, and as a result of its regular activities during these years, the Task Force on Air Pollution and Climate Change of the Italian Society of Allergology, Asthma and Clinical Immunology (SIAAIC) has proposed a National Healthcare Program to help the cities' public administrations in choosing non allergenic trees in public parks. The "DECALOGUE: ALLERGY SAFE TREE" document suggests how to use non allergenic trees in gardens and public parks [81, 82] (Fig. 1).

As the subtitle indicates, the Decalogue plans to carry out a prevention campaign to reduce the amount of pollen in the air without sacrificing public green areas. To this end, the document adopted by the SIAAIC TF proposes "simple actions" concerning the management and care of plants, targeting several factors affecting allergen concentrations, including the "pollen calendar," namely the recording of seasonal peaks of airborne pollen concentrations. The SIAAIC TF believes that compliance with the provisions of the Decalogue can help meet the campaign goal, that is, reducing the concentrations of airborne allergenic pollen in the cities. Among the forthcoming activities, the TF is preparing aerobiology courses, as well as the creation of a national SIAAIC aerobiology network for the monitoring of allergies across the country.

Behind the initiatives of the SIAAIC TF on "Air Pollution and Climate Change," there is the authors' opinion, which is supported by recent studies, that the prevention of allergies can be implemented by public administrations through a careful choice of non allergenic trees and plants. Likewise, a careful selection of ornamental plants can contribute to reduce pollen levels in the private sector (condos, sports, malls and industrial green areas) [77]. These aspects are of high relevance as parks and gardens are primarily visited by both children and elderly people, who are susceptible to allergic sensitisation and respiratory diseases. Finally, allergen exposure within the parks is particularly dangerous when combined with climate conditions characterized by rising temperatures that can promote pollen production, taking into account the fact that urbanization and high levels of vehicle emissions correlate with a higher frequency of pollen-induced respiratory allergy [4].

Conclusion

The effects of global warming on human health are supported by many official documents which emphasize the importance of air pollution on the rising incidence of many respiratory diseases. Climate change, by modifying major climatic variables, influences directly and indirectly the formation of air pollutants. Both global warming and solar radiation contribute to the formation of secondary pollutants in the atmosphere, especially tropospheric ozone. All these factors can explain, at least partly, the increasing incidence of respiratory and allergic diseases in different parts of the world. Recent forecasts suggest that climate change will persist for several decades (IPCC 2013). It is likely that we will face the impact of climate change for at least the next 50 years. The effects of climate change are already here and their negative consequences cannot be easily avoided or prevented. In many patients with respiratory diseases like asthma, symptomatic treatment with bronchodilators or inhaled corticosteroids is sufficient to control disease. However, there are patients who do not achieve control despite treatment with the best current therapy. This heterogeneity of asthma and allergic diseases is increasingly appreciated based primarily on recent cluster analyses, molecular phenotyping, biomarkers and differential

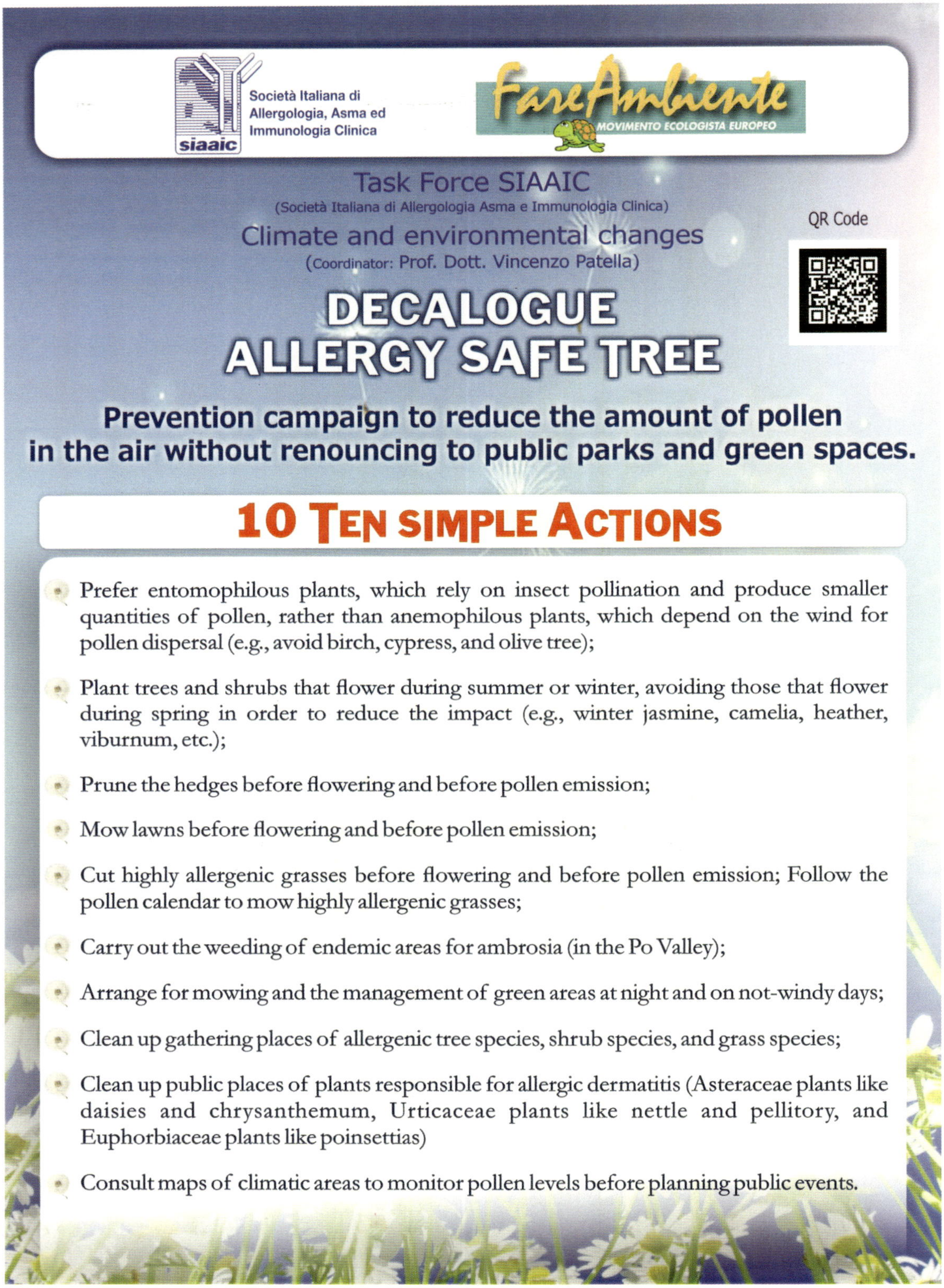

Fig. 1 Prevention campaign to reduce the amount of pollen in the air without renouncing to public parks and green spaces

responses to targeted and non-targeted therapies [83]. This can be explained, at least in part, by different patient exposure to climate change and air pollution. A joint effort among scientists of different disciplines together with public administrations is highly desirable to limit present and future harm to human health as a result of interaction between climate change and air pollution.

Authors' contributions

VP, GF, DM, AG, MAC, DDB, AG, MP, AP, ER, CS, MTV, AZ have been partecipated equally participate in the review, drafting, and final approval of the manuscript. All authors read and approved the final manuscript.

Author details

[1] Division Allergy and Clinical Immunology, Department of Medicine ASL Salerno, "Santa Maria della Speranza" Hospital, Battipaglia, Salerno, Italy. [2] Postgraduate Program in Allergy and Clinical Immunology–University of Naples Federico II, Naples, Italy. [3] Air Pollution and Climate Change Task Force of the Italian Society of Allergology, Asthma and Clinical Immunology (SIAAIC), Milan, Italy. [4] Laboratory of Environmental Analysis, Department of Public Health, ASL Salerno, Salerno, Italy. [5] Department of Cardiac, Thoracic and Vascular Sciences, University of Padua, Padua, Italy. [6] Association of International Culture, Athena of Paestum, Capaccio-Paestum, Salerno, Italy. [7] Former Primary of Unit of Pediatry, Hospital of Eboli, Salerno, Italy. [8] International Court of the Environment Foundation (ICEF), Rome, Italy. [9] Department of Medicine and Surgery, University of Parma, Parma, Italy. [10] Unit of Internal Medicine, Department of Experimental and Clinical Medicine, University of Florence, Florence, Italy. [11] Department of Interdisciplinary Medicine, University of Bari, Bari, Italy. [12] Department of Studies and Researches, Movimento Ecologista Europeo FareAmbiente, Rome, Italy.

Funding

The Authors declare that they did not receive any funding for this manuscript.

References

1. World Health Organization: WHO. Air quality guidelines for particulate matter, ozone, nitrogen dioxide and sulphur dioxide. Global Update 2005. In summary of risk assessment. http://apps.who.int/iris/bitstream/handle/10665/69477/WHO_SDE_PHE_OEH_06.02_eng.pdf;jsessionid=21948A7B88EA2D5BFB55A5F84629FF39sequence=1.
2. European Environment Agency (EEA) report. EEA Report No 28/2016. https://www.eea.europa.eu/data-and-maps/figures/percentage-of-the-eu-urban.
3. US Environmental Protection Agency: National ambient air quality standards (NAAQS). http://www.epa.gov/air/criteria.html.
4. D'Amato G, Holgate ST, Pawankar R, Ledford DK, Cecchi L, Al-Ahmad M, Al-Enezi F, Al-Muhsen S, Ansotegui I, Baena-Cagnani CE, Baker DJ, Bayram H, Bergmann KC, Boulet LP, Buters JT, D'Amato M, Dorsano S, Douwes J, Finlay SE, Garrasi D, Gómez M, Haahtela T, Halwani R, Hassani Y, Mahboub B, Marks G, Michelozzi P, Montagni M, Nunes C, Oh JJ, Popov TA, Portnoy J, Ridolo E, Rosário N, Rottem M, Sánchez-Borges M, Sibanda E, Sienra-Monge JJ, Vitale C, Annesi-Maesano. Meteorological conditions, climate change, new emerging factors, and asthma and related allergic disorders. A statement of the World Allergy Organization. World Allergy Organ J. 2015;8(1):1–52. https://doi.org/10.1186/s40413-015-0073-0.
5. de Hartog JJ, Hoek G, Mirme A, Tuch T, Kos GP, ten Brink HM, Brunekreef B, Cyrys J, Heinrich J, Pitz M, Lanki T, Vallius M, Pekkanen J, Kreyling WG. Relationship between different size classes of particulate matter and meteorology in three European cities. J Environ Monit. 2005;7:302–10.
6. Donaldson K, Stone V, Clouter A, Renwick L, MacNee W. Ultrafine particles. Occup Environ Med. 2001;58(211–216):199.
7. Pekkanen J, Kulmala M. Exposure assessment of ultrafine particles in epidemiologic time-series studies. Scand J Work Environ Health. 2004;30(Suppl 2):9–18.
8. D'Amato G, Baena-Cagnani CE, Cecchi L, Annesi-Maesano I, Nunes C, Ansotegui I, D'Amato M, Liccardi G, Sofia M, Canonica WG. Climate change, air pollution and extreme events leading to increasing prevalence of allergic respiratory diseases. Multidiscip Respir Med. 2013;8(1):12. https://doi.org/10.1186/2049-6958-8-12.
9. Bai Y, Sun Q. Fine particulate matter air pollution and atherosclerosis: mechanistic insights. Biochim Biophys Acta. 2016;4165(16):30150–7. https://doi.org/10.1016/j.bbagen.2016.04.030.
10. Yitshak Sade M, Novack V, Ifergane G, Horev A, Kloog I. Air pollution and ischemic stroke among young adults. Stroke. 2015;46(12):3348–53. https://doi.org/10.1161/STROKEAHA.115.010992.
11. Mirowsky JE, Peltier RE, Lippmann M, Thurston G, Chen LC, Neas L, Diaz-Sanchez D, Laumbach R, Carter JD, Gordon T. Repeated measures of inflammation, blood pressure, and heart rate variability associated with traffic exposures in healthy adults. Environ Health. 2015;15(14):66. https://doi.org/10.1186/s12940-015-0049-0.
12. Franchini M, Guida A, Tufano A, Coppola A. Air pollution, vascular disease and thrombosis: linking clinical data and pathogenic mechanisms. J Thromb Haemost. 2012;10(12):2438–51. https://doi.org/10.1111/jth.12006.
13. Global Climate Change and Extreme Weather Events. Understanding the contributions to infectious disease emergence: workshop summary institute of medicine (US) forum on microbial threats. Washington (DC): National Academies Press; 2008.
14. Pietrogrande MC, Abbaszade G, Schnelle-Kreis J, et al. Seasonal variation and source estimation of organic compounds in urban aerosol of Augsburg, Germany. Environ Pollut. 2011;159(7):1861–8. https://doi.org/10.1016/j.envpol.2011.03.023
15. Sprovieri F, Pirrone N. Particle size distributions and elemental composition of atmospheric particulate matter in southern Italy. J Air Waste Manag Assoc. 2008;58(6):797–805.
16. D'Amato G, Cecchi L, D'Amato M, Annesi-Maesano I. Climate change and respiratory diseases. Eur Respir Rev. 2014;23:161–9.
17. D'Amato G, Rottem M, Dahl R, Blaiss M, Ridolo E, Cecchi L, Rosario N, Motala C, Ansotegui I, Annesi-Maesano I, WAO Special Committee on Climate Change and Allergy. Climate change, migration, and allergic respiratory diseases: an update for the allergist. World Allergy Organ J. 2011;4(7):120–5. https://doi.org/10.1097/wox.0b013e3182260a57.
18. D'Amato G. Effects of climatic changes and urban air pollution on the rising trends of respiratory allergy and asthma. Multidiscip Respir Med. 2011;6(1):28–37. https://doi.org/10.1186/2049-6958-6-1-28.
19. D'Amato G, Annesi-Maesano I, Vaghi A, Cecchi L, D'Amato M. How do storms affect asthma? Curr Allergy Asthma Rep. 2018;18(4):24. https://doi.org/10.1007/s11882-018-0775-9.
20. Chan AW, Hon KL, Leung TF, Ho MH, Rosa Duque JS, Lee TH. The effects of global warming on allergic diseases. Hong Kong Med J. 2018;24(3):277–84. https://doi.org/10.12809/hkmj177046.
21. Turillazzi S, Turillazzi F. Climate changes and hymenoptera venom allergy: are there some connections? Curr Opin Allergy Clin Immunol. 2017;17(5):344–9.

22. Baylis M. Potential impact of climate change on emerging vector-borne and other infections in the UK. Environ Health. 2017;16(Suppl 1):112. https://doi.org/10.1186/s12940-017-0326-1.
23. Semenza JC, Suk JE. Vector-borne diseases and climate change: a European perspective. FEMS Microbiol Lett. 2018;365(2):fnx244. https://doi.org/10.1093/femsle/fnx244.
24. Hansel NN, McCormack MC, Kim V. the effects of air pollution and temperature on COPD. COPD. 2016;13(3):372–9. https://doi.org/10.3109/15412555.2015.1089846.
25. de Groot PM, Wu CC, Carter BW, Munden RF. The epidemiology of lung cancer. Transl Lung Cancer Res. 2018;7(3):220–33. https://doi.org/10.21037/tlcr.2018.05.06.
26. Brook RD. Cardiovascular effects of air pollution. Clin Sci (Lond). 2008;115:175–87.
27. Nogueira JB. Air pollution and cardiovascular disease. Rev Port Cardiol. 2009;28(6):715–33.
28. Calderón-Garcidueñas L, Torres-Jardón R, Kulesza RJ, Park S-B, D'Angiulli A. Air pollution and detrimental effects on children's brain. The need for a multidisciplinary approach to the issue complexity and challenges. Fron Hum Neurosci. 2014;8:613.
29. Calderon-Garcidueñas L, Kavanaugh M, Block M, D'Angiulli A, Delgado-Chavez R, Torres-Jardon R, Gonzalez-Maciel A, Reynoso-Robles R, Osnaya N, Villarreal-Calderon R, et al. Neuroinflammation, hyperphosphorylated tau, diffuse amyloid plaques, and down-regulation of the cellular prion protein in air pollution exposed children and young adults. J Alzheimers Dis. 2012;28:93–107.
30. Calderón-Garcidueñas L, Franco-Lira M, Mora-Tiscareño A, Medina-Cortina H, Torres-Jardón R, Kavanaugh M. Early Alzheimer's and Parkinson's disease pathology in urban children: friend versus Foe responses–it is time to face the evidence. Biomed Res Int. 2013;2013:161687. https://doi.org/10.1155/2013/161687.
31. Hutton G, Menne B. Economic evidence on the health impacts of climate change in Europe. Environ Health Insights. 2014;8:43–52. https://doi.org/10.4137/EHI.S16486.
32. Schmitt LHM, Graham HM, White PCL. Economic evaluations of the health impacts of weather-related extreme events: a scoping review. Int J Environ Res Public Health. 2016;13(11):1105. https://doi.org/10.3390/ijerph13111105.
33. Knowlton K, Rotkin-Ellman M, Geballe L, Max W, Solomon GM. Six climate change-related events in the United States accounted for about USD 14 billion in lost lives and health costs. Health Aff. 2011;30:2167–76. https://doi.org/10.1377/hlthaff.2011.0229.
34. Silva RA, Adelman Z, Fry MM, West JJ. The impact of individual anthropogenic emissions sectors on the global burden of human mortality due to ambient air pollution. Environ Health Perspect. 2016;124(11):1776–84.
35. Brunekreef B, Holgate S. Air pollution and health. Lancet. 2002;360:1233–42.
36. Main CE. Aerobiological, ecological, and health linkages. Environ Int. 2003;29(2–3):347–9.
37. Ghio AJ, Carraway MS, Madden MC. Composition of air pollution particles and oxidative stress in cells, tissues, and living systems. J Toxicol Environ Health B Crit Rev. 2012;15(1):1–21. https://doi.org/10.1080/10937404.2012.632359.
38. Gandhi VD, Vliagoftis H. Airway epithelium interactions with aeroallergens: role of secreted cytokines and chemokines in innate immunity. Front Immunol. 2015;2(6):147. https://doi.org/10.3389/fimmu.2015.00147.eCollection2015.Review.
39. Ghiani A, Aina R, Asero R, Bellotto E, Citterio S. Ragweed pollen collected along high-traffic roads shows a higher allergenicity than pollen sampled in vegetated areas. Allergy. 2012;67(7):887–94.
40. Alexis NE, Carlsten C. Interplay of air pollution and asthma immunopathogenesis: a focused review of diesel exhaust and ozone. Int Immunopharmacol. 2014;23(1):347–55. https://doi.org/10.1016/j.intimp.2014.08.009
41. Lee SI, le Pham D, Shin YS, Suh DH, Park HS. Environmental changes could enhance the biological effect of Hop J pollens on human airway epithelial cells. J Allergy Clin Immunol. 2014;134(2):470. https://doi.org/10.1016/j.jaci.2014.01.034.
42. Diaz-Sanchez D, Tsien A, Fleming J, Saxon A. Combined diesel exhaust particulate and ragweed allergen challenge markedly enhances human in vivo nasal ragweed-specific IgE and skews cytokine production to a T helper cell 2-type pattern. J Immunol. 1997;158(5):2406–13.
43. Durham A, Chou PC, Kirkham P, Adcock IM. Epigenetics in asthma and other inflammatory lung diseases. Epigenomics. 2010;2(4):523–37. https://doi.org/10.2217/epi.10.27.
44. Liang L, Willis-Owen SA, Laprise C, Wong KC, Davies GA, Hudson TJ, Binia A, Hopkin JM, Yang IV, Grundberg E, Busche S. An epigenome-wide association study of total serum immunoglobulin E concentration. Nature. 2015;520(7549):670. https://doi.org/10.1038/nature14125.
45. Mortaz E, Masjedi MR, Barnes PJ, Adcock IM. Epigenetics and chromatin remodeling play a role in lung disease. Tanaffos. 2011;10(4):7–16.
46. Irusen E, Matthews JG, Takahashi A, Barnes PJ, Chung KF, Adcock IM. p38Mitogen-activated protein kinase-induced glucocorticoid receptor phosphorylation reduces its activity: role in steroid-insensitive asthma. J Allergy Clin Immunol. 2002;109(4):649–57.
47. Paganelli R, Petrarca C, Di Gioacchino M. Biological clocks: their relevance to immune-allergic diseases. Clin Mol Allergy. 2018;10(16):1.
48. Alexis NE, Huang YC, Rappold AG, Kehrl H, Devlin R, Peden DB. Patients with asthma demonstrate airway inflammation after exposure to concentrated ambient particulate matter. Am J Respir Crit Care Med. 2014;190(2):235–7.
49. Hernandez M, Brickey WJ, Alexis NE, Fry RC, Rager JE, Zhou B, et al. Airway cells from atopic asthmatic patients exposed to ozone display an enhanced innate immune gene profile. J Allergy Clin Immunol. 2012;129(1):259–61.
50. Geiser M, Lay JC, Bennett WD, Zhou H, Wang X, Peden DB, et al. Effects of ex vivo γ-tocopherol on airway macrophage function in healthy and mild allergic asthmatics. J Innate Immun. 2013;5(6):613–24.
51. Simoni M, Baldacci S, Maio S, Cerrai S, Sarno G, Viegi G. Adverse effects of outdoor pollution in the elderly. J Thorac Dis. 2015;7(1):34–45. https://doi.org/10.3978/j.issn.2072-1439.2014.12.10.
52. Bentayeb M, Simoni M, Baiz N, Norback D, Baldacci S, Maio S, Viegi G, Annesi-Maesano I, Geriatric Study in Europe on Health Effects of Air Quality in Nursing Homes Group. Adverse respiratory effects of outdoor air pollution in the elderly. Int J Tuberc Lung Dis. 2012;16(9):1149–61. https://doi.org/10.5588/ijtld.11.0666.
53. Bell ML, Zanobetti A, Dominici F. Evidence on vulnerability and susceptibility to health risks associated with short-term exposure to particulate matter: a systematic review and meta-analysis. Am J Epidemiol. 2013;178(6):865–76. https://doi.org/10.1093/aje/kwt090.
54. Bell ML, Zanobetti A, Dominici F. Who is more affected by ozone pollution? A systematic review and meta-analysis. Am J Epidemiol. 2014;180(1):15–28. https://doi.org/10.1093/aje/kwu115.
55. Gouveia N, Fletcher T. Time series analysis of air pollution and mortality: effects by cause, age and socioeconomic status. J Epidemiol Community Health. 2000;54(10):750–5.
56. Ho HC, Wong MS, Yang L, Chan TC, Bilal M. Influences of socioeconomic vulnerability and intra-urban air pollution exposure on short-term mortality during extreme dust events. Environ Pollut. 2018;235:155–62. https://doi.org/10.1016/j.envpol.2017.12.047
57. Pearson C, Littlewood E, Douglas P, Robertson S, Gant TW, Hansell AL. Exposures and health outcomes in relation to bioaerosol emissions from composting facilities: a systematic review of occupational and community studies. J Toxicol Environ Health B Crit Rev. 2015;18(1):43–69. https://doi.org/10.1080/10937404.2015.1009961.
58. Larbi A, Franceschi C, Mazzatti D, Solana R, Wikby A. Pawelec G Aging of the immune system as a prognostic factor for human longevity. Physiology. 2008. https://doi.org/10.1152/physiol.00040.2007
59. McElhaney JE, Effros RB. Immunosenescence: what does it mean to health outcomes in older adults? Curr Opin Immunol. 2009;21(4):418–24. https://doi.org/10.1016/j.coi.2009.05.023.
60. Fülöp T, Dupuis G, Witkowski JM, Larbi A. The Role of Immunosenescence in the development of age-related diseases. Rev Invest Clin. 2016;68(2):84–91.
61. Brunekreef B, Holgate ST. Air pollution and health. Lancet. 2002;360(9341):1233–42.
62. Anderson HR, Favarato G, Atkinson RW. Long-term exposure to air pollution and the incidence of asthma: metaanalysis of cohort studies. Air Qual Atmos Health. 2013;6(1):47–56.

63. Curtis L, Rea W, Smith-Willis P, Fenyves E, Pan Y. Adverse health effects of outdoor air pollutants. Environ Int. 2006;32(6):815–30.
64. Medina S, Plasencia A, Ballester F, Mücke HG, Schwartz J. Apheis: public health impact of PM10 in 19 European cities. J Epidemiol Community Health. 2004;58(10):831–6.
65. Peng RD, Dominici F, Pastor-Barriuso R, Zeger SL, Samet JM. Seasonal analyses of air pollution and mortality in 100 US cities. Am J Epidemiol. 2005;161(6):585–94.
66. Kannan JA, Bernstein DI, Bernstein CK, Ryan PH, Bernstein JA, Villareal MS, Smith AM, Lenz PH, Epstein TG. Significant predictors of poor quality of life in older asthmatics. Ann Allergy Asthma Immunol. 2015;115(3):198–204. https://doi.org/10.1016/j.anai.2015.06.021.
67. Epstein TG, Ryan PH, LeMasters GK, Bernstein CK, Levin LS, Bernstein JA, Villareal MS, Bernstein DI. Poor asthma control and exposure to traffic pollutants and obesity in older adults. Ann Allergy Asthma Immunol. 2012;108(6):423–8. https://doi.org/10.1016/j.anai.2012.04.009.
68. Bobb JF, Obermeyer Z, Wang Y, Dominici F. Cause-specific risk of hospital admission related to extreme heat in older adults. JAMA. 2014;312(24):2659–67. https://doi.org/10.1001/jama.2014.15715.
69. Shaposhnikov D, Revich B, Bellander T, Bedada GB, Bottai M, Kharkova T, Kvasha E, Lezina E, Lind T, Semutnikova E, Pershagen G. Mortality related to air pollution with the Moscow heat wave and wildfire of 2010. Epidemiology. 2014;25(3):359–64. https://doi.org/10.1097/EDE.0000000000000090.
70. Brook RD, Franklin B, Cascio W, Hong Y, Howard G, Lipsett M, Luepker R, Mittleman M, Samet J, Smith SC Jr. Tager I;. Air pollution and cardiovascular disease: a statement for healthcare professionals from the expert panel on population and prevention science of the American Heart Association. Circulation. 2004;109:2655–71.
71. Burte E, Nadif R, Jacquemin B. Susceptibility factors relevant for the association between long-term air pollution exposure and incident asthma. Curr Environ Health Rep. 2016;3(1):23–39. https://doi.org/10.1007/s40572-016-0084-1.
72. Guibas GV, Manios Y, Xepapadaki P, Moschonis G, Douladiris N, Mavrogianni C, Papadopoulos NG. The obesity-asthma link in different ages and the role of body mass index in its investigation: findings from the Genesis and Healthy Growth Studies. Allergy. 2013;68(10):1298–305. https://doi.org/10.1111/all.12245
73. Longobardi G, Napolitano G, Simonetti DM, Palmieri M. Parental smoking and asthma in childhood. Eur J Pediatr. 1990;149(10):738–40.
74. Janson C, Kalm-Stephens P, Foucard T, Alving K, Nordvall SL. Risk factors associated with allergic and non-allergic asthma in adolescents. Clin Respir J. 2007;1(1):16–22. https://doi.org/10.1111/j.1752-699X.2007.00001.
75. Yang M, Pan X. Time-series analysis of air pollution and cardiovascular mortality in Beijing, China. J Environ Health. 2008;25:294–7.
76. Van Eeden SF, Sin DD. Oxidative stress in chronic obstructive pulmonary disease: a lung and systemic process. Can Respir J. 2013;20(1):27–9.
77. Crimmins A, Balbus J, Gamble JL, Beard CB, Bell JE, Dodgen D, Eisen RJ, Fann N, Hawkins MD, Herring SC, Jantarasami L, Mills DM, Saha S, Sarofim MC, Trtanj J, Ziska L. Impacts of Climate change on human health in the united states: a scientific assessment. Washington, DC: US Global Change Research Program, USGCRP; 2016. p. 312. https://doi.org/10.7930/j0r49nqx.
78. Bezirtzoglou C, Dekas K, Charvalos E. Climate changes, environment and infection: facts, scenarios and growing awareness from the public health community within Europe. Anaerobe. 2011;17(6):337–40. https://doi.org/10.1016/j.anaerobe.2011.05.016
79. Barata M, Ligeti E, De Simone G, Dickinson T, Jack D, Penney J, Rahman M, Zimmerman R. Climate change and human health in cities. In: Rosenzweig C, Solecki WD, Hammer SA, Mehrotra S, editors. Climate change and cities: first assessment report of the urban climate change research network. Cambridge: Cambridge University Press; 2011. p. 179–213.
80. Hurst JR, Vestbo J, Anzueto A, Locantore N, Mullerova H, Tal-Singer R, Miller B, Lomas DA, Agusti A, Macnee W, Calverley P, Rennard S, Wouters EF, Wedzicha JA. Susceptibility to exacerbation in chronic obstructive pulmonary disease. N Engl J Med. 2010;363:1128–38.
81. Frenguelli G, Passaleva A. La scelta delle piante destinate al verde ornamentale. Ital J Allergy Clin Immunol. 2003;13:177–91.
82. Patella V. Decalogo SIAAIC allergy safe tree. 2015. http://www.siaaic.eu/notizia.php?id=12.
83. Fajt ML, Wenzel SE. Asthma phenotypes and the use of biologic medications in asthma and allergic disease: the next steps toward personalized care. J Allergy Clin Immunol. 2015. https://doi.org/10.1016/j.jaci.2014.12.1871.

19

Bench to bedside review of myositis autoantibodies

Boaz Palterer*, Gianfranco Vitiello, Alessia Carraresi, Maria Grazia Giudizi, Daniele Cammelli and Paola Parronchi

Abstract

Idiopathic inflammatory myopathies represent a heterogeneous group of autoimmune diseases with systemic involvement. Even though numerous specific autoantibodies have been recognized, they have not been included, with the only exception of anti-Jo-1, into the 2017 Classification Criteria, thus perpetuating a clinical-serologic gap. The lack of homogeneous grouping based on the antibody profile deeply impacts the diagnostic approach, therapeutic choices and prognostic stratification of these patients. This review is intended to highlight the comprehensive scenario regarding myositis-related autoantibodies, from the molecular characterization and biological significance to target antigens, from the detection tools, with a special focus on immunofluorescence patterns on HEp-2 cells, to their relative prevalence and ethnic diversity, from the clinical presentation to prognosis. If, on the one hand, a notable body of literature is present, on the other data are fragmented, retrospectively based and collected from small case series, so that they do not sufficiently support the decision-making process (i.e. therapeutic approach) into the clinics.

Keywords: Myositis, Autoantibodies, Immunofluorescence, Anti-nuclear antibodies, Dermatomyositis, Polymyositis, Immune-mediated necrotizing myopathy, Inclusion body myositis, MDA5, HMGCR

Background

The detection of autoantibodies in autoimmune diseases, either systemic or organ specific, can have both diagnostic and prognostic importance. Some autoantibodies have a clear pathogenic role, such as anti-erythrocyte membrane proteins antibodies in autoimmune hemolytic anemia and anti-dsDNA in Systemic Lupus Erythematosus (SLE). However, the presence of autoantibodies is more frequently considered to be an epiphenomenon, even though their detection plays a critical role for the diagnosis of some connective tissue diseases (CTDs), [i.e. anti-SSA/Ro in Sjögren syndrome (SjS) and anti-Sm in SLE], as included into the classification criteria of CTDs [1, 2]. Repeated serum sampling might be informative about the clinical course of the disease and response to immunosuppressive therapy, as in the case of anti-dsDNA antibodies in SLE. Furthermore, the presence of some autoantibodies could help to discriminate specific clinical patterns within the same disease, as with diffuse and limited cutaneous systemic sclerosis (SSc) and their relationship with anti-Scl-70 and anti-centromere, respectively.

In idiopathic inflammatory myopathies (IIMs), albeit anti-Jo-1 autoantibody was discovered more than thirty years ago, the percentage of patients in whom an autoantibody could not be recognized (the so called "serologic gap") was still high until recently. IIMs have been historically divided in polymyositis (PM) and dermatomyositis (DM) on a purely clinical basis despite phenotypic variability.

Due to this heterogeneity, the numerous autoantibodies and unavailability of reliable assays in all the laboratories, the clinical use of serology lagged behind and autoantibodies are not part of the most recent IIM Classification Criteria [3].

A comprehensive review regarding the clinical features, diagnostic work-up and relationship to some peculiar autoantibodies has been recently published by Milone [4].

*Correspondence: boaz.palterer@unifi.it
Experimental and Clinical Medicine Department, University of Florence, Largo Brambilla 3, 50134 Florence, Italy

Myositis-specific and –associated autoantibodies: definitions

Autoantibodies found in IIM patients have been classified into two main categories: myositis-specific autoantibodies (MSAs), which can be found in IIMs exclusively, and myositis-associated autoantibodies (MAAs), which can also be found in other CTDs [5, 6]. MSAs and MAAs are summarized in Table 1.

There is no agreement about the attribution of rare and newly discovered autoantibodies to either MSAs or MAAs group [7]. Anti-synthetase autoantibodies (ARS) themselves, especially anti-PL-7, PL-12 and KS, often detected in interstitial pneumonia with autoimmune features (IPAF) patients, independently from muscular involvement, are still discussed as MSAs [8].

The MAAs group contains Anti-Pm-Scl, U1/U2RNP and Ku, which are associated with overlap syndromes with muscular involvement [9]. Anti-fibrillarin and anti-U1-snRNP are sometimes considered as MAAs, even though they are more specific for the diagnosis of SSc and mixed connective tissue disease (MCTD), respectively [10, 11]. Anti-Ro52 are usually considered a MAA, even though they are more frequently found in association with other MSA (ARS, anti-MDA5 and anti-SRP, in particular) [12], and define a peculiar clinical spectrum in which the lung involvement is more common than the muscular one [13].

Detection methods

There are several methods to test for MSAs and MAAs, with variable sensibility, specificity, costs, complexity and feasibility in clinical and research settings. Indirect immuno-fluorescence (IIF) on HEp-2 cells, counter-immuno-electrophoresis (CIE), immuno-diffusion (ID) and immuno-enzymatic assays such as enzyme-linked immunosorbent assay (ELISA), fluorescent enzyme-linked assay (FEIA) and chemiluminescent immuno-assay (CLIA) are the most commonly adopted systems in diagnostic laboratories. However, immuno-precipitation (IP) of RNAs with silver staining and/or protein IP of cellular lysates (usually K562 cells) radiolabeled with ^{35}S-methionin, is the gold standard for most antibodies. In order to streamline the detection of many autoantibodies at the same time in a cost/effective manner, recent multiplex assays, like immunoblots (IB) and Addressable Laser Beads Immuno Assay (ALBIA) have been developed [14].

Anti-nuclear autoantibodies (ANA) determination by IIF is virtually universally available and it can be considered an accessible screening method for many MSAs and MAAs [15]. Furthermore, the recognition of particular IIF patterns can hint to some specific autoantibodies. However, using ANA IIF as the sole screening method for MSAs/MAAs, is not recommended because of low sensitivity, very low specificity and/or lack of antigen expression by HEp-2 cells [16]. In addition to this, ANA IIF is burdened by reproducibility issues due to the operator-dependent recognition of rare patterns and variation among different commercial HEp-2 substrates [17].

CIE and ID have historically been the first methods to detect specific MSAs/MAAs. Even though they identify numerous specificities within a single assay, they are semi-quantitative, work-intensive and scarcely sensitive [14]. For all those reasons, they have been largely substituted by immunoenzymatic tests.

The main advantages of ELISAs are standardization, large-scale reproducibility and quantitative results. The disadvantage of the conjugation of antigens to a substrate resides on the possible loss of conformational epitopes and/or the formation of neo-epitopes, which may in turn impact the test performance [14].

Immunoblot (IB) assays can simultaneously test for many autoantibodies, albeit the denaturation of proteins during gel preparation implicates the recognition of linear epitopes only [14].

Commercial multiplex IBs, like dot blots or line blot assays (LIA), based on recombinant or synthetic peptides have been increasingly available, benefitting from pure antigens not requiring a gel passage [18, 19].

IP is the gold standard as it evaluates the binding of the autoantibodies to the RNA and protein complexes in their native conformation, yielding the best sensitivity and specificity [20]. The major limitations of IP are due to technical difficulties, costs and use of radioactive reagents [20]. In addition, interpretation may be complex because the target antigen can co-precipitate with non-target complexed proteins, with the consequence of multiple IP bands [20]. Thus, a comparison with reference sera or further purification and characterization with other methods (i.e. mass spectrometry) is necessary [14]. Quantitative PCR of reverse transcribed RNA components extracted from standard IP can be also used as a detection method for autoantibodies binding ribonucleoproteic complexes [21].

Myositis-specific autoantibodies

Anti-synthetases autoantibodies

ARS are a group of autoantibodies directed against the aminoacyl transfer RNA (tRNA) synthetases, which are amino acid-charging enzymes. Autoantibodies to eight tRNA synthetases have been discovered so far: histidyl (Jo-1), threonyl (PL-7), alanyl (PL-12), glycyl (EJ), isoleucyl (OJ), asparaginyl (KS), phenylalanyl (ZO), and tyrosyl (YRS/HA) tRNA synthetases [22].

Anti-Jo-1 antibodies were identified by double immune-diffusion (DID) of calf thymus extract in 1980

Table 1 Summary of the main features of MSAs and MAAs

Antibody	Antigen	IP		IIF	Clinical association
		Proteins (kDa)	RNA	HEp-2	
Myositis-specific autoantibodies (MSAs)					
Anti-Jo-1	Histidyl-tRNA synthetase	50	$tRNA^{His}$	Cytoplasmic fine speckled	Classic anti-synthetase syndrome with more frequent muscle involvement
Anti-PL-7	Threonyl-tRNA synthetase	80	$tRNA^{Thr}$	Cytoplasmic dense fine speckled	Anti-synthetase syndrome with prevalent ILD
Anti-PL-12	Alanyl-tRNA synthetase	110	$tRNA^{Ala}$	Cytoplasmic dense fine speckled	Anti-synthetase syndrome with prevalent ILD
Anti-EJ	Glycyl-tRNA synthetase	75	$tRNA^{Gly}$	Cytoplasmic speckled	Anti-synthetase syndrome
Anti-OJ	Isoleucyl-tRNA synthetase	150 + 170/130/75	$tRNA^{Iso}$	Cytoplasmic speckled	ILD alone or anti-synthetase syndrome
Anti-KS	Asparaginyl-tRNA synthetase	65	$tRNA^{Asp}$	Cytoplasmic speckled	ILD alone or anti-synthetase syndrome
Anti-Zo	Phenylalanyl-tRNA synthetase	60/70	$tRNA^{Phe}$	Cytoplasmic speckled	Myositis
Anti-YRS/HA	Tyrosyl-tRNA synthetase	59	$tRNA^{Tyr}$	Cytoplasmic speckled	Myositis
Anti-Mi-2	Nucleosome Remodelling Deacetylase (NuRD) (Mi-2α/β)	240 + 200/150/75/65/63/50/34		Fine speckled	Classical DM
Anti-SAE	Small ubiquitin-like modifier activating enzyme (SAE1/2)	40/90		Fine speckled	Severe cutaneous disease that classically precede DM with severe dysphagia and systemic symptoms
Anti-MDA5 (anti-CADM140)	Melanoma Differentiation-Associated gene 5 (MDA5)	140		Negative or Cytoplasmic speckled	Hypo-amyopathic, ILD with possible RP-ILD and severe and peculiar skin involvement
Anti-TIF1γ/α (anti-p155/p140)	Transcription intermediary factor 1 (TIF1γ/α)	155/140		Fine speckled	Juvenile DM. Cancer-associated hypo-myopathic DM
Anti-TIF1β	Transcription intermediary factor 1β	120		Fine speckled	DM
Anti-NXP2 (anti-MJ)	Nuclear matrix protein (NXP-2)	140		Fine speckled and/or multiple nuclear dots	Juvenile DM, diffused calcinosis. Cancer-associated DM
Anti-SRP	Signal recognition particle	72/68/54/19/14/9	7SL	Cytoplasmic dense fine speckled	IMNM with frequent esophageal involvement. Possible ILD
Anti-HMGCR	HMG-CoA reductase	200/100		Negative or Cytoplasmic speckled	IMNM with or without history of statin exposure
Myositis-associated autoantibodies(MAAs)					
Anti-PM-Scl	Exosome protein complex (PM/Scl75/100)	75/100		Nucleolar homogeneous	Overlap PM/SSc
Anti-C1D	Exosome associated protein				Overlap PM/SSc
Anti-U1-RNP	U1 small nuclear RNP	11–70	U1	Coarse speckled	MCTD
Anti-fibrillarin (anti-U3-snRNP)	Fibrillarin	34	U3	Nucleolar clumpy	SSc
Anti-Ku	DNA-PK regulatory subunit	70/80		Fine speckled	PM/SSc. Potentially severe ILD

Table 1 continued

Antibody	Antigen	IP		IIF	Clinical association
		Proteins (kDa)	RNA	HEp-2	
Anti-Ro52	Ro-52/TRIM21	52		Negative, fine speckled or cytoplasmic speckled	ILD. Frequently coupled with other MSA
Anti-Ro60/SSA	Ro-60/SS-A	60		Fine speckled	SjS, SLE
Anti-La/SSB	SS-B	48		Fine speckled	SjS, SLE
Anti-cN-1A (anti-Mup44)	Cytosolic 5′nucleotidase 1A				sIBM
Miscellaneous					
Anti-RuvBL1/2	RuvBL1/2 complex	48/49		Speckled	SSc, PM, Morphea
Anti-Su/Ago2	Argonaute 2	100/102 and 200		Cytoplasmic discrete dots	ILD in absence of cancer. Frequently coupled with MSA, Ro-52 and other antibodies
Anti-SMN	Survival of Motor Neuron	38 + 130/120/33		Few nuclear dots	PM/SSc
Anti-NUP	Nup358/RanBP2, gp210, Nup90, p200/p130, Nup62	\		Punctate nuclear envelope	Subgroup of PM/SSc patients (so called NUP-syndrome). PBC
Anti-mitochondrial (AMA-M2)	Branched-chain α-ketoacid dehydrogenase complex			Cytoplasmic reticular/AMA	Long-lasting myositis with muscle atrophy and cardiac involvement. PBC
Anti-KJ	Translocation factor	30/43		Cytoplasmic speckled	Anti-synthetase-like syndrome
Anti-Fer (anti-eEF1)	Eukaryotic elongation factor 1				Anti-synthetase-like syndrome
Anti-Wa		48		Cytoplasmic speckled	Anti-synthetase-like syndrome
Anti-Mas	selenocysteine seryl-tRNA-protein complex	48	$tRNA^{[Ser]Sec}$	Cytoplasmic speckled	Non-immune mediated rhabdomyolysis. Autoimmune hepatitis
Anti-PMS	DNA repair mismatch enzyme (PMS1, PMS2, MLH1)				Mild myositis
Anti-cortactin	Cortactin	68			PM. Myasthenia gravis
Anti-FHL1	Four-and-a-Half LIM domain 1				Myositis and muscular atrophy with severe systemic involvement

and were the first MSAs described [23]. IP represents the gold standard for their identification with the following protein bands: Jo-1 50 kDa, PL-7 80 kDa, PL-12 110 kDa, EJ 75 kDa, OJ 150 kDa and a multi-enzyme complex of 170, 130, and 75 kDa, KS 65 kDa, ZO 60/70 kDa, YRS/HA 59 kDa [22].

IIF on HEp-2 cells usually demonstrates a cytoplasmic pattern, ranging from fine (Jo-1) to dense fine speckled or homogeneous (PL-7, PL-12) whereas the nucleoplasm is usually negative (Fig. 1a–e) [24]. In these cases, also patients without muscular involvement should be assessed for ARS especially when interstitial lung disease (ILD), arthritis or scleroderma features are present [25].

Anti-Jo-1 is the only autoantibody routinely tested as widely available in most commercial ENA screening assays. An ELISA screening test has been recently developed to identify ARS, with high sensibility and specificity if compared to IP [26] and some commercially available IBs can identify some non-Jo-1 anti-synthetase antibodies [20, 25].

Anti-Jo-1 was first discovered in the ‘80ies in patients with PM [23]. Larger cohorts later demonstrated that its presence was associated with the classical triad of arthritis, myositis and ILD in the majority of patients, in addition to Raynaud's phenomenon, mechanic's hands and fever. This clinical presentation together with anti-Jo-1 autoantibodies, led to the description of the

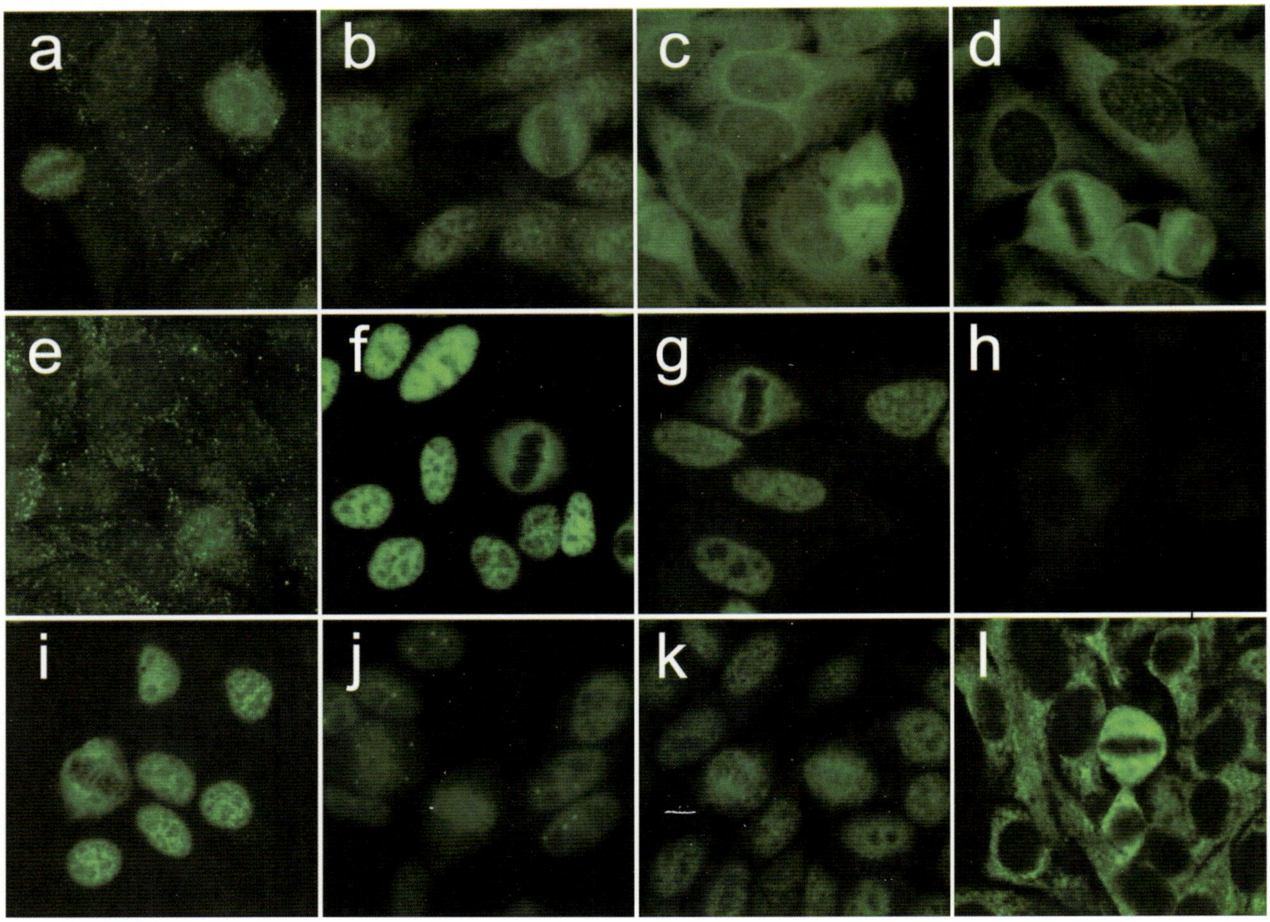

Fig. 1 IIF on HEp-2 ANA slides of myositis-specific autoantibodies from patients with IIMs (EUROIMMUN, Lübeck, Germany). **a** Anti-Jo-1 and **b** anti-Jo-1 and anti-Ro52, **c** anti-PL-7, **d** anti-PL-12, **e** anti-KS, **f** anti-Mi-2, **g** anti-SAE-1, **h** anti-MDA5, **i** anti-NXP-2 and **j** anti-NXP-2 with coiled bodies, **k** anti-TIF1γ, **l** anti-SRP

antisynthetase syndrome (ASSD), the first attempt to phenotype IIMs in clinical-serologic syndromes [27]. Anti-Jo-1 is detected in 15-25% of patients with polymyositis/dermatomyositis (PM/DM), whereas the other ARS are rarer (anti-PL-7 4-12%, PL-12 < 5%, EJ < 5%, OJ < 5% and only few cases reported with anti-KS, ZO e HA/YRS) [22]. In two-third of the cases, high titers of anti-Ro52 antibodies can be also detected and have been associated with an higher risk of ILD [28].

Clinically, anti-PL-7 patients more frequently present hypo-myopathic features [29, 30], whereas in anti-PL-12 and anti-KS patients the disease can be limited to the lung [31–33]. In a quarter of anti-Jo-1 patients, a symmetrical polyarthritis mimicking rheumatoid arthritis is the main presenting finding and, in some of them, anti-cyclic citrullinated peptide antibodies and rheumatoid factors can be also detected [34].

Regardless of clinical characteristics at presentation (arthritis, myositis and ILD) every patient tends to develop the other features of ASSD when not properly treated [34]. Of note, the lower esophageal sphincter is involved more frequently if compared to the other IIMs [35]. ASSD is histopathologically classified within perimysial immune-myopathies in which perimysium fragmentation and muscle fiber necrosis are the main feature, differently from other DM biopsically characterized by atrophy and vasculopathy [36]. Type I interferon-signature in ASSD is responsible for MHC class I upregulation [37] and MHC class II perifascicular expression [38].

Anti-Mi-2

Anti-Mi-2 antibodies were the first autoantibodies specific for DM recognized by DID using calf thymus extract [39]. Mi-2 is a helicase of the Nucleosome Remodeling

Deacetylase (NuRD) multi-protein complex with nucleosome remodeling and histone deacetylase/demethylase activities [40]. Anti-Mi-2 autoantibodies immunoprecipitate a major protein of 240 kDa, composed by two proteins, Mi-2α and Mi-2β of 220 and 218 kDa, respectively. Other NuRD complex proteins co-precipitate at 200, 150, 75, 65, 63, 50 and 34 kDa [41, 42]. IIF on HEp-2 cells reveals a characteristic fine speckled ANA pattern; during metaphase, chromatin mass is not stained but the nucleoplasm presents the same fine tiny speckles (Fig. 1f). Commercial ELISA and immunoblot kits identify anti-Mi-2 autoantibodies. Anti-Mi-2 are commonly detected in DM patients, either in adults (11–59%) or in children (4–10%), with a great variability among the studies. Their presence in PM and sporadic inclusion body myositis (sIBM) is rarer [40].

The Mi-2 protein is over-regulated during muscle regeneration in DM patients and thought to be related to UV rays exposition, sex and HLA (DRB1*0302 and DRB1*0701) [43–45]. Anti-Mi-2 positive DM patients usually exhibit mild myopathy despite high creatine kinase (CK) levels, without lung involvement and/or cancer [43]. Overall, anti-Mi2 positive is associated with a positive prognosis and a good response to corticosteroids [43].

Anti-SAE

Small Ubiquitin-like Modifiers (SUMOs) have a key role in post-transcriptional modification of specific proteins in a ubiquitin-like fashion. This process is controlled by the SUMO-Activating Enzyme (SAE), a heterodimer composed of two subunits, SAE-1 and SAE-2 [46], representing the targets of anti-SAE autoantibodies. IP characteristically shows two bands of 40 and 90 kDa, respectively [46, 47]. The IIF ANA pattern is coarse or fine speckled and nucleoli are typically not stained (Fig. 1g) [47].

Anti-SAE are associated with a typical DM phenotype with different prevalence in European (4-10%) and Asian (1–3%) cohorts [48–50], probably due to the strict association with HLADRB1*04-DQA1*03-DQB1*03 haplotypes [51].

The cutaneous involvement is usually severe and typically precedes the muscular involvement. Other clinical relationships cannot be excluded because of the few described cases. However, ILD seems to be rare, whereas severe dysphagia and systemic symptoms have been reported [47]. Only one case series claimed an association with cancer [52].

Anti-MDA5

Melanoma Differentiation-Associated gene 5 (MDA5) or Interferon-induced helicase C domain-containing protein 1 (IFIH1), is an innate cytosolic sensor, member of the retinoic acid-inducible gene I (RIG-I)-like receptors family (RLRs). MDA5 is able to recognize double-stranded RNA and to initiate signaling events leading to type I interferons production [53].

Anti-MDA5 autoantibodies were firstly detected in IP as a 140 kDa band in a Japanese case series of patients with clinically amyopathic dermatomyositis (CADM) and rapidly progressive interstitial lung disease (RP-ILD). For this reason, they were initially called anti-CADM-140 autoantibodies [54]. Nowadays, ELISA and IB tests are commercially available.

IIF on HEp-2 cells is usually negative. In our experience, a faint fine speckled cytoplasmic fluorescence may be detected in scattered cells (unpublished data) (Fig. 1h).

Clinically, DM anti-MDA5 positive patients present low grade/absent muscle inflammation and acute or subacute RP-ILD [55, 56], which is considered the major negative prognostic factor of this subgroup [57].

MDA5 represents the most frequent target antigen in DM patients of Asian ancestry (10–48% of cases) [58] whereas its prevalence in Europe and USA ranges from 0 to 13%, with great variability among the studies [59–61] and a different clinical presentation. A forthcoming European case series is going to be presented at the European League Against Rheumatism 2018 Congress by Cavagna et al. (unpublished data). A seasonal pattern of CADM has been proposed by Muro et al. [62], suggesting the influence of environmental factors and HLA-DRB1*04:01 and *12:02 have been proposed as further predisposing factors [63].

In addition to classic DM-related cutaneous manifestations, skin involvement is usually severe and characterized by the so called "inverse Gottron papules", which are tender palmar papules that tend to evolve towards ulcerated-necrotic lesions, with or without digital pulp ulcers [64, 65]. In addition, polyarthritis, recurrent oral aphtosis and diffuse alopecia have been described [66]. A juvenile DM with anti-MDA5 autoantibodies has been also described [67]. No association with malignancies has been demonstrated so far. Macrophage activation syndrome have been described in CADM associated RP-ILD patients. Particularly, a ferritin level of above 1500 ng/mL has been claimed as a predictor of death [68, 69]. Anti-MDA5 autoantibodies titer seems to correlate with disease activity and response to therapy [69].

Anti-TIF-1

The transcription intermediary factors-1 (TIF-1) family belongs to the tripartite motif-containing proteins (TRIM) superfamily and is involved in multiple biological processes, such as cycle regulation, mitosis and innate immunity [70].

Targoff et al. and Kaji et al. [71, 72] independently described two antibodies directed against a 155 and 140 kDa, rapidly identified as TIF-1γ (TRIM33) and TIF-1α (TRIM24), respectively. Subsequently, a third 120 kDa band, partially overlapping with anti-PL-12, was identified as TIF1β (TRIM28) [73].

IIF on HEp-2 cells demonstrates a fine speckled nuclear pattern (Fig. 1i). ELISA and IB, compared to IP, are reliable test for the detection of anti-TIF-1γ autoantibodies [74]. Two-thirds of the patients present anti-TIF-1γ and anti-TIF-1α autoantibodies, whereas the remaining one-third is positive for anti-TIF-1γ autoantibodies exclusively [70]. Albeit MSAs are claimed to be mutually exclusive, double-positive patients for anti-TIF-1α/Mi-2 autoantibodies have been described [75].

Hyper-expression of TIF-1γ has been found in tumors [76] and regenerating myofibres of DM patients [77]. A meta-analysis demonstrated that anti-TIF-1γ has a 78% sensitivity and 89% specificity for the diagnosis of cancer-associated myositis, with a 58% positive and 95% negative predictive value [78]. The risk of malignancy is higher in patients with anti-TIF-1γ/α than in those with anti-TIF-1γ alone [70].

Clinically, anti-TIF-1 positive patients can be classified in two age groups: (1) younger than 40-year-old patients, with a classical DM at presentation and (2) older than 40-year-old patients, with cancer-associated myositis [70]. Solid tumors, like ovary, lung and breast cancer are the most commonly associated neoplasia, but hematologic disorders and malignancies have been described as well [79]. In general anti-TIF-1γ patients exhibit a hypomyopathic DM with reduced prevalence of systemic involvement, namely ILD, Raynaud's phenomenon and arthritis [80]. Conversely, nutcracker esophagus is three times more frequent in anti-TIF-1γ patients than other IIMs [35]. Widespread cutaneous involvement is associated with unique features, such as palmar hyper-keratotic papules, psoriatic-like dermatitis and atrophic hypo-pigmented patches with telangiectasias [80]. An ovoid palatal patch may be present in about one half of patients, more frequently females with cancer-associated amyopathic disease [81].

Anti-NXP-2

Nuclear matrix protein 2 (NXP-2), encoded by the microrchidia 3 gene, is a 140 kDa protein involved in epigenetic regulation, RNA metabolism and preservation of nuclear chromatin architecture [82]. Anti-NXP-2 autoantibodies were found in a cohort of juvenile DM patients as a 140 kDa protein firstly named anti-MJ [83].

IIF on HEp-2 cells reveals a fine speckled nuclear pattern (Fig. 1k). Moreover, a nuclear dots pattern is detectable in 60% of sera [84], due to co-localization of NXP-2 with pro-myelocitic leukemia (PML) bodies [85] (Fig. 1j).

Anti-NXP-2 antibodies have been initially associated with a severe juvenile DM complicated by calcinosis, polyarthritis and intestinal vasculitis [86]. More recently, they have been also found in adult patients, with variable prevalence from 1.6 to 17% [87–89]. Anti-NXP-2 autoantibodies show a bimodal spectrum of clinical association, with calcinosis being more frequent in younger patients and cancer more common in the elderly [90], especially in male gender [88], even though with a lower prevalence when compared to anti-TIF-1 [87, 88].

Anti-SRP

The signal recognition particle (SRP) is a complex of six proteins (9, 14, 19, 54, 68 and 72 kDa) and a 300 nucleotides long RNA (7SL RNA) involved in the recognition and transportation of proteins to the endoplasmic reticulum [91]. Anti-SRP autoantibodies are more frequently directed against the SRP-54 fragment, albeit anti-SRP-68, anti-SRP-72 and anti-7SL RNA autoantibodies have been also described [91].

A dense fine speckled cytoplasmic pattern has been associated with the presence of anti-SRP (Fig. 2a); moreover, IIF on stomach–liver–kidney rat sections demonstrates a cytoplasmic staining of gastric chief cells (Fig. 2b) and hepatocytes (Fig. 2c) [92].

Anti-SRP-54 autoantibodies ELISA tests are commercially available, but they are less sensitive than IP [93]. Anti-SRP antibodies can also be tested on LIA assays, however careful temperature control is necessary in order to avoid false positive results [19].

These autoantibodies are strongly associated with immune-mediated necrotizing myositis (IMNM) where they may play a pathogenic role [94]. Histopathologically, they are characterized by scarce inflammatory CD8+ endomysial infiltrate, class I MHC upregulation, necrosis and myofiber regeneration [36] with poor response to therapy, mimicking muscular dystrophy [95]. Being strongly associated to HLA-DR5, the prevalence of anti-SRP autoantibodies is higher in Asian (8–13%) than in European patients [96]. Prevalence of anti-SRP in IMNM is highly variable among studies, ranging from 0 to 54%, because of differences regarding the type of assay (IB vs IP), low number of patients and genetic background [97–100]. In addition, esophageal involvement is common [101], whereas the possibility of a prominent cardiac involvement has not been yet confirmed [99, 102]. Lung involvement has been reported in a few cases [103], as well as an overlap with anti-synthetase antibodies like PL-12 and anti-Jo-1 [104, 105]. Intriguingly,

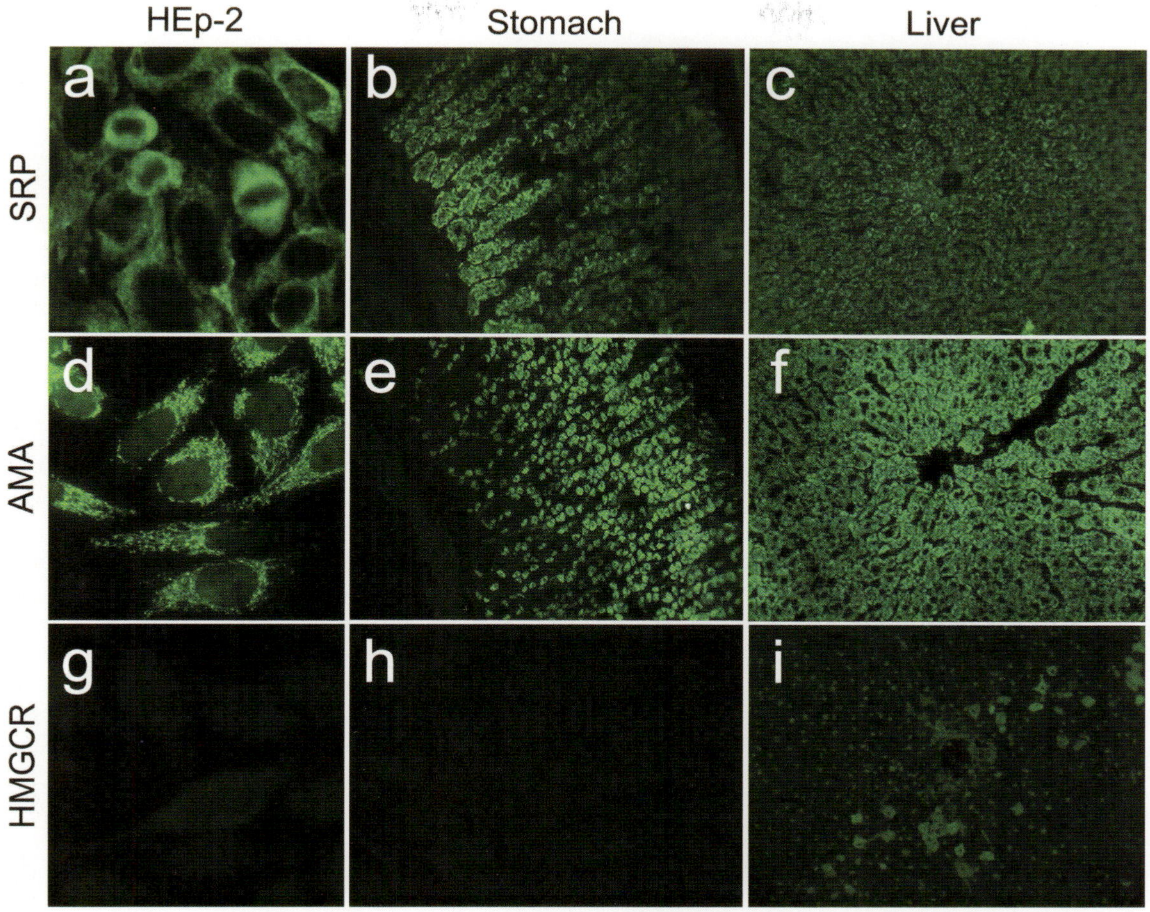

Fig. 2 Immunofluorescence patterns from patients with IMNMs with anti-SRP and anti-HMGCR antibodies on HEp-2 ANA slides (EUROIMMUN, Lübeck, Germany) and rat liver and stomach slides (DiaSorin, Italy), compared to AMA-M2 antibodies. **a** Anti-SRP cytoplasmic dense fine speckled pattern on HEp-2, **b** chief cells on stomach and **c** fine granular liver staining; **d** AMA-M2 cytoplasmic reticular on HEp-2, **e** granular staining of parietal stomach cells and **f** diffused fluorescence of hepatocytes; **g** Anti-HMGCR faint cytoplasmic fluorescence on few numbers of HEp-2 cells, **h** negative stomach and **i** fine cytoplasmic fluorescence of scattered hepatocytes around the biliary ducts

autoantibodies level correlates to disease activity, CK levels and response to therapy [106].

Anti-HMGCR

The 3-hydroxy-3-methylglutaryl-coenzyme A reductase (HMGCR) is the rate-controlling enzyme of the mevalonate pathway, bringing to the production of cholesterol. Of note, HMGCR is the same enzyme targeted by statins. Autoantibodies towards a complex 200/100 kDa band were first described in patients with IMNM, and only after identified as anti-HMGCR autoantibodies [107].

IIF pattern is difficult to recognize. In a minority of cases finely granular cytoplasmic staining with a perinuclear reinforcement is visible on a small number of scattered cells (3% of the total cellularity) (Fig. 2g). On rat liver, a scattered cytoplasmic staining of hepatocytes around the liver lobules, namely anti-HMGCR Antibody Associated Liver Immunofluorescence Pattern (HALIP), can be noted (Fig. 2i) [108, 109]. Anti-HMGCR antibodies can be identified with different immunoenzymatic technologies, such as ELISA, CLIA, IB or ALBIA [110].

A history of statin exposure is not mandatory to develop anti-HMGCR positive IMNM, being of some relevance only in patients older than 50 [111, 112]. Anti-HMGCR antibodies are not found in self-limiting statin associated myopathy [113], albeit they may be associated with an increased risk of cancer [114]. An association with the DRB1*11:01 haplotype has been demonstrated, whereas DQA1 and DQB1 seem to have a protective role [115].

Anti-HMGCR positive patients present with a typical IMNM, responds well to immunosuppressive therapy and intravenous immunoglobulins [116], but tend to relapse after tapering [111]. Younger patients experience more severe disease with worse prognosis [117]. Autoantibody titers seem to correlate with CK levels, muscular weakness and response to therapy [111].

Myositis-associated autoantibodies

Numerous MAAs have been described so far. Characteristically, they can be found in IIMs, albeit not specific as found in other CTDs [118].

Anti-PM-Scl

Anti-PM-Scl autoantibodies are directed against the exosome, a macromolecular nucleolar complex composed by 11–16 proteins (from 20 to 110 kDa) that degrades mRNA. The two pivotal proteins of the complex are PM-Scl-75 and PM-Scl-100. IP represents the gold standard for their determination. Historically, an ID test after positive nucleolar staining in IIF was used to confirm anti-PM-Scl reactivity.

PM-Scl-100 and PM-Scl-75 were identified in 1992 and, in the following years, the immuno-dominant epitope PM1α was cloned and employed to develop reliable and specific ELISA tests [119]. PM1α ELISA and PM-Scl-100 LIA tests show concordance with IP at high level (> 90 and 98.3%, respectively), whereas PM-Scl-75 LIA has a lower specificity, especially when considering PM/SSc overlap syndromes [120]. Single positivity against PM-Scl-75 or -100 can be detected and associates with different disease phenotypes. HEp-2 IIF typically shows a mixed homogeneous nucleolar and fine speckled nuclear pattern when anti-PM-Scl-100 are present, whilst anti-PM1-α and PM-Scl-75 may show both nucleolar and non-nucleolar patterns (Fig. 3a, b).

PM-Scl autoantibodies are found in 4–12% of adult patients with myositis [121, 122] with low prevalence in Asiatic and paediatric cohorts [123]. Their presence has been associated with HLA-DQA1*0501, DQB1*02 and DRB1*0301 alleles [122].

Despite their presence in many connective tissue diseases, these autoantibodies are typically present in PM/SSc overlap syndromes with an increased risk of Raynaud's phenomenon, arthritis, mechanic's hands and ILD [124]. In detail, isolated anti-PM-Scl-75 have been more frequently found in patients with joint contractures and SSc, higher CK levels associate with anti-PM-Scl-100, whereas the simultaneous presence of anti-PM-Scl-75 and -100 are linked to muscle involvement, digital ulcers and ILD but lower prevalence of lung hypertension [125].

Autoantibodies directed against C1D, an exosome associated protein, were detected by ELISA and Western blot analysis in 23% of a PM/SSc overlap syndrome cohort, with frequencies comparable to anti-PM/Scl antibodies [126].

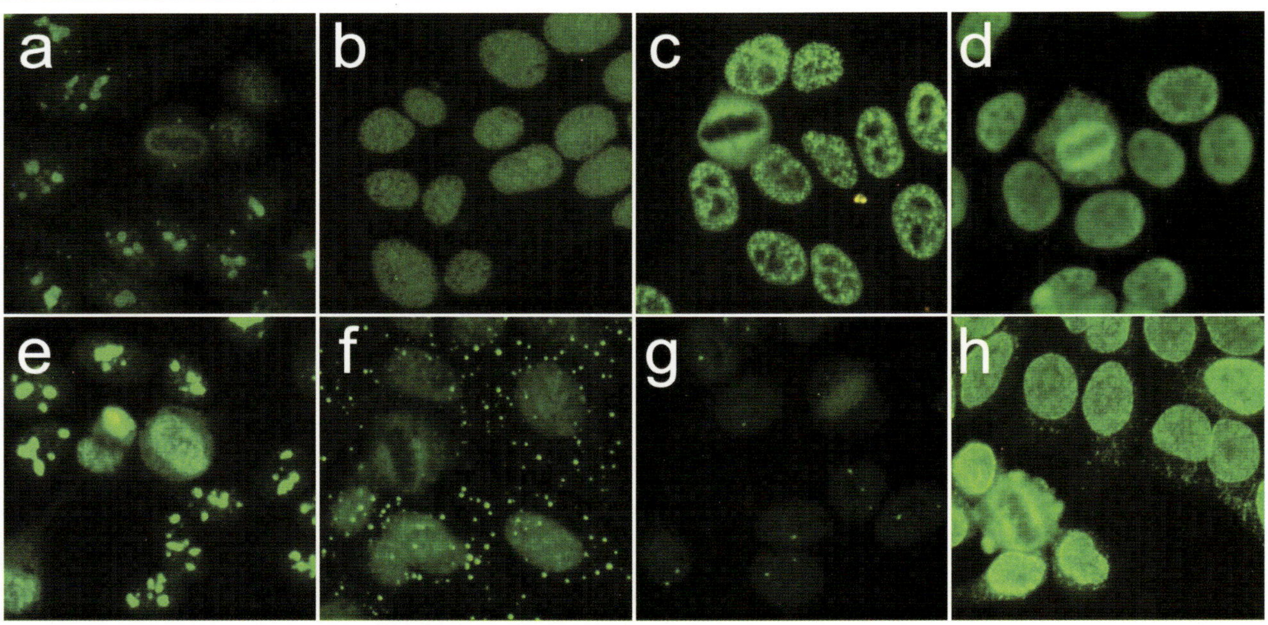

Fig. 3 Myositis-associated autoantibodies and some peculiar IIF pattern on HEp-2 ANA slides (EUROIMMUN, Lübeck, Germany). **a** anti-PM-Scl-100, **b** anti-PM-Scl-75, **c** anti-U1-snRNP, **d** anti-Ku, **e** anti-fibrillarin, **f** cytoplasmic discrete dots as seen in anti-Su/Ago2, **g** nuclear few nuclear dots as seen in anti-SMN, **h** punctate nuclear envelope as seen in anti-NUP

Anti-RNP

The RNP/Sm complex comprises several proteins (70 kD, A, A′, B, B′, B″, C, D, E, F, G) and five RNA (U1, U2, U4, U5 and U6). U1 RNA interacts with 70 kD, A and C to create the U1-snRNP [127]. High-titre anti-U1-snRNP and in particular when targeting the 70kD protein are considered specific markers of mixed connective tissue disease (MTCD), whereas low titres can be found in other CTDs [127].

Many home-made or commercial assays can detect anti-RNP autoantibodies, with differences among immunoassays depending on the immobilized antigen [127]. Usually, anti-U1-snRNP (more often the 70k subunit) and the anti-Sm (typically the D subunit) are the only autoantibodies tested in clinical practice. Large speckled and large coarse speckled are the most frequent HEp-2 IIF patterns observed (Fig. 3c).

Patients with myositis may exhibit anti-U1-snRNP positivity, especially those with a mild disease [128, 129]. They are usually steroid-responsive, even though ILD and/or neurological involvement may be part of the clinical presentation [128, 129]. Whether the only presence of anti-U1-snRNP and myositis has to be considered an incomplete form of MTCD or a true myositis, is still a matter of debate [128, 129]. In addition, anti-U2-RNP [130], U5-RNP [131] and anti-U4/U6-RNP [132] have been described in patients with PM/SSc overlap syndrome.

Anti-fibrillarin

Fibrillarin, a highly conserved nucleolar 34 kDa protein involved in the processing of ribosomal RNA, is part of the U3-small nucleolar (sno)-RNP complex together with other proteins and U3 RNA. Fibrillarin is the primary target of anti-U3-snoRNP autoantibodies [133]. IP is the gold standard for its detection showing good concordance with IB assays that use the recombinant protein [134].

HEp-2 IIF demonstrates a typical "clumpy" nucleolar pattern, with jagged staining of the nucleoli, coiled bodies and peri-chromosomal staining at the metaphase plates [135] (Fig. 3e).

Anti-fibrillarin antibodies are detected in a small percentage of SSc patients and rarely in SLE, primary Raynaud's phenomenon and myositis [136]. In detail, they identify a subset of SSc patients more often of African origin, with serious cutaneous and visceral involvement and a higher prevalence of myositis [137, 138].

Anti-Ku

The Ku protein, involved in the canonical non-homologous end-joining pathway of the DNA repair, is a heterodimer consisting of the two subunits, 70 and 80 kDa [139]. Anti-Ku can be identified with numerous assays, such as ELISA, CIE or IB. IIF demonstrates a fine speckled nuclear pattern with a peculiar ring beam surrounding the metaphase on HEp-2 cells and a clumpy speckled pattern on primate's liver [140] (Fig. 3d).

Anti-Ku autoantibodies have been identified in 9-19% of the patients with PM/SSc overlap syndromes and SLE, being associated with arthralgia, Raynaud's phenomenon and ILD [141, 142]. Of note, whilst muscular involvement seems to be steroid-sensitive, ILD is more frequently progressive, severe and steroid-resistant [143].

Anti-Ro

Antibodies directed against the ribonucleoproteic complex SSA/Ro and SSB/La have been originally identified in SjS and SLE. Actually, antigen Ro is made by two separate complexes of 52 and 60 kDa called Ro52/TRIM21 and SSA/Ro60, respectively. Antigen SSB/La has a molecular weight of 48 kDa [144].

ANA may result falsely negative on traditional HEp-2 cells when isolate anti-Ro are present, because Ro52 is a cytoplasmic antigen and Ro60 may be lost during the preparation. For this reason, human SSA/Ro60-transfected HEp-2 cells (HEp-2000) are sometimes used [145, 146]. Otherwise, a characteristic pattern defined as "myriad discrete fine speckled" may be observed [147]. Anti-SSB autoantibodies show a similar pattern [148].

Anti-Ro52 can be found in IIMs [149] and are frequently associated with other MSAs, in particular anti-synthetase [28], anti-MDA5 [61] and anti-SRP autoantibodies [12].

They are known to be a negative prognostic factor regarding systemic involvement such as ILD, whereas their role in the severity of muscular involvement has not been identified [13]. Anti-Ro52 autoantibodies are known to be associated with atrioventricular congenital heart block [150].

Anti-cN-1A

Cytosolic 5′nucleotidase 1A (cN-1A o NT5C1A) is a protein involved in the hydrolysis of adenosine monophosphate, controlling energy and metabolic cell balance [151]. Anti-cN-1A autoantibodies, first called anti-Mup44, were simultaneously described by Salajegheh et al. and Pluk et al. [152, 153] as targeting a 44 kDa protein in patients with sIBM.

These autoantibodies were initially detected by immunoblotting from purified skeletal muscle extracts [153]. A novel standardized IgG ELISA is now available [154]. In addition to IgG, circulating IgA and IgM anti-cN-1A autoantibodies have been recognized [155]. IIF ANA pattern is still undefined.

Anti-cN-1A autoantibodies are demonstrated in one-third of the patients with sIBM and in less than 5% with other IIMs or neuromuscular diseases [151]. A recent study demonstrated that positive anti-cN-1A sIBM patients are included in a more severe sIBM subtype and represent a homogeneous group as exhibiting higher mortality risk, less proximal upper limb weakness (not typical of sIBMs) and a cytochrome oxidase deficiency in muscular fibers, when compared to negative patients [156].

It is not known whether they have to be considered as MSAs or MAAs as also demonstrated in other autoimmune diseases, such as SjS (30%) and SLE (20%) [157]. Furthermore, they have been recently demonstrated in a cohort of severe juvenile myositis with lung involvement, juvenile idiopathic arthritis, but also in 12% of healthy children [158].

Despite low sensitivity, anti-cN-1A autoantibodies are high specific and highly predictive of sIBM [159] thus being of particular importance when bioptic specimens are not diagnostic.

Miscellaneous autoantibodies in IIM

Several other autoantibodies have been identified as associated with IIMs, but little is known about their clinical relevance. In fact, they are not routinely determined because easy-to-perform routine specific immunoassays still lack and they are rarely found.

Anti-RuvBL1/2

RuvBL1 (49kD) and RuvBL2 (48kD) constitute a nuclear complex involved into DNA repair and transcription. Two distinct bands of approximately 50 kDa are found in IP [160]. By means of ELISA and/or IB techniques, anti-RuvBL1/2 have been found in several CTDs, but those involved in SSc and myositis recognize different conformational epitopes identified by IP exclusively [160]. On HEp-2 cells, a fine speckled pattern is associated with these antibodies, with increased fluorescence in prophase and decreased in metaphase. Additionally, a fine speckled pattern can be found in the cytoplasm of about 40% positive sera [160]. Anti-RuvBL1/2 antibodies are highly specific for SSc, are associated with PM/SSc overlaps with diffuse cutaneous sclerosis and more frequently found in older patients of male sex [160–162] or, less frequently, in necrotizing polymyositis with morphea [162].

Anti-Su/Ago2

Anti-Su/Argonaute-2 (anti-Su/Ago2) autoantibodies have been originally identified in SLE patients by means of immunodiffusion technique in the late '80ies [163]. Although their high prevalence in CTDs, few studies are available.

By IP, two distinct 100 and 102 kDa adjacent bands can be seen in addition to a further 200 kDa band [164]. Argonaute-2 protein constitutes the 100 kDa band and plays a key role in miRNA and interference RNA maturation and metabolism [163]. Argonaute-2 colocalized with GW bodies, a cytoplasmic organelle associated with RNA metabolism [164]. Its location and function is responsible for the particular cytoplasmic pattern of these autoantibodies also known as "GW-bodies-like" or "cytoplasmic discrete dots" (Fig. 3f) [164].

Anti-Su/Ago2 autoantibodies are frequently associated with other MSA or MAA antibodies, in particular ARS, anti-TIF-1γ and anti-MDA5 [165]; anti-Ro52 antibodies are found in almost one half of the patients [166]. It has been reported that anti-Su/Ago2 antibodies can be demonstrated in about 7.5% of the patients of Japanese origin. Apparently, there is no statistical difference between anti-Su/Ago2 positive and negative patients; however, a correlation seems to exist with ILD and absence of cancers [165].

Anti-SMN

The Survival of Motor Neuron (SMN) is a multi-ribonucleoproteic complex able to interact with the RNP-complex related D–E–F-G proteins. The SMN complex is involved into the assembly of snRNPs and co-localizes with Cajal bodies. These autoantibodies have been first described in a small number of PM patients negative for anti-U1-snRNP and/or anti-Sm but positive for RNP D–E–F-G bands by IP. This observation was indeed responsible for the identification of other SMN-complex components, namely Gemin 2 (33 kDa), Gemin 3 (130 kDa), Gemin 4 (120 kDa) and SMN itself (38 kDa) [167].

Anti-SMN antibodies typically exhibit a few nuclear dots pattern on HEp-2 cells with well distinguished 2–7 nuclear dots, similarly to anti-p80-coilin, anti-NXP2 and anti-PML pattern, seldom associated to cytoplasmic or nuclear speckled patterns (Fig. 3g).

It is not clear whether positive patients exhibit distinct clinical features. Anyhow, in the original small group of positive patients [167] and a small Italian cohort [20], a PM/SSc overlap syndrome was present. It is of note that SMN-complex genetic mutations are frequently found in neuromuscular degenerative diseases such as spinal-muscle atrophy. That is why anti-SMN autoantibodies are of relevance in basic research [168].

Anti-NPC

Nuclear pore complex (NPC) regulates protein and RNA trafficking to the nucleus. It is constituted by a complex of several proteins including Nup358/RanBP2, Nup90, Nup62 and gp210 [169]. Anti-NPC autoantibodies, and, in particular, anti gp210 are typically associated to Primary Biliary Cholangitis (PBC) and Autoimmune Hepatitis (AIH) [170]. In a cohort study from Canada, anti-NPC antibodies were found in a PM/SSc overlap syndrome and called anti-NUP Syndrome, which was found to be associated with HLA-DQ1*0501. In this case, a typical nuclear speckled laminar pattern on HEp-2 cells was observed [171] (Fig. 3h).

AMA-M2

Among the ten different anti-mitochondrial antibodies (AMA), called M1–M10, anti-M2 antibodies (AMA-M2) are the hallmark of PBC [172]. However, they can be also found in 7–12% of IIM patients without PBC [173]. AMA antibodies are readily detectable on HEp-2 cells as they display a pathognomonic cytoplasmic reticular pattern, and in triple tissue slides (Fig. 2d–f). In a Japanese study, the presence of AMA-M2 in the course of IIM was associated with muscle atrophy, granuloma formation [173] and heart involvement with high risk of supraventricular arrhythmias [174]. A distinct inflammatory phenotype associated with chronic skeletal muscle disease and severe cardiac involvement was also found in a North American cohort [175]. These associations have not been confirmed in an European series [176].

Other antibodies

Several cytoplasmic autoantibodies are described in IIM patients such as anti-KJ towards a 30/43 kDa translocation factor [177], anti-Fer directed against the elongation factor 1 and anti-Wa recognizing a 48 kDa cytoplasmic protein with still unknown function [132]. All these antibodies are typically found in anti-synthetase-like syndromes. Anti-Mas antibodies are directed against a selenocysteine-containing tRNA complex lacking any tRNA-synthetase activity but involved in protein translocation. The band of precipitation is found at 48 kDa [178]. These antibodies have been described in AIH and in a single patient with non-immune mediated rhabdomyolysis [178].

DNA-repairing complexes, especially mismatch-repair complexes such as PMS1, PMS2 and MLH1, are frequently recognized as target antigens in IIMs [179]. Initially defined as MSAs, they do indeed frequently associate with other MSAs, in particular anti-Mi-2, but they can also be found in other non-muscular diseases, such as SLE. They generally mark mild disease [180].

Anti-cortactin antibodies have been initially found in IIM patients characterized by the simultaneous presence of anti-MDA5 or anti-HMGCR antibodies by ELISA [181]. As blot confirming assay identified an unexpected 68 kDa band, it was then found that MDA5 and HMGCR extracts used in the ELISA tests were contaminated by cortactin [181]. Anti-cortactin antibodies were originally found in myasthenia gravis [182] and later in IIM patients (about 20%) and other systemic connective tissue diseases [181].

Anti-Four-and-a-Half LIM domain 1 (FHL1) antibodies were identified in about 25% of IIM patients. These antibodies associated with a severe prognosis, muscle atrophy, vasculitis, dysphagia and advanced muscular damage. Curiously, FHL1 mutations cause hereditary X-linked congenital myopathies [183].

Conclusions

Although autoantibodies are considered to be epiphenomenon in autoimmunity, their presence frequently plays a pivotal role for the diagnosis of these diseases. Indeed, several of them exhibit a pathogenethic role in IIMs. Despite this, there is still a gap between bench and bedside because the intense basic research efforts have not been translated in clinical practice, as already futuristically underlined more than 20 years ago [96, 184]. As a fact, only anti-Jo-1 have been included into the 2017 Classification Criteria for Adult and Juvenile IIMs [3].

Remarkably, in the context of heterogeneously grouped diseases such as myositis, they should be even more appreciated as able to clinically stratify patients in terms of diagnostic work-up, histological patterns, peculiar organ involvement, severity, and, therefore, treatment intensity and prognosis. This process could be accomplished by a laboratory auto-immunologist [185] well-trained in recognition of IIF ANA nuclear and, also, cytoplasmic patterns, in strict collaboration with the clinical doctor, as a decision-maker for running in-depth analysis towards the identification of the culprit autoantibody.

In addition, multicentric studies with a multidisciplinary approach may help bridging the divide of the selection bias depending on the setting where patients are initially screened (i.e. pneumologic vs. dermatologic vs. immuno-rheumatologic vs. neurologic outpatient clinics).

Abbreviations

SLE: systemic lupus erythematosus; CTD: connective tissue disease; SjS: Sjögren syndrome; SSc: systemic sclerosis; IIM: idiopathic inflammatory myopathies; PM: polymyositis; DM: dermatomyositis; MSA: myositis-specific autoantibodies; MAA: myositis-associated autoantibodies; ARS: anti-synthetase autoantibodies; IPAF: interstitial pneumonia with autoimmune features; IIF: indirect immuno-fluorescence; CIE: counter-immuno-electrophoresis; ID: immuno-diffusion; ELISA: enzyme-linked immunosorbent assay; FEIA: fluorescent enzyme-linked assay; CLIA: chemiluminescent immuno-assay; IP: immuno-precipitation; ALBIA: addressable laser beads immunoassay; ANA: anti-nuclear autoantibodies; IB: immunoblot; LIA: line blot assays; tRNA: transfer RNA; DID: double immune-diffusion; ILD: interstitial lung disease; ASSD: antisynthetase syndrome; PM/DM: polymyositis/dermatomyositis; NuRD: nucleosome remodelling deacetylase; sIBM: sporadic inclusion body myositis; CK: creatine kinase; SUMOs: small ubiquitin-like modifiers; SAE:

SUMO-activating enzyme; MDA5: Melanoma Differentiation-Associated gene 5; RIG-I: retinoic acid-inducible gene I; RLR: RIG-I-like receptors family; RP-ILD: rapidly progressive interstitial lung disease; CADM: clinically amyopathic dermatomyositis; TIF1: transcription intermediary factors-1; TRIM: tripartite motif-containing proteins; NXP-2: nuclear matrix protein 2; PML: pro-myelocitic leukaemia bodies; SRP: signal recognition particle; IMNM: immune-mediated necrotizing myositis; HMGCR: 3-hydroxy-3-methylglutaryl-coenzime A reductase; HALIP: anti-HMGCR antibody associated liver immunofluorescence pattern; MTCD: mixed connective tissue disease; sno: small nucleolar; cN-1A: cytosolic 5′nucleotidase; SMN: survival of motor neuron; NPC: nuclear pore complex; PBC: primary biliary cholangitis; AIH: autoimmune hepatitis; FHL1: anti-four-and-a-half LIM domain 1; AMA: anti-mitochondrial antibodies.

Authors' contributions

BP and GV drafted the manuscript. All authors read and approved the final manuscript.

Acknowledgements

We thank the team of Immunoallergology Laboratory, AOU-Careggi, Florence for the great deal of teamwork and constant readiness to our requests.

Funding

This research received no specific grant from any funding agency in the pub lic, commercial, or not-for-profit sectors.

References

1. Petri M, Orbai A-M, Alarcón GS, Gordon C, Merrill JT, Fortin PR, et al. Derivation and validation of the Systemic Lupus International Collaborating Clinics classification criteria for systemic lupus erythematosus. Arthritis Rheum. 2012;64:2677–86.
2. Shiboski CH, Shiboski SC, Seror R, Criswell LA, Labetoulle M, Lietman TM, et al. 2016 American College of Rheumatology/European League Against Rheumatism classification criteria for primary Sjögren's syndrome. Ann Rheum Dis. 2017;76:9–16.
3. Lundberg IE, Tjärnlund A, Bottai M, Werth VP, Pilkington C, de Visser M, et al. 2017 European League Against Rheumatism/American College of Rheumatology classification criteria for adult and juvenile idiopathic inflammatory myopathies and their major subgroups. Ann Rheum Dis. 2017;76:1955–64.
4. Milone M. Diagnosis and Management of Immune-Mediated Myopathies. Mayo Clin Proc. 2017;92:826–37.
5. Targoff IN. Autoantibodies in polymyositis. Rheum Dis Clin North Am. 1992;18:455–82.
6. Targoff IN. Idiopathic inflammatory myopathy: autoantibody update. Curr Rheumatol Rep. 2002;4:434–41.
7. Satoh M, Tanaka S, Ceribelli A, Calise SJ, Chan EKL. A comprehensive overview on myositis-specific antibodies: new and old biomarkers in idiopathic inflammatory myopathy. Clin Rev Allergy Immunol. 2015;52:1–9.
8. Nakashima R, Imura Y, Hosono Y, Seto M, Murakami A, Watanabe K, et al. The multicenter study of a new assay for simultaneous detection of multiple anti-aminoacyl-tRNA synthetases in myositis and interstitial pneumonia. PLoS ONE. 2014;9:e85062.
9. Colafrancesco S, Priori R, Valesini G. Inflammatory myopathies and overlap syndromes: update on histological and serological profile. Best Pract Res Clin Rheumatol. 2015;29:810–25.
10. Gunawardena H, Betteridge ZE, McHugh NJ. Myositis-specific autoantibodies: their clinical and pathogenic significance in disease expression. Rheumatology (Oxford). 2009;48:607–12.
11. Chinoy H, Fertig N, Oddis CV, Ollier WER, Cooper RG. The diagnostic utility of myositis autoantibody testing for predicting the risk of cancer-associated myositis. Ann Rheum Dis. 2007;66:1345–9.
12. Frank MB, McCubbin V, Trieu E, Wu Y, Isenberg DA, Targoff IN. The association of anti-Ro52 autoantibodies with myositis and scleroderma autoantibodies. J Autoimmun. 1999;12:137–42.
13. Ferreira JP, Almeida I, Marinho A, Cerveira C, Vasconcelos C. Anti-ro52 antibodies and interstitial lung disease in connective tissue diseases excluding scleroderma. ISRN Rheumatol. 2012;2012:415272.
14. van Dooren SHJ, van Venrooij WJ, Pruijn GJM. Myositis-specific autoantibodies: detection and clinical associations. Autoimmun Highlights. 2011;2:5–20.
15. Chan EKL, Damoiseaux J, Carballo OG, Conrad K, de Melo Cruvinel W, Francescantonio PLC, et al. Report of the first international consensus on standardized nomenclature of antinuclear antibody HEp-2 cell patterns 2014–2015. Front Immunol. 2015;6:412.
16. García-DeLaTorre I. Clinical usefulness of autoantibodies in idiopathic inflammatory myositis. Front Immunol. 2015;6:331.
17. Damoiseaux J, von Mühlen CA, Garcia-De La Torre I, Carballo OG, de Melo Cruvinel W, Francescantonio PLC, et al. International consensus on ANA patterns (ICAP): the bumpy road towards a consensus on reporting ANA results. Autoimmun Highlights. 2016;7:1–8.
18. Ghirardello A, Bendo R, Rampudda ME, Bassi N, Zampieri S, Doria A. Commercial blot assays in the diagnosis of systemic rheumatic diseases. Autoimmun Rev. 2009;8:645–9.
19. Rönnelid J, Barbasso Helmers S, Storfors H, Grip K, Rönnblom L, Franck-Larsson K, et al. Use of a commercial line blot assay as a screening test for autoantibodies in inflammatory myopathies. Autoimmun Rev. 2009;9:58–61.
20. Cavazzana I, Fredi M, Ceribelli A, Mordenti C, Ferrari F, Carabellese N, et al. Testing for myositis specific autoantibodies: comparison between line blot and immunoprecipitation assays in 57 myositis sera. J Immunol Methods. 2016;433:1–5.
21. Ceribelli A, Satoh M, Chan EK. A new immunoprecipitation-real time quantitative PCR assay for anti-Th/To and anti-U3RNP antibody detection in systemic sclerosis. Arthritis Res Ther. 2012;14:R128.
22. Mahler M, Miller FW, Fritzler MJ. Idiopathic inflammatory myopathies and the anti-synthetase syndrome: a comprehensive review. Autoimmun Rev. 2014;13:367–71.
23. Nishikai M, Reichlin M. Heterogeneity of precipitating antibodies in polymyositis and dermatomyositis. Characterization of the Jo-1 antibody system. Arthritis Rheum. 1980;23:881–8.
24. Agmon-Levin N, Damoiseaux J, Kallenberg C, Sack U, Witte T, Herold M, et al. International recommendations for the assessment of autoantibodies to cellular antigens referred to as anti-nuclear antibodies. Ann Rheum Dis. 2014;73:17–23.
25. Infantino M, Palterer B, Biagiotti R, et al. Reflex testing of speckled cytoplasmic patterns observed in routine ANA HEp-2 indirect immunofluorescence with a multiplex anti-synthetase dot-blot assay: a multicentric pilot study. Immunol Res. 2018;66(1):74–8.
26. Abe T, Tsunoda S, Nishioka A, Azuma K, Tsuboi K, Ogita C, et al. Reliability and clinical utility of enzyme-linked immunosorbent assay for detection of anti-aminoacyl-tRNA synthetase antibody. Nihon Rinsho Meneki Gakkai Kaishi. 2016;39:140–4.
27. Yoshida S, Akizuki M, Mimori T, Yamagata H, Inada S, Homma M. The precipitating antibody to an acidic nuclear protein antigen, the Jo-1, in connective tissue diseases. A marker for a subset of polymyositis with interstitial pulmonary fibrosis. Arthritis Rheum. 1983;26:604–11.

28. Yamasaki Y, Satoh M, Mizushima M, Okazaki T, Nagafuchi H, Ooka S, et al. Clinical subsets associated with different anti-aminoacyl transfer RNA synthetase antibodies and their association with coexisting anti-Ro52. Mod Rheumatol. 2016;26:403–9.
29. Yamasaki Y, Yamada H, Nozaki T, Akaogi J, Nichols C, Lyons R, et al. Unusually high frequency of autoantibodies to PL-7 associated with milder muscle disease in Japanese patients with polymyositis/dermatomyositis. Arthritis Rheum. 2006;54:2004–9.
30. Marie I, Josse S, Decaux O, Diot E, Landron C, Roblot P, et al. Clinical manifestations and outcome of anti-PL7 positive patients with antisynthetase syndrome. Eur J Intern Med. 2013;24:474–9.
31. Targoff IN, Arnett FC. Clinical manifestations in patients with antibody to PL-12 antigen (alanyl-tRNA synthetase). Am J Med. 1990;88:241–51.
32. Hirakata M, Suwa A, Nagai S, Kron MA, Trieu EP, Mimori T, et al. Anti-KS: identification of autoantibodies to asparaginyl-transfer RNA synthetase associated with interstitial lung disease. J Immunol. 1999;162:2315–20.
33. Scirè CA, Gonzalez-Gay MA, Selva-O'Callaghan A, Cavagna L, Selva-O'Callaghan A, Cavagna L. Clinical spectrum time course of interstitial pneumonia with autoimmune features in patients positive for antisynthetase antibodies. Respir Med. 2017;132:265–6.
34. Cavagna L, Nuño L, Scirè CA, Govoni M, Longo FJL, Franceschini F, et al. Clinical spectrum time course in anti Jo-1 positive antisynthetase syndrome: results from an international retrospective multicenter study. Medicine (Baltimore). 2015;94:e1144.
35. Casal-Dominguez M, Pinal-Fernandez I, Mego M, Accarino A, Jubany L, Azpiroz F, et al. High-resolution manometry in patients with idiopathic inflammatory myopathy: Elevated prevalence of esophageal involvement and differences according to autoantibody status and clinical subset. Muscle Nerve. 2016;45(suppl_4):iv18–21.
36. Pestronk A. Acquired immune and inflammatory myopathies. Curr Opin Rheumatol. 2011;23:595–604.
37. Mescam-Mancini L, Allenbach Y, Hervier B, Devilliers H, Mariampillay K, Dubourg O, et al. Anti-Jo-1 antibody-positive patients show a characteristic necrotizing perifascicular myositis. Brain. 2015;138(Pt 9):2485–92.
38. Aouizerate J, De Antonio M, Bassez G, Gherardi RK, Berenbaum F, Guillevin L, et al. Myofiber HLA-DR expression is a distinctive biomarker for antisynthetase-associated myopathy. Acta Neuropathol Commun. 2014;2:154.
39. Targoff IN, Reichlin M. The association between Mi-2 antibodies and dermatomyositis. Arthritis Rheum. 1985;28:796–803.
40. Ghirardello A, Zampieri S, Iaccarino L, Tarricone E, Bendo R, Gambari PF, et al. Anti-Mi-2 antibodies. Autoimmunity. 2005;38:79–83.
41. Nilasena DS, Trieu EP, Targoff IN. Analysis of the Mi-2 autoantigen of dermatomyositis. Arthritis Rheum. 1995;38:123–8.
42. Zhang Y, LeRoy G, Seelig HP, Lane WS, Reinberg D. The dermatomyositis-specific autoantigen Mi2 is a component of a complex containing histone deacetylase and nucleosome remodeling activities. Cell. 1998;95:279–89.
43. Petri MH, Satoh M, Martin-Marquez BT, Vargas-Ramírez R, Jara LJ, Saavedra MA, et al. Implications in the difference of anti-Mi-2 and -p155/140 autoantibody prevalence in two dermatomyositis cohorts from Mexico City and Guadalajara. Arthritis Res Ther. 2013;15:R48.
44. Love LA, Weinberg CR, McConnaughey DR, Oddis CV, Medsger TA, Reveille JD, et al. Ultraviolet radiation intensity predicts the relative distribution of dermatomyositis and anti-Mi-2 autoantibodies in women. Arthritis Rheum. 2009;60:2499–504.
45. Prieto S, Grau JM. The geoepidemiology of autoimmune muscle disease. Autoimmun Rev. 2010;9:A330–4.
46. Tarricone E, Ghirardello A, Rampudda M, Bassi N, Punzi L, Doria A. Anti-SAE antibodies in autoimmune myositis: identification by unlabelled protein immunoprecipitation in an Italian patient cohort. J Immunol Methods. 2012;384:128–34.
47. Betteridge Z, Gunawardena H, North J, Slinn J, McHugh N. Identification of a novel autoantibody directed against small ubiquitin-like modifier activating enzyme in dermatomyositis. Arthritis Rheum. 2007;56:3132–7.
48. Ge Y, Lu X, Shu X, Peng Q, Wang G. Clinical characteristics of anti-SAE antibodies in Chinese patients with dermatomyositis in comparison with different patient cohorts. Sci Rep. 2017;7:188.
49. Muro Y, Sugiura K, Akiyama M. Low prevalence of anti-small ubiquitin-like modifier activating enzyme antibodies in dermatomyositis patients. Autoimmunity. 2013;46:279–84.
50. Fujimoto M, Matsushita T, Hamaguchi Y, Kaji K, Asano Y, Ogawa F, et al. Autoantibodies to small ubiquitin-like modifier activating enzymes in Japanese patients with dermatomyositis: comparison with a UK Caucasian cohort. Ann Rheum Dis. 2013;72:151–3.
51. Betteridge ZE, Gunawardena H, Chinoy H, North J, Ollier WER, Cooper RG, et al. Clinical and human leucocyte antigen class II haplotype associations of autoantibodies to small ubiquitin-like modifier enzyme, a dermatomyositis-specific autoantigen target, in UK Caucasian adult-onset myositis. Ann Rheum Dis. 2009;68:1621–5.
52. Muro Y, Sugiura K, Nara M, Sakamoto I, Suzuki N, Akiyama M. High incidence of cancer in anti-small ubiquitin-like modifier activating enzyme antibody-positive dermatomyositis. Rheumatology (Oxford). 2015;54:1745–7.
53. Nakashima R, Imura Y, Kobayashi S, Yukawa N, Yoshifuji H, Nojima T, et al. The RIG-I-like receptor IFIH1/MDA5 is a dermatomyositis-specific autoantigen identified by the anti-CADM-140 antibody. Rheumatology (Oxford). 2010;49:433–40.
54. Sato S, Hirakata M, Kuwana M, Suwa A, Inada S, Mimori T, et al. Autoantibodies to a 140-kd polypeptide, CADM-140, in Japanese patients with clinically amyopathic dermatomyositis. Arthritis Rheum. 2005;52:1571–6.
55. Sato S, Hoshino K, Satoh T, Fujita T, Kawakami Y, Fujita T, et al. RNA helicase encoded by melanoma differentiation-associated gene 5 is a major autoantigen in patients with clinically amyopathic dermatomyositis: association with rapidly progressive interstitial lung disease. Arthritis Rheum. 2009;60:2193–200.
56. Parronchi P, Radice A, Palterer B, Liotta F, Scaletti C. MDA5-positive dermatomyositis: an uncommon entity in Europe with variable clinical presentations. Clin Mol Allergy. 2015;13:22.
57. Zhang L, Wu G, Gao D, Liu G, Pan L, Ni L, et al. Factors Associated with interstitial lung disease in patients with polymyositis and dermatomyositis: a systematic review and meta-analysis. PLoS ONE. 2016;11:e0155381.
58. Chen Z, Hu W, Wang Y, Guo Z, Sun L, Kuwana M. Distinct profiles of myositis-specific autoantibodies in Chinese and Japanese patients with polymyositis/dermatomyositis. Clin Rheumatol. 2015;34:1627–31.
59. Ceribelli A, Fredi M, Taraborelli M, Cavazzana I, Tincani A, Selmi C, et al. Prevalence and clinical significance of anti-MDA5 antibodies in European patients with polymyositis/dermatomyositis. Clin Exp Rheumatol. 2014;32:891–7.
60. Labrador-Horrillo M, Martinez MA, Selva-O'Callaghan A, Trallero-Araguas E, Balada E, Vilardell-Tarres M, et al. Anti-MDA5 antibodies in a large Mediterranean population of adults with dermatomyositis. J Immunol Res. 2014;2014:290797.
61. Hall JC, Casciola-Rosen L, Samedy L-A, Werner J, Owoyemi K, Danoff SK, et al. Anti-melanoma differentiation-associated protein 5-associated dermatomyositis: expanding the clinical spectrum. Arthritis Care Res (Hoboken). 2013;65:1307–15.
62. Muro Y, Sugiura K, Hoshino K, Akiyama M, Tamakoshi K. Epidemiologic study of clinically amyopathic dermatomyositis and anti-melanoma differentiation-associated gene 5 antibodies in central Japan. Arthritis Res Ther. 2011;13:R214.
63. Chen Z, Wang Y, Kuwana M, Xu X, Hu W, Feng X, et al. HLA-DRB1 alleles as genetic risk factors for the development of anti-MDA5 antibodies in patients with dermatomyositis. J Rheumatol. 2017;44:1389–93.
64. Ward I, Hiles P, Arroyo R, Downs W, Bell D. Digital pulp ulcerations and inverse gottron papules in melanoma differentiation-associated gene 5-related dermatomyositis. J Clin Rheumatol. 2016;22:274–5.
65. Cao H, Xia Q, Pan M, Zhao X, Li X, Shi R, et al. Gottron papules and gottron sign with ulceration: a distinctive cutaneous feature in a subset of patients with classic dermatomyositis and clinically amyopathic dermatomyositis. J Rheumatol. 2016;43:1735–42.
66. Fiorentino D, Chung L, Zwerner J, Rosen A, Casciola-Rosen L. The mucocutaneous and systemic phenotype of dermatomyositis patients with antibodies to MDA5 (CADM-140): a retrospective study. J Am Acad Dermatol. 2011;65:25–34.
67. Tansley SL, Simou S, Shaddick G, Betteridge ZE, Almeida B, Gunawardena H, et al. Autoantibodies in juvenile-onset myositis: their

diagnostic value and associated clinical phenotype in a large UK cohort. J Autoimmun. 2017;84:55–64.
68. Gono T, Kawaguchi Y, Hara M, Masuda I, Katsumata Y, Shinozaki M, et al. Increased ferritin predicts development and severity of acute interstitial lung disease as a complication of dermatomyositis. Rheumatology (Oxford). 2010;49:1354–60.
69. Muro Y, Sugiura K, Akiyama M. Limitations of a single-point evaluation of anti-MDA5 antibody, ferritin, and IL-18 in predicting the prognosis of interstitial lung disease with anti-MDA5 antibody-positive dermatomyositis. Clin Rheumatol. 2013;32:395–8.
70. Fujimoto M, Hamaguchi Y, Kaji K, Matsushita T, Ichimura Y, Kodera M, et al. Myositis-specific anti-155/140 autoantibodies target transcription intermediary factor 1 family proteins. Arthritis Rheum. 2012;64:513–22.
71. Targoff IN, Mamyrova G, Trieu EP, Perurena O, Koneru B, O'Hanlon TP, et al. A novel autoantibody to a 155-kd protein is associated with dermatomyositis. Arthritis Rheum. 2006;54:3682–9.
72. Kaji K, Fujimoto M, Hasegawa M, Kondo M, Saito Y, Komura K, et al. Identification of a novel autoantibody reactive with 155 and 140 kDa nuclear proteins in patients with dermatomyositis: an association with malignancy. Rheumatology (Oxford). 2007;46:25–8.
73. Satoh M, Chan JYF, Ross SJ, Li Y, Yamasaki Y, Yamada H, et al. Autoantibodies to transcription intermediary factor TIF1β associated with dermatomyositis. Arthritis Res Ther. 2012;14:R79.
74. Labrador-Horrillo M, Martínez MA, Selva-O'Callaghan A, Trallero-Araguás E, Balada E, Vilardell-Tarrés M, et al. Anti-TIF1γ antibodies (anti-p155) in adult patients with dermatomyositis: comparison of different diagnostic assays. Ann Rheum Dis. 2012;71:993–6.
75. Muro Y, Ishikawa A, Sugiura K, Akiyama M. Clinical features of anti-TIF1-α antibody-positive dermatomyositis patients are closely associated with coexistent dermatomyositis-specific autoantibodies and anti-TIF1-γ or anti-Mi-2 autoantibodies. Rheumatology (Oxford). 2012;51:1508–13.
76. Kasuya A, Hamaguchi Y, Fujimoto M, Tokura Y. TIF1γ-overexpressing, highly progressive endometrial carcinoma in a patient with dermatomyositis positive for malignancy-associated anti-p155/140 autoantibody. Acta Derm Venereol. 2013;93:715–6.
77. Mohassel P, Rosen P, Casciola-Rosen L, Pak K, Mammen AL. Expression of the dermatomyositis autoantigen transcription intermediary factor 1γ in regenerating muscle. Arthritis Rheumatol. 2015;67:266–72.
78. Trallero-Araguás E, Rodrigo-Pendás JÁ, Selva-O'Callaghan A, Martínez-Gõmez X, Bosch X, Labrador-Horrillo M, et al. Usefulness of anti-p155 autoantibody for diagnosing cancer-associated dermatomyositis: a systematic review and meta-analysis. Arthritis Rheum. 2012;64:523–32.
79. Palterer B, Vitiello G, Cammelli D. First report of anti-TIF1γ dermatomyositis in a patient with myelodysplastic syndrome. Reumatismo. 2017;69:75–7.
80. Fiorentino DF, Kuo K, Chung L, Zaba L, Li S, Casciola-Rosen L. Distinctive cutaneous and systemic features associated with antitranscriptional intermediary factor-1γ antibodies in adults with dermatomyositis. J Am Acad Dermatol. 2015;72:449–55.
81. Bernet LL, Lewis MA, Rieger KE, Casciola-Rosen L, Fiorentino DF. Ovoid palatal patch in dermatomyositis: a novel finding associated with anti-TIF1γ (p155) antibodies. JAMA Dermatol. 2016;152:1049–51.
82. Kimura Y, Sakai F, Nakano O, Kisaki O, Sugimoto H, Sawamura T, et al. The newly identified human nuclear protein NXP-2 possesses three distinct domains, the nuclear matrix-binding, RNA-binding, and coiled-coil domains. J Biol Chem. 2002;277:20611–7.
83. Targoff IN, Trieu EP, Levy-Neto M. Sera with autoantibodies to the MJ antigen react with NXP2. Arthritis Rheum. 2007;56:S787.
84. Fredi M, Bartoli F, Cavazzana I, Ceribelli A, Carabellese N, Tincani A, et al. Calcinosis in poly-dermatomyositis: clinical and laboratory predictors and treatment options. Clin Exp Rheumatol. 2017;35:303–8.
85. Mimura Y, Takahashi K, Kawata K, Akazawa T, Inoue N. Two-step colocalization of MORC3 with PML nuclear bodies. J Cell Sci. 2010;123(Pt 12):2014–24.
86. Espada G, Maldonado Cocco JA, Fertig N, Oddis CV. Clinical and serologic characterization of an Argentine pediatric myositis cohort: identification of a novel autoantibody (anti-MJ) to a 142-kDa protein. J Rheumatol. 2009;36:2547–51.
87. Ichimura Y, Matsushita T, Hamaguchi Y, Kaji K, Hasegawa M, Tanino Y, et al. Anti-NXP2 autoantibodies in adult patients with idiopathic inflammatory myopathies: possible association with malignancy. Ann Rheum Dis. 2012;71:710–3.
88. Fiorentino DF, Chung LS, Christopher-Stine L, Zaba L, Li S, Mammen AL, et al. Most patients with cancer-associated dermatomyositis have antibodies to nuclear matrix protein NXP-2 or transcription intermediary factor 1γ. Arthritis Rheum. 2013;65:2954–62.
89. Ceribelli A, Fredi M, Taraborelli M, Cavazzana I, Franceschini F, Quinzanini M, et al. Anti-MJ/NXP-2 autoantibody specificity in a cohort of adult Italian patients with polymyositis/dermatomyositis. Arthritis Res Ther. 2012;14:R97.
90. Tansley SL, Betteridge ZE, Shaddick G, Gunawardena H, Arnold K, Wedderburn LR, et al. Calcinosis in juvenile dermatomyositis is influenced by both anti-NXP2 autoantibody status and age at disease onset. Rheumatology (Oxford). 2014;53:2204–8.
91. Reeves WH, Nigam SK, Blobel G. Human autoantibodies reactive with the signal-recognition particle. Proc Natl Acad Sci USA. 1986;83:9507–11.
92. Picard C, Vincent T, Lega J-CC, Hue S, Fortenfant F, Lakomy D, et al. Heterogeneous clinical spectrum of anti-SRP myositis and importance of the methods of detection of anti-SRP autoantibodies: a multicentric study. Immunol Res. 2016;64:677–86.
93. Suzuki S, Nishikawa A, Kuwana M, Nishimura H, Watanabe Y, Nakahara J, et al. Inflammatory myopathy with anti-signal recognition particle antibodies: case series of 100 patients. Orphanet J Rare Dis. 2015;10:61.
94. Allenbach Y, Arouche-Delaperche L, Preusse C, et al. Necrosis in anti-SRP+ and anti-HMGCR+myopathies: role of autoantibodies and complement. Neurology. 2018;90(6):e507–17.
95. Ikeda K, Mori-Yoshimura M, Yamamoto T, Sonoo M, Suzuki S, Kondo Y, et al. Chronic myopathy associated with anti-signal recognition particle antibodies can be misdiagnosed as facioscapulohumeral muscular dystrophy. J Clin Neuromuscul Dis. 2016;17:197–206.
96. Love LA, Leff RL, Fraser DD, Targoff IN, Dalakas M, Plotz PH, et al. A new approach to the classification of idiopathic inflammatory myopathy: myositis-specific autoantibodies define useful homogeneous patient groups. Medicine (Baltimore). 1991;70:360–74.
97. Aggarwal R, Oddis CV, Goudeau D, Fertig N, Metes I, Stephens C, et al. Anti-signal recognition particle autoantibody ELISA validation and clinical associations. Rheumatology. 2015;54:1194–9.
98. Suzuki S, Yonekawa T, Kuwana M, Hayashi YK, Okazaki Y, Kawaguchi Y, et al. Clinical and histological findings associated with autoantibodies detected by RNA immunoprecipitation in inflammatory myopathies. J Neuroimmunol. 2014;274:202–8.
99. Wang L, Liu L, Hao H, Gao F, Liu X, Wang Z, et al. Myopathy with anti-signal recognition particle antibodies: clinical and histopathological features in Chinese patients. Neuromuscul Disord. 2014;24:335–41.
100. Ellis E, Ann Tan J, Lester S, Tucker G, Blumbergs P, Roberts-Thomson P, et al. Necrotizing myopathy: clinicoserologic associations. Muscle Nerve. 2012;45:189–94.
101. Kao AH, Lacomis D, Lucas M, Fertig N, Oddis CV. Anti-signal recognition particle autoantibody in patients with and patients without idiopathic inflammatory myopathy. Arthritis Rheum. 2004;50:209–15.
102. Takada T, Hirakata M, Suwa A, Kaneko Y, Kuwana M, Ishihara T, et al. Clinical and histopathological features of myopathies in Japanese patients with anti-SRP autoantibodies. Mod Rheumatol. 2009;19:156–64.
103. Togawa R, Tanino Y, Nikaido T, Fukuhara N, Uematsu M, Misa K, et al. Three cases of interstitial pneumonia with anti-signal recognition particle antibody. Allergol Int. 2017;66:485–7.
104. Sugie K, Tonomura Y, Ueno S. Characterization of dermatomyositis with coexistence of anti-Jo-1 and anti-SRP antibodies. Intern Med. 2012;51:799–802.
105. Malkan A, Cappelen-Smith C, Beran R, Griffith N, Toong C, Wang M-X, et al. Anti-synthetase syndrome associated with anti PL-12 and anti-Signal recognition particle antibodies and a necrotizing auto-immune myositis. J Clin Neurosci. 2015;22:396–8.
106. Benveniste O, Drouot L, Jouen F, Charuel J-L, Bloch-Queyrat C, Behin A, et al. Correlation of anti-signal recognition particle autoantibody levels with creatine kinase activity in patients with necrotizing myopathy. Arthritis Rheum. 2011;63:1961–71.
107. Christopher-Stine L, Casciola-Rosen LA, Hong G, Chung T, Corse AM, Mammen AL. A novel autoantibody recognizing 200-kd and 100-kd

proteins is associated with an immune-mediated necrotizing myopathy. Arthritis Rheum. 2010;62:2757–66.
108. Alvarado-Cardenas M, Marin-Sánchez A, Martínez MA, Martínez-Martínez L, Pinal-Fernandez I, Labrador-Horrillo M, et al. Statin-associated autoimmune myopathy: a distinct new IFL pattern can increase the rate of HMGCR antibody detection by clinical laboratories. Autoimmun Rev. 2016;15:1161–6.
109. Palterer B, Cammelli D, Vitiello G, Giudizi MGMG, Cammelli D, Giudizi MGMG, et al. Anti-HMGCR and anti-DFS70 antibodies immunofluorescence patterns. Autoimmune Dis. 2017;16:321–2.
110. Musset L, Miyara M, Benveniste O, Charuel J-L, Shikhman A, Boyer O, et al. Analysis of autoantibodies to 3-hydroxy-3-methylglutaryl-coenzyme A reductase using different technologies. J Immunol Res. 2014;2014:1–8.
111. Musset L, Allenbach Y, Benveniste O, Boyer O, Bossuyt X, Bentow C, et al. Anti-HMGCR antibodies as a biomarker for immune-mediated necrotizing myopathies: a history of statins and experience from a large international multi-center study. Autoimmun Rev. 2016;15:983–93.
112. Alshehri A, Choksi R, Bucelli R, Pestronk A. Myopathy with anti-HMGCR antibodies. Neurol Neuroimmunol Neuroinflamm. 2015;2:e124.
113. Keating P, Young J, George P, Florkowski C, Spellerberg M, Kennedy N. Anti-HMGCR autoantibodies in self-limiting statin-induced myopathy. Int J Rheum Dis. 2017;20:2179–81.
114. Kadoya M, Hida A, Hashimoto Maeda M, Taira K, Ikenaga C, Uchio N, et al. Cancer association as a risk factor for anti-HMGCR antibody-positive myopathy. Neurol Neuroimmunol Neuroinflamm. 2016;3:e290.
115. Mammen AL, Gaudet D, Brisson D, Christopher-Stine L, Lloyd TE, Leffell MS, et al. Increased frequency of DRB1*11:01 in anti-HMG-CoA reductase-associated autoimmune myopathy. Arthritis Care Res (Hoboken). 2012;64:1233–7.
116. Giudizi M, Cammelli D, Vivarelli E, Biagiotti R, Ferraro A, Bentow C, et al. Anti-HMGCR antibody-associated necrotizing myopathy: diagnosis and treatment illustrated using a case report. Scand J Rheumatol. 2016;45:427–9.
117. Tiniakou E, Pinal-Fernandez I, Lloyd TE, Albayda J, Paik J, Werner JL, et al. More severe disease and slower recovery in younger patients with anti-3-hydroxy-3-methylglutaryl-coenzyme A reductase-associated autoimmune myopathy. Rheumatology (Oxford). 2017;56:787–94.
118. Rider LG, Shah M, Mamyrova G, Huber AM, Rice MM, Targoff IN, et al. The myositis autoantibody phenotypes of the juvenile idiopathic inflammatory myopathies. Medicine (Baltimore). 2013;92:223–43.
119. Mahler M, Fritzler MJ. PM1-Alpha ELISA: the assay of choice for the detection of anti-PM/Scl autoantibodies? Autoimmun Rev. 2009;8:373–8.
120. Jaskowski TD, Wilson A, Hill HR, Tebo AE. Diagnostic assays for Anti-PM/Scl IgG antibodies: heterogeneity in antibody response or lack of standardization? Clin Chim Acta. 2011;412:1100–5.
121. Lega J-CC, Fabien N, Reynaud Q, Durieu I, Durupt SS, Dutertre M, et al. The clinical phenotype associated with myositis-specific and associated autoantibodies: a meta-analysis revisiting the so-called antisynthetase syndrome. Autoimmun Rev. 2014;13:883–91.
122. Mahler M, Raijmakers R. Novel aspects of autoantibodies to the PM/Scl complex: clinical, genetic and diagnostic insights. Autoimmun Rev. 2007;6:432–7.
123. Muro Y, Hosono Y, Sugiura K, Ogawa Y, Mimori T, Akiyama M. Anti-PM/Scl antibodies are found in Japanese patients with various systemic autoimmune conditions besides myositis and scleroderma. Arthritis Res Ther. 2015;17:57.
124. Aguila LA, Lopes MRU, Pretti FZ, Sampaio-Barros PD, Carlos De Souza FH, Borba EF, et al. Clinical and laboratory features of overlap syndromes of idiopathic inflammatory myopathies associated with systemic lupus erythematosus, systemic sclerosis, or rheumatoid arthritis. Clin Rheumatol. 2014;33:1093–8.
125. Hanke K, Brückner CS, Dähnrich C, Huscher D, Komorowski L, Meyer W, et al. Antibodies against PM/Scl-75 and PM/Scl-100 are independent markers for different subsets of systemic sclerosis patients. Arthritis Res Ther. 2009;11:R22.
126. Schilders G, Egberts WV, Raijmakers R, Pruijn GJM. C1D is a major autoantibody target in patients with the polymyositis-scleroderma overlap syndrome. Arthritis Rheum. 2007;56:2449–54.
127. Migliorini P, Baldini C, Rocchi V, Bombardieri S. Anti-Sm and anti-RNP antibodies. Autoimmunity. 2005;38:47–54.
128. Lundberg I, Nennesmo I, Hedfors E. A clinical, serological, and histopathological study of myositis patients with and without anti-RNP antibodies. Semin Arthritis Rheum. 1992;22:127–38.
129. Coppo P, Clauvel JP, Bengoufa D, Oksenhendler E, Lacroix C, Lassoued K. Inflammatory myositis associated with anti-U1-small nuclear ribonucleoprotein antibodies: a subset of myositis associated with a favourable outcome. Rheumatology (Oxford). 2002;41:1040–6.
130. Craft J, Mimori T, Olsen TL, Hardin JA. The U2 small nuclear ribonucleoprotein particle as an autoantigen. Analysis with sera from patients with overlap syndromes. J Clin Invest. 1988;81:1716–24.
131. Kubo M, Ihn H, Kuwana M, Asano Y, Tamaki T, Yamane K, et al. Anti-U5 snRNP antibody as a possible serological marker for scleroderma-polymyositis overlap. Rheumatology (Oxford). 2002;41:531–4.
132. Sibilia J, Chatelus E, Meyer A, Gottenberg J-E, Sordet C, Goetz J. How can we diagnose and better understand inflammatory myopathies? The usefulness of auto-antibodies. Presse Med. 2010;39:1010–25.
133. Van Eenennaam H, Vogelzangs JHP, Bisschops L, Te Boome LCJ, Seelig HP, Renz M, et al. Autoantibodies against small nucleolar ribonucleoprotein complexes and their clinical associations. Clin Exp Immunol. 2002;130:532–40.
134. Peterson LK, Jaskowski TD, Mayes MD, Tebo AE. Detection of anti-U3-RNP/fibrillarin IgG antibodies by line immunoblot assay has comparable clinical significance to immunoprecipitation testing in systemic sclerosis. Immunol Res. 2016;64:483–8.
135. Reimer G, Steen VD, Penning CA, Medsger TA, Tan EM. Correlates between autoantibodies to nucleolar antigens and clinical features in patients with systemic sclerosis (scleroderma). Arthritis Rheum. 1988;31:525–32.
136. Murata K-Y, Nakatani K, Yananeki M, Nakanishi I, Ito H. Anti-U3 ribonucleoprotein antibody-positive inflammatory myopathy: a case report. J Med Case Rep. 2016;10:169.
137. Tall F, Dechomet M, Riviere S, Cottin V, Ballot E, Tiev KP, et al. The clinical relevance of antifibrillarin (anti-U3-RNP) autoantibodies in systemic sclerosis. Scand J Immunol. 2017;85:73–9.
138. Tormey VJ, Bunn CC, Denton CP, Black CM. Anti-fibrillarin antibodies in systemic sclerosis. Rheumatology (Oxford). 2001;40:1157–62.
139. Belizna C, Henrion D, Beucher A, Lavigne C, Ghaali A, Lévesque H. Anti-Ku antibodies: clinical, genetic and diagnostic insights. Autoimmun Rev. 2010;9:691–4.
140. Cooley HM, Melny BJ, Gleeson R, Greco T, Kay TW. Clinical and serological associations of anti-Ku antibody. J Rheumatol. 1999;26:563–7.
141. Mimori T, Hardin JA, Steitz JA. Characterization of the DNA-binding protein antigen Ku recognized by autoantibodies from patients with rheumatic disorders. J Biol Chem. 1986;261:2274–8.
142. Cavazzana I, Ceribelli A, Quinzanini M, Scarsi M, Airò P, Cattaneo R, et al. Prevalence and clinical associations of anti-Ku antibodies in systemic autoimmune diseases. Lupus. 2008;17:727–32.
143. Rigolet A, Musset L, Dubourg O, Maisonobe T, Grenier P, Charuel J-L, et al. Inflammatory myopathies with anti-Ku antibodies: a prognosis dependent on associated lung disease. Medicine (Baltimore). 2012;91:95–102.
144. Franceschini F, Cavazzana I. Anti-Ro/SSA and La/SSB antibodies. Autoimmunity. 2005;38:55–63.
145. Pollock W, Toh BH. Routine immunofluorescence detection of Ro/SS-A autoantibody using HEp-2 cells transfected with human 60 kDa Ro/SS-A. J Clin Pathol. 1999;52:684–7.
146. Fritzler MJ, Hanson C, Miller J, Eystathioy T. Specificity of autoantibodies to SS-A/Ro on a transfected and overexpressed human 60 kDa Ro autoantigen substrate. J Clin Lab Anal. 2002;16:103–8.
147. Dellavance A, Alvarenga RR, Rodrigues SSH, Barbosa SH, Camilo ACP, Shiguedomi HSO, et al. Autoantibodies to 60 kDa SS-A/Ro yield a specific nuclear myriad discrete fine speckled immunofluorescence pattern. J Immunol Methods. 2013;390:35–40.
148. Defendenti C, Atzeni F, Spina MF, Grosso S, Cereda A, Guercilena G, et al. Clinical and laboratory aspects of Ro/SSA-52 autoantibodies. Autoimmun Rev. 2011;10:150–4.
149. Ghillani P, André C, Toly C, Rouquette AM, Bengoufa D, Nicaise P, et al. Clinical significance of anti-Ro52 (TRIM21) antibodies non-associated

with anti-SSA 60 kDa antibodies: results of a multicentric study. Autoimmun Rev. 2011;10:509–13.
150. Sonesson S-E, Hedlund M, Ambrosi A, Wahren-Herlenius M. Factors influencing fetal cardiac conduction in anti-Ro/SSA-positive pregnancies. Rheumatology (Oxford). 2017;56:1755–62.
151. Lloyd TE, Christopher-Stine L, Pinal-Fernandez I, Tiniakou E, Petri M, Baer A, et al. Cytosolic 5′-nucleotidase 1A As a target of circulating autoantibodies in autoimmune diseases. Arthritis Care Res (Hoboken). 2016;68:66–71.
152. Salajegheh M, Lam T, Greenberg SA. Autoantibodies against a 43 KDa muscle protein in inclusion body myositis. PLoS ONE. 2011;6:e20266.
153. Pluk H, van Hoeve BJA, van Dooren SHJ, Stammen-Vogelzangs J, van der Heijden A, Schelhaas HJ, et al. Autoantibodies to cytosolic 5′-nucleotidase 1A in inclusion body myositis. Ann Neurol. 2013;73:397–407.
154. Kramp SL, Karayev D, Shen G, Metzger AL, Morris RI, Karayev E, et al. Development and evaluation of a standardized ELISA for the determination of autoantibodies against cN-1A (Mup44, NT5C1A) in sporadic inclusion body myositis. Auto Immun highlights. 2016;7:16.
155. Greenberg SA. Cytoplasmic 5′-nucleotidase autoantibodies in inclusion body myositis: isotypes and diagnostic utility. Muscle Nerve. 2014;50:488–92.
156. Lilleker JB, Rietveld A, Pye SR, Mariampillai K, Benveniste O, Peeters MTJ, et al. Cytosolic 5′-nucleotidase 1A autoantibody profile and clinical characteristics in inclusion body myositis. Ann Rheum Dis. 2017;76:862–8.
157. Herbert MK, Stammen-Vogelzangs J, Verbeek MM, Rietveld A, Lundberg IE, Chinoy H, et al. Disease specificity of autoantibodies to cytosolic 5′-nucleotidase 1A in sporadic inclusion body myositis versus known autoimmune diseases. Ann Rheum Dis. 2016;75:696–701.
158. Yeker RM, Pinal-Fernandez I, Kishi T, Pak K, Targoff IN, Miller FW, et al. Anti-NT5C1A autoantibodies are associated with more severe disease in patients with juvenile myositis. Ann Rheum Dis. 2018. https://doi.org/10.1136/annrheumdis-2017-212436.
159. Herbert MK, Pruijn GJM. Novel serology testing for sporadic inclusion body myositis: disease-specificity and diagnostic utility. Curr Opin Rheumatol. 2015;27:595–600.
160. Kaji K, Fertig N, Medsger TA, Satoh T, Hoshino K, Hamaguchi Y, et al. Autoantibodies to RuvBL1 and RuvBL2: a novel systemic sclerosis-related antibody associated with diffuse cutaneous and skeletal muscle involvement. Arthritis Care Res. 2014;66:575–84.
161. Pauling JD, Salazar G, Lu H, Betteridge ZE, Assassi S, Mayes MD, et al. Presence of anti-eukaryotic initiation factor-2B, anti-RuvBL1/2 and anti-synthetase antibodies in patients with anti-nuclear antibody negative systemic sclerosis. Rheumatology. 2017.
162. Takahashi T, Nakanishi T, Hamaguchi Y, Tanaka T, Fujimoto N. Case of anti-RuvBL1/2 antibody-positive morphea and polymyositis. J Dermatol. 2017:44:1188–90.
163. Satoh M, Langdon JJ, Chou C-H, McCauliffe DP, Treadwell EL, Ogasawara T, et al. Characterization of the Su antigen, a macromolecular complex of 100/102 and 200-kDa proteins recognized by autoantibodies in systemic rheumatic diseases. Clin Immunol Immunopathol. 1994;73:132–41.
164. Satoh M, Chan JYF, Ceribelli A, Vazquez del-Mercado M, EKL A. Autoantibodies to argonaute 2 (Su antigen). Adv Exp Med Biol. 2013;768:45–59.
165. Ogawa-Momohara M, Muro Y, Satoh M, Akiyama M. Autoantibodies to Su/Argonaute 2 in Japanese patients with inflammatory myopathy. Clin Chim Acta. 2017;471:304–7.
166. Bhanji RA, Eystathioy T, Chan EKL, Bloch DB, Fritzler MJ. Clinical and serological features of patients with autoantibodies to GW/P bodies. Clin Immunol. 2007;125:247–56.
167. Satoh M, Chan JYF, Ross SJ, Ceribelli A, Cavazzana I, Franceschini F, et al. Autoantibodies to survival of motor neuron complex in patients with polymyositis: immunoprecipitation of D, E, F, and G proteins without other components of small nuclear ribonucleoproteins. Arthritis Rheum. 2011;63:1972–8.
168. Cobben JM, de Visser M, Scheffer H. From gene to disease; "survival" motor neuron protein and hereditary proximal spinal muscle atrophy. Ned Tijdschr Geneeskd. 2001;145:2525–7.
169. Enarson P, Rattner JB, Ou Y, Miyachi K, Horigome T, Fritzler MJ. Autoantigens of the nuclear pore complex. J Mol Med (Berl). 2004;82:423–33.
170. Nishio A, Water J, Leung PS, Joplin R, Neuberger JM, Lake J, et al. Comparative studies of antimitochondrial autoantibodies in sera and bile in primary biliary cirrhosis. Hepatology. 1997;25:1085–9.
171. Senécal J-L, Isabelle C, Fritzler MJ, Targoff IN, Goldstein R, Gagné M, et al. An autoimmune myositis-overlap syndrome associated with autoantibodies to nuclear pore complexes. Medicine (Baltimore). 2014;93:383–94.
172. Lleo A, Marzorati S, Anaya J-M, Gershwin ME. Primary biliary cholangitis: a comprehensive overview. Hepatol Int. 2017;11:485–99.
173. Maeda MH, Tsuji S, Shimizu J. Inflammatory myopathies associated with anti-mitochondrial antibodies. Brain. 2012;135(Pt 6):1767–77.
174. Konishi H, Fukuzawa K, Mori S, Satomi-Kobayashi S, Kiuchi K, Suzuki A, et al. Anti-mitochondrial M2 antibodies enhance the risk of supraventricular arrhythmias in patients with elevated hepatobiliary enzyme levels. Intern Med. 2017;56:1771–9.
175. Albayda J, Khan A, Casciola-Rosen L, Corse AM, Paik JJ, Christopher-Stine L. Inflammatory myopathy associated with anti-mitochondrial antibodies: a distinct phenotype with cardiac involvement. Semin Arthritis Rheum. 2018;47:552–6.
176. Mauhin W, Mariampillai K, Allenbach Y, Charuel J-L, Musset L, Benveniste O. Anti-mitochondrial antibodies are not a hallmark of severity in idiopathic inflammatory myopathies. Joint Bone Spine. 2017. https://doi.org/10.1016/j.jbspin.2017.04.004.
177. Targoff IN, Arnett FC, Berman L, O'Brien C, Reichlin M. Anti-KJ: a new antibody associated with the syndrome of polymyositis and interstitial lung disease. J Clin Invest. 1989;84:162–72.
178. Gelpi C, Sontheimer EJ, Rodriguez-Sanchez JL. Autoantibodies against a serine tRNA-protein complex implicated in cotranslational selenocysteine insertion. Proc Natl Acad Sci USA. 1992;89:9739–43.
179. Casciola-Rosen LA, Pluta AF, Plotz PH, Cox AE, Morris S, Wigley FM, et al. The DNA mismatch repair enzyme PMS1 is a myositis-specific autoantigen. Arthritis Rheum. 2001;44:389–96.
180. Muro Y, Nakashima R, Hosono Y, Sugiura K, Mimori T, Akiyama M. Autoantibodies to DNA mismatch repair enzymes in polymyositis/dermatomyositis and other autoimmune diseases: a possible marker of favorable prognosis. Arthritis Rheumatol (Hoboken, NJ). 2014;66:3457–62.
181. Labrador-Horrillo M, Martínez MA, Selva-O'Callaghan A, Trallero-Araguás E, Grau-Junyent JM, Vilardell-Tarrés M, et al. Identification of a novel myositis-associated antibody directed against cortactin. Autoimmun Rev. 2014;13:1008–12.
182. Berrih-Aknin S. Cortactin: a new target in autoimmune myositis and myasthenia gravis. Autoimmun Rev. 2014;13:1001–2.
183. Albrecht I, Wick C, Hallgren Å, Tjärnlund A, Nagaraju K, Andrade F, et al. Development of autoantibodies against muscle-specific FHL1 in severe inflammatory myopathies. J Clin Invest. 2015;125:4612–24.
184. Amato AA, Griggs RC. Unicorns, dragons, polymyositis, and other mythological beasts. Neurology. 2003;61:288–9.
185. Tozzoli R, Villalta D, Bizzaro N. Challenges in the standardization of autoantibody testing: a comprehensive review. Clin Rev Allergy Immunol. 2017;53:68–77.

20

House dust mite-related respiratory allergies and probiotics

Filippo Fassio[1*] and Fabio Guagnini[2]

Abstract

The socio-economic burden of allergic respiratory conditions on continental Europe is even higher than that of mainstream diseases, such as diabetes and cardiovascular disease, as allergic rhinitis alone accounts for billions of Euros in healthcare expenses across Europe. House dust mites (HDM) are one of the most common triggers behind allergic rhinitis and asthma. The role of probiotics in the treatment and prevention of some allergic conditions, such as atopic dermatitis, is already well recognized, whereas evidence about their efficacy in patients with respiratory allergies—while increasing—is still limited. Here the current evidence for the use of probiotics in patients with allergic rhinitis and/or asthma is discussed.

Keywords: House dust mite, Allergy, Probiotics

Background

Allergies and asthma are health conditions that have become highly prevalent across the globe, triggering respiratory symptoms—such as runny nose and sneezing, shortness of breath, and wheezing—in affected individuals. One of the most common triggers behind such allergic reactions are the allergens of house dust mites (HDMs). HDMs, which thrive in warm and humid household conditions, are classified as Arachnids and form a very diverse class in the Animalia kingdom. While mites are associated with a wide range of pathological and parasitic conditions in plants and animals, HDMs are rather unique as they can trigger a type I hypersensitivity reaction in predisposed persons, which can lead to severe allergic manifestations [1]. The organism is microscopic in nature, approximately 0.2–0.4 mm in size, and proliferates well in the presence of skin cells and moulds, especially when conditions are moist and humid [1]. High HDM content can be detected in bedding materials, as mites feed on skin and hair, and it becomes natural that people inhale the allergen in large volumes when they sleep.

The geographical distribution of different subspecies of HDMs is truly multi continental, as numerous research studies have indicated their prevalence across all continents except for Antarctica [2]. In regard to their ideal thriving conditions, temperatures in the range of 18–24 °C together with humidity levels of 70% and above are perfect for the organism, whereas the prevalence of various subspecies of HDMs is relatively low in environments with less than 50% relative humidity [2]. The effect of humidity on HDM proliferation is clearly visible in regions of British Columbia, Canada, in which high moisture content in the air supports high prevalence and proliferation of the organism. However, as altitude increases, and humidity levels decrease, the mite infestation rate decreases significantly. It also must be noted that altitude alone is not the only limiting factor that affects the proliferation of HDM as seen in the high-altitude regions of the Andes in South America, where the distribution of the organism is extensive [2]. Figure 1 presents a schematic representation of the distribution of 6 subspecies of HDMs across different regions of the globe [2].

History of HDMs in medicine

HDMs belong to the taxonomic group called Astigmata and were established as a prominent source of indoor allergens with the discovery of the house mite species *Dermatophagoides pteronyssinus* in 1967 [1].

*Correspondence: filippo.fassio@uslcentro.toscana.it
[1] SOC Allergologia e Immunologica Clinica, Azienda USL Toscana Centro, Nuovo Ospedale S. Giovanni di Dio, Via di Torregalli, 3, 50143 Florence, Italy
Full list of author information is available at the end of the article

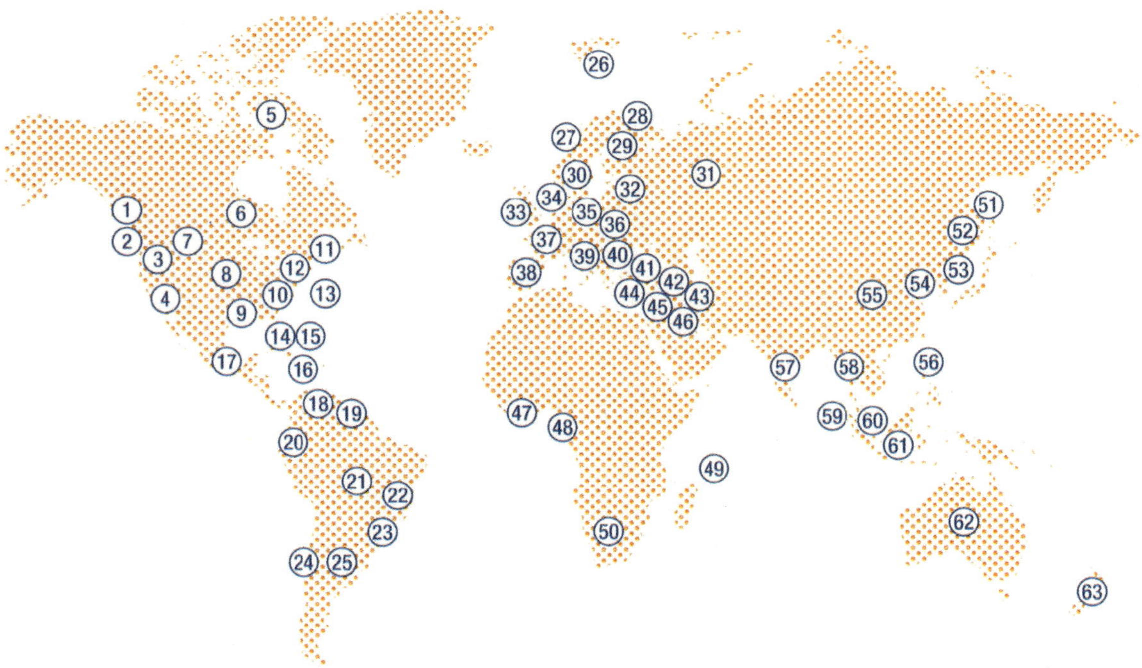

1 Vancouver Dp	10 Louisiana Dp	19 Venezuela Dp	28 Finland Dp	37 France DpDf	46 Saudi Arabia Dp(Df)	55 China DpDf
2 Seattle Dp	11 North East Df(Dp)	20 Ecuador DpDf	29 Sweden DfDp	38 Spain Dp(Df)	47 Ghana Dp	56 Philippines Dp
3 Los Angeles DfDp	12 Virginia DfDp	21 Inland Brazil DfDp	30 Denmark DfDp	39 Italy Df	48 Nigeria Dp	57 India Dp(Df)
4 San Diego Dp	13 Florida Dp	22 Salvador Dp	31 Moscow Dp	40 Croatia Dp	49 Mauritius Dp	58 Thailand Dp(Df)
5 Nunavut NIL	14 Cuba DsDf	23 Sao Paulo Dp	32 Germany DfDp	41 Turkey Dp	50 South Africa Dp(Df)	59 Singapore Dp
6 Midwest DfDp	15 Puerto Rico Dp	24 Chile Dp	33 England Dp	42 Kuwait Dp	51 Japan DpDf	60 Malaysia Dp
7 Rockies Df	16 Barbados Dp	25 Argentina DpDf	34 Netherlands DpDf	43 Iran Dp	52 Korea Df(Dp)	61 Indonesia DfDp
8 Arizona DfDp	17 Mexico DpDf	26 Iceland NIL	35 Belgium DfDp	44 Israel Dp	53 Taiwan Dp(Df)	62 Australia Dp
9 Texas Dp	18 Colombia Dp	27 Norway Dp	36 Switzerland Df	45 Palestine Dp	54 Hong Kong Dp	63 New Zealand Dp

Fig. 1 Geographical distribution of 6 subspecies of *Dermatophagoides* spp. Dp: *D. pteronyssinus* predominant; Df: *D. farinae* predominant; DpDf: mixed with more *D. pteronyssinus* than *D. farinae*; DfDp: mixed with more *D. farinae* than *D. pteronyssinus*; Ds: *D. siboney*. Parentheses indicate low levels (modified from [2])

While Prof. Reindert Voorhorst is well recognized for presenting the organism to the global scientific community in that year, other prominent contributors dating back to the early 20's and 30's laid the foundation for research on house dust mite-related allergies in humans. Prominent examples include Prof. Willem Storm van Leeuwen, who observed that housing conditions with high moisture content was not conducive for patients suffering from asthma, and researcher Marise Spieksma-Boezeman, who identified and even cultured mite samples belonging to the genus *Dermatophagoides* in samples of house dust during her research. At that time, however, the organism had no research significance regarding its role as an allergen in humans [3].

Epidemiology

It can be estimated that approximately 1–2% of the general population worldwide has allergic sensitization towards HDMs with significant variability depending on the cohort being studied [4]. In developed countries, this rate is much higher: in Europe, HDM allergic sensitization is above 20%; it is rising up to 40% in some cohorts in North America and to over 80% in a cohort of paediatric patients in Taiwan [4].

This result demonstrates that substantial diversity in HDM allergic sensitization prevalence exists and depends on factors such as ethnicity, socio-economic conditions, geographical variations and even the diagnostic paradigm that is adopted. For this reason, a wide range of confounding factors need to be considered to understand the epidemiology of HDM-mediated allergies [5].

A very common manifestation of HDM allergic sensitization is rhinitis, the symptoms of which include sneezing, and stuffy and running nose. These symptoms may not appear to be very serious and thus people often ignore them until the conditions become unbearable. However, a recent research article stated that the socio-economic burden of allergic rhinitis on continental Europe is even higher than that of mainstream health conditions, such as diabetes and cardiovascular disease [6]. When scaled in terms of cost to the continental economy, allergic rhinitis accounts for billions of Euros in healthcare expenses across Europe [6]. When this statistic is seen in context of the fact that allergy prevalence is rising (more than 50% of Europeans will suffer from allergic rhinitis in 10 years), the economic burden from the entire European Union's perspective is enormous, to put it mildly [7].

Pathogenic mechanism of HDM-related allergies

Due to the rising prevalence of different allergic conditions in recent decades, there has been a massive surge in research endeavours towards understanding their underlying pathogenic mechanisms and clinical implications [8]. Research studies have clearly shown that allergic manifestations increase significantly in individuals when there is a disruption in the T helper balance with polarization toward a Th2 phenotype, and that the dynamics of the gut microbiota has a role in maintaining this immune response balance [8]. Multiple immunological research studies have stated that a healthy gut microbiota helps in building and maintaining a well-balanced immune system in humans. Moreover, the World Health Organization has emphasized on the role of probiotic agents in enriching intestinal microflora.

A study by Calderon et al. [4] described a direct correlation between HDM-mediated allergies and the level of exposure to the organism itself during the early life of an individual. This study stated that young children in their first 3 years of life have the highest chance of contracting the allergy when exposed to HDM allergens, such as Der p 1 and Der f 1, at levels of 10 mcg/g of carpet dust. The study further added that a prior family history of allergy positively affects development of the allergy in these young children [4]. When exposure to the HDM allergens is as low as 0.1 mcg/g of dust, the probability of contracting HDM allergy is significantly reduced. While there appears to be a linear relationship between the level of exposure to allergens and HDM allergy, a wide range of scientific studies state otherwise. There are reports of low prevalence of HDM allergy in young children who are either exposed to very high or low levels of HDM allergens in their first 5 years of life. This non-linear association may be explained in terms of the high dose tolerance phenomenon that is observed in the case of cat allergens, but there is still no conclusive scientific evidence in this regard [9]. Different allergens from HDMs vary significantly in size, and this aspect can significantly impact the way that they are inhaled. Allergens that are smaller in size can penetrate deep into the lungs, but their rate of inhalation is less than that of large allergens, which can trigger an early phase immune response and elicit rather mild clinical symptoms [10]. As allergens are inhaled by the exposed individual, they enter the epithelial linings of the lungs and trigger the spread of dendritic cells into the lymph nodes. This stage is followed by the triggering of Th2 cell-mediated immunity and consequent inflammation of the lung's epithelial linings [11]. Calderon et al. [4] further added that the efficacy of HDM allergens in eliciting a powerful allergic reaction is compounded by stimulation of the innate immune system along with the Th2 cell-mediated immune response.

Therapeutic role of probiotics against respiratory allergies

Considering the massive socio-economic burden of different allergic conditions on global healthcare resources, there is a considerable research impetus towards finding pioneering therapeutic and preventive interventions. In this regard, the role of the gut microbiota in shaping the immune response against conditions such as HDM allergy was anticipated in a previous section. Following up, there are new findings that suggest that the dynamics of gut colonization in infants play a critical role in shaping the immune system, and there is a possibility of enriching the gut microflora using probiotics that could contribute towards the prevention of allergic conditions in later life [12, 13]. The microbiome bacteria can affect T helper responses by eliciting T helper-1 (Th1) cytokine production and/or by inducing T regulatory cells (Treg) [14], thereby suppressing Th2 responses. *Lactobacillus* bacteria affect Treg cells by generating semi-mature dendritic cells and increasing the expression of CD40; they are capable of inhibiting Interleukin (IL)-4 and IL-5 while inducing specific regulatory cytokines, such as transforming growth factor (TGF-β) and IL-10 [15]. Probiotics can also enhance local IgA production, which directly affects mucosal defences [15], and they have been involved in the maturation of adaptive T cell immunity by stimulating the production of IL-17 [16].

One of the first observations about the role of probiotic supplementation for the prevention of atopic eczema dates to 2001, when Kalliomaki et al. [17] found a significant reduction in the probability of developing atopic eczema by age 2 when supplementation of *Lactobacillus rhamnosus* was given for 2–4 weeks prenatally and 6 months postnatally; these results were confirmed in two subsequent follow-up studies in which a minor incidence of atopic disease was confirmed after 4 and after 7 years, respectively [18, 19].

A recent systematic review and meta-analysis of the literature that documented the use of probiotic agents for the prevention of allergic conditions in early life was carried out by Zuccotti et al. [12]. The authors analysed 29 RCTs on a total of 4755 children and found a significant reduction (odds ratio 0.78, CI 0.69–0.89) in the development of AD when dietary probiotic supplementation was added during pregnancy and early infancy with an even more prominent effect when a probiotic mixture was employed [12]. They concluded that the current literature demonstrates an overall benefit of probiotic supplementation for the prevention of eczema in high-risk infants. The same study further highlighted that lower diversity of the gut microbiota is associated with an increased risk of type I hypersensitivity reactions in young children [12]. It may be possible that when probiotic supplementation is given to these susceptible individuals, it results in a more favourable "allergy-protecting" gut microbiota.

In regard to the role of probiotic supplementation in patients with allergic rhinitis, Vilà-Nadal et al. [20], recently reviewed this topic [21]. Table 1 highlights different probiotic strains that have been evaluated in allergic rhinitis caused by allergens such as pollen and HDMs in adults and children.

The authors of this review conclude that probiotics appear to have beneficial therapeutic effects in allergic response as improvements in symptom scores and quality of life have been observed in these patients. In contrast, no positive impact was shown for the prevention of asthma and respiratory diseases [21].

In another systematic review on the effect of probiotics in AR, Zajac et al. [22] considered 23 randomized controlled trials on a total 1919 patients; quantitative analysis found a positive significant effect of probiotics on rhinitis-related quality of life (RQLQ Global Score and RQLQ Nose Score), whereas a positive but non-significant effect was found regarding symptom scores. Despite the lack of evidence for an improvement of symptom scores and the significant heterogeneity of these RCTs, the authors concluded that probiotics may have beneficial effects in patients affected by AR and that further studies are needed to adequately address this question [22].

It has to be underlined that probiotics effects must be considered strain-specific; therefore, future studies are required to investigate which strain(s) can be considered the most suitable in order to achieve the best immunomodulatory effect in patients affected by allergic respiratory diseases [23].

Table 1 Different probiotic strains that were evaluated in patients with allergic rhinitis. Modified from [21]

Probiotic agent	Study population	N	Type of allergic rhinitis/allergen	Primary end point	Statistical significance	References
L. acidophilus and *B. lactis*	Children	47	Birch pollen	Symptoms score	$p = 0.078$	[41]
E. coli strain Nissle 1917	Adults	34	Grass pollen	Symptoms score	$p = 0.257$	[42]
L. johnsonii EM	Children	63	Perennial rhinitis	Symptoms score	$p = 0.09$	[43]
B. longum BB536	Adults	40	Japanese cedar pollen	Ocular symptoms score	$p = 0.04$	[44]
L. paracasei (LP-33)	Children	80	Perennial	Quality of life	$p = 0.037$	[45]
L. paracasei	Children	90	House dust mites	Quality of life	$p < 0.0001$	[27]
L. paracasei KW3110	Adults	126	Japanese cedar pollen	Symptoms score	$p < 0.05$	[46]
L. paracasei ST-11	Adults	31	Grass pollen	Nasal provocation test	Ns	[47]
L. paracasei NCC2461	Adults	28	Grass pollen	Nasal congestion	Ns	[48]
L. paracasei 33	Adults	425	Grass pollen	Rhinitis quality of life (RQLQ score)	$p = 0.0255$	[49]

Role of probiotics in HDM-related allergic conditions

Scientific evidence assessing the role of probiotics in the treatment of HDM-related respiratory allergies, while limited, is increasing.

The potential capacity of *Lactobacillus plantarum* NCIMB8826 to reduce the allergic response in HDM allergic patients was evaluated in vivo and in vitro. In this study [24], it was shown that the co-application of *L. plantarum* and Der p 1 induced a Th1-shift in the immune response with upregulation of IgG and Th1-cytokine (IFN-γ and IL-12) production, moderate stimulation of IL-10, reduction of bronchoalveolar lavage eosinophilia after allergen challenge and suppression of allergen-specific IgE-response.

In one study on 29 patients affected by allergic asthma and HDM sensitization, a 4-week treatment with synbiotics significantly reduced the systemic production of Th2-cytokines (namely, IL-5) after allergen challenge and improved peak expiratory flow, despite a lack of any observed effects on bronchial inflammation markers [25].

Another recent and interesting approach consists of probiotic-impregnated bedding material. In the first pilot RCT in which 20 patients with AR and HDM sensitization used such materials for 8 weeks, no differences were found in HDM allergen levels compared to the placebo, whereas a significant improvement was reported by patients in terms of rhinitis-related symptom reduction and quality of life [26].

Of interest, it has been shown that even heat-killed lactic acid bacteria can be of help in the treatment of patients with respiratory allergy and HDM sensitization. Peng et al. [27] showed that heat-killed *Lactobacillus paracasei* supplementation significantly improved rhinitis-related quality of life scores in a group of 90 children with HDM sensitization.

The therapeutic potential of probiotic strains against allergic conditions was also explored by an observational study published in 2014. This study focused on the efficacy of two different symbiotic formulations (*Lactobacillus acidophilus* NCFM, *Bifidobacterium lactis* BL-04 and fructo-oligosaccharide (FOS); *Lactobacillus plantarum* LP01, *Lactobacillus paracasei* LPC00 and FOS) in the management of seasonal allergic rhinitis (SAR) and perennial allergic rhinitis (PAR) [28]. Aspects such as total nasal symptoms score, ARIA classification [29] for AR severity and data on the concomitant treatments were collected at the beginning of the study and evaluated at two different time points, 1 and 2 months after the beginning of the supplementation period. The results of this study highlighted a decrease in the total nasal symptoms score and an improvement in the AR severity according to the ARIA classification of rhinitis at both the time points. The reduction in the symptom score was statistically significant for the probiotic combination of *Lactobacillus plantarum* and *Lactobacillus paracasei* in patients with PAR, whereas the symbiotic combination against SAR showed a statistically significant improvement at only the first timepoint. However, a concomitant decrease in the consumption of symptomatic medications, such as antihistamine, and corticosteroids drugs significantly and progressively decreased after 2 and 4 months of treatment.

The observed decrease in the utilization of co-administered oral antihistamine drugs and oral corticosteroid drugs during the study period with this symbiotic multistrain combination may represent additional evidence of the beneficial effect of probiotics in the management of allergic rhinitis [28].

As it has already been mentioned before, identification of the most suitable probiotic strains in order to achieve a significant immunomodulatory effect in patients with HDM-related allergic conditions, will be one main challenge in this research field in the near future. Moreover, more research and effort are needed to improve the formulation of probiotic products (e.g. resistance to gastrointestinal conditions; drops—especially for pediatric use) to assure higher efficacy.

Future perspectives on the role of probiotics as adjuvants in allergen immunotherapy

Allergen-specific immunotherapy (AIT) is a well-established treatment option for allergic rhinitis, including HDM-triggered AR [30]. AIT triggers immunoregulatory mechanisms, including Treg cell activation, leading to the suppression of Th2 responses in favour of tolerance towards the allergen [31].

Adjuvants have been shown to amplify the effect of AIT by modulating the immune response to this therapy, thus increasing both its efficacy and safety [32].

In recent times, it has been hypothesized that probiotics, which stimulate innate immunity via toll-like receptor activation, could be used as adjuvants in AIT.

The effectiveness of probiotics as potential adjuvants in sublingual AIT (SLIT) has been studied in animal models; multiple lactic acid bacteria strains were found to act as Th1/possibly Treg inducers, and therefore—in the authors' opinion—they could represent valid candidates for adjuvants in SLIT [33].

In a murine model of mite allergy, immunotherapy with a recombinant Der p 1 allergen plus a probiotic strain (*E. coli* Nissle 1917) prevented the development of allergic symptoms after an airway challenge with mite extracts; moreover, it was observed that it contributed to the upregulation of allergen-specific IgG2a production, down-regulation of specific IgE production and induction of a strong reduction of IL-5 secretion by allergen-restimulated splenocytes [34].

In such preclinical models, probiotics acting as pure Th1 adjuvants did not seem to improve the efficacy of SLIT, whereas probiotic strains acting as Th1/Treg adjuvants (stimulating both IL-12 and IL-10 secretion by DCs) significantly enhanced SLIT efficacy [35].

In a study by Jerzynska et al. [36] on children with AR and grass sensitization, the addition of probiotics (*Lactobacillus rhamnosus* GG) to SLIT improved symptom scores and the induction of T regulatory cells after 5 months of treatment relative to children treated with SLIT alone or placebo.

In one study, *Lactobacillus acidophilus* and *Bifidobacterium lactis* contributed to improved asthma control test (ACT) scores in children with allergic asthma undergoing AIT for HDM; the effect was additive relative to the sole effect of AIT [37].

Clostridium butyricum coadministration with AIT has shown to improve the efficacy of AIT in patients with AR and asthma [38, 39]; this effect has been attributed to an increase in allergen-specific regulatory B cells.

Recently, in an observational real-life study, Rossi et al. [40] showed that supplementation with a symbiotic (consisting of *Lactobacillus rhamnosus, Bifidobacterium lactis* and FOS) during AIT for AR may act synergistically to improve the clinical efficacy of sublingual allergen immunotherapy. After 2 and 4 months of treatment, patients who were administered AIT plus probiotics showed a trend towards the reduction of symptoms scores together with a significant improvement in medication scores, number of "well days"; and no relevant local or systemic adverse reactions [40].

Conclusion

The use of probiotics in the treatment of allergic diseases is very promising, thanks to increasing evidence of their immunomodulatory effects. Their role in the treatment and prevention of some allergic conditions, such as atopic dermatitis, is already well recognized, whereas evidence about their efficacy in patients with respiratory allergies—while increasing—is still limited.

The prospective of employing probiotics as novel adjuvants for AIT is intriguing and already supported by a number of interesting studies.

Future research is needed to improve our understanding of the use of probiotics in the treatment of allergic conditions and as an adjuvant in immunotherapy; in particular, we need to better understand which probiotic strains are the most suitable for these purposes and which immunologic mechanisms are involved. Moreover, evidence is still lacking regarding which formulations will guarantee the best results, what are the best timing and duration for probiotic administration in order to prevent/modulate HDM-related allergic conditions, and if a critical dose (beside the 10^9 colony forming units generally considered) exists.

Authors' contributions

FF and FG reviewed the relevant literature and prepared the manuscript. Both authors read and approved the final manuscript.

Author details

[1] SOC Allergologia e Immunologica Clinica, Azienda USL Toscana Centro, Nuovo Ospedale S. Giovanni di Dio, Via di Torregalli, 3, 50143 Florence, Italy. [2] Allergy Therapeutics Italia, via IV Novembre 76, 20019 Settimo Milanese, Milan, Italy.

References

1. Portnoy J, Miller JD, Williams PB, Chew GL, Miller JD, Zaitoun F, et al. Environmental assessment and exposure control of dust mites: a practice parameter. Ann Allergy Asthma Immunol. 2013;111:465–507.
2. Thomas WR. Geography of house dust mite allergens. Asian Pac J Allergy Immunol. 2010;28:211–24.
3. Spieksma FT, Dieges PH. The history of the finding of the house dust mite. J Allergy Clin Immunol. 2004;113:573–6.
4. Calderón MA, Linneberg A, Kleine-Tebbe J, De Blay F, De Rojas DHF, Virchow JC, et al. Respiratory allergy caused by house dust mites: what do we really know? J Allergy Clin Immunol. 2015;136:38–48.
5. Bousquet PJ, Chinn S, Janson C, Kogevinas M, Burney P, Jarvis D, et al. Geographical variation in the prevalence of positive skin tests to environmental aeroallergens in the European community respiratory health survey I. Allergy. 2007;62:301–9.
6. Rossi O, Massaro I, Caminati M, Quecchia C, Fassio F, Heffler E, et al. Escaping the trap of allergic rhinitis. Clin Mol Allergy. 2015;13:17.
7. Calderon MA, Demoly P, Gerth van Wijk R, Bousquet J, Sheikh A, Frew A, et al. EAACI: a European declaration on immunotherapy. Designing the future of allergen specific immunotherapy. Clin Transl Allergy. 2012;2:20.
8. Fassio F, Guagnini F. Probiotics, gut microbiota and immunomodulation: is this the key to counteract the allergy epidemics? J Pharm Nutr Sci. 2016;6:83–8.
9. Platts-Mills T, Vaughan J, Squillace S, Woodfolk J, Sporik R. Sensitisation, asthma, and a modified Th2 response in children exposed to cat allergen: a population-based cross-sectional study. Lancet. 2001;357:752–6.
10. Custovic A, Woodcock H, Craven M, Hassall R, Hadley E, Simpson A, et al. Dust mite allergens are carried on not only large particles. Pediatr Allergy Immunol. 1999;10:258–60.
11. Lambrecht BN, Hammad H. The role of dendritic and epithelial cells as master regulators of allergic airway inflammation. Lancet. 2010;376:835–43.
12. Zuccotti G, Meneghin F, Aceti A, Barone G, Callegari ML, Di Mauro A, et al. Probiotics for prevention of atopic diseases in infants: systematic review and meta-analysis. Allergy. 2015;70:1356–71.
13. Ismail IH, Licciardi PV, Tang MLK. Probiotic effects in allergic disease. J Paediatr Child Health. 2013;49:709–15.
14. Smith-Norowitz TA, Bluth MH. Probiotics and diseases of altered IgE regulation: a short review. J Immunotoxicol. 2016;13:136–40.
15. Campeotto F, Suau A, Kapel N, Magne F, Viallon V, Ferraris L, et al. A fermented formula in pre-term infants: clinical tolerance, gut microbiota, down-regulation of faecal calprotectin and up-regulation of faecal secretory IgA. Br J Nutr. 2011;105:1843–51.

16. Isailovic N, Daigo K, Mantovani A, Selmi C. Interleukin-17 and innate immunity in infections and chronic inflammation. J Autoimmun. 2015;60:1–11.
17. Kalliomäki M, Salminen S, Arvilommi H, Kero P, Koskinen P, Isolauri E. Probiotics in primary prevention of atopic disease: a randomised placebo-controlled trial. Lancet. 2001;357:1076–9.
18. Kalliomäki M, Salminen S, Poussa T, Arvilommi H, Isolauri E. Probiotics and prevention of atopic disease: 4-year follow-up of a randomised placebo-controlled trial. Lancet. 2003;361:1869–71.
19. Kalliomäki M, Salminen S, Poussa T, Isolauri E. Probiotics during the first 7 years of life: a cumulative risk reduction of eczema in a randomized, placebo-controlled trial. J Allergy Clin Immunol. 2007;119:1019–21.
20. Vilà-Nadal G, Phillips-Anglés E, Domínguez-Ortega J. The use of probiotics in respiratory allergy. J Pharm Nutr Sci. 2016;6:89–94
21. Domínguez-Ortega J, Phillips-Anglés E. The use of probiotics in respiratory allergy. J Pharm Nutr Sci. 2016;6:89–94.
22. Zajac AE, Adams AS, Turner JH. A systematic review and meta-analysis of probiotics for the treatment of allergic rhinitis. Int Forum Allergy Rhinol. 2015;5:524–32.
23. Toscano M, De Grandi R, Pastorelli L, Vecchi M, Drago L. A consumer's guide for probiotics: 10 golden rules for a correct use. Dig Liver Dis. 2017;49:1177–84.
24. Hisbergues M, Magi M, Rigaux P, Steuve J, Garcia L, Goudercourt D, et al. In vivo and in vitro immunomodulation of der p 1 allergen-specific response by *Lactobacillus plantarum* bacteria. Clin Exp Allergy. 2007;37:1286–95.
25. Van De Pol MA, Lutter R, Smids BS, Weersink EJM, Van Der Zee JS. Synbiotics reduce allergen-induced T-helper 2 response and improve peak expiratory flow in allergic asthmatics. Allergy. 2011;66:39–47.
26. Berings M, Jult A, Vermeulen H, De Ruyck N, Derycke L, Ucar H, et al. Probiotics-impregnated bedding covers for house dust mite allergic rhinitis: a pilot randomized clinical trial. Clin Exp Allergy. 2017;47:1092–6.
27. Peng GC, Hsu CH. The efficacy and safety of heat-killed *Lactobacillus paracasei* for treatment of perennial allergic rhinitis induced by house-dust mite. Pediatr Allergy Immunol. 2005;16:433–8.
28. Manzotti G, Heffler E, Fassio F. Multi-strain symbiotic preparations as a novel adjuvant approach to allergic rhinitis. JCI. 2014;1:67–80.
29. Brozek JL, Bousquet J, Baena-Cagnani CE, Bonini S, Canonica GW, Casale TB, et al. Allergic rhinitis and its impact on asthma (ARIA) guidelines: 2010 revision. J Allergy Clin Immunol. 2010;126:466–76.
30. Eifan AO, Calderon MA, Durham SR. Allergen immunotherapy for house dust mite: clinical efficacy and immunological mechanisms in allergic rhinitis and asthma. Expert Opin Biol Ther. 2013;13:1543–56.
31. Fujita H, Meyer N, Akdis M, Akdis CA. Mechanisms of immune tolerance to allergens. Chem Immunol Allergy. 2012;96:30–8.
32. Pfaar O, Cazan D, Klimek L, Larenas-Linnemann D, Calderon MA. Adjuvants for immunotherapy. Curr Opin Allergy Clin Immunol. 2012;12:648–57.
33. Van Overtvelt L, Moussu H, Horiot S, Samson S, Lombardi V, Mascarell L, et al. Lactic acid bacteria as adjuvants for sublingual allergy vaccines. Vaccine. 2010;28:2986–92.
34. Adam E, Delbrassine L, Bouillot C, Reynders V, Mailleux AC, Muraille E, et al. Probiotic *Escherichia coli* Nissle 1917 activates DC and prevents house dust mite allergy through a TLR4-dependent pathway. Eur J Immunol. 2010;40:1995–2005.
35. Moingeon P, Lombardi V, Baron-Bodo V, Mascarell L. Enhancing allergen-presentation platforms for sublingual immunotherapy. J Allergy Clin Immunol Pract. 2017;5:23–31.
36. Jerzynska J, Stelmach W, Balcerak J, Woicka-Kolejwa K, Rychlik B, Blauz A, et al. Effect of Lactobacillus rhamnosus GG and vitamin D supplementation on the immunologic effectiveness of grass-specific sublingual immunotherapy in children with allergy. Allergy Asthma Proc. 2016;37:324–34.
37. Kardani AK, Fitri LE, Barlianto W, Olivianto E, Kusuma C. The effect of house dust mite immunotherapy, probiotic and *Nigella sativa* in the number of Th17 cell and asthma control test score. IOSR J Dent Med Sci. 2013;6:2279–861.
38. Liu J, Chen FH, Qiu SQ, Yang LT, Zhang HP, Liu JQ, et al. Probiotics enhance the effect of allergy immunotherapy on regulating antigen specific B cell activity in asthma patients. Am J Transl Res. 2016;8:5256–70.
39. Xu LZ, Yang LT, Qiu SQ, Yang G, Luo XQ, Miao BP, et al. Combination of specific allergen and probiotics induces specific regulatory B cells and enhances specific immunotherapy effect on allergic rhinitis. Oncotarget. 2016;7:54360–9.
40. Rossi R, Monasterolo G. Combination of probiotics and sublingual immunotherapy in allergic rhinitis: a real-life study. J Pharm Nutr Sci. 2016;6:98–104.
41. Ouwehand AC, Nermes M, Collado MC, Rautonen N, Salminen S, Isolauri E. Specific probiotics alleviate allergic rhinitis during the birch pollen season. World J Gastroenterol. 2009;15:3261–8.
42. Dölle S, Berg J, Rasche C, Worm M. Tolerability and clinical outcome of coseasonal treatment with *Escherichia coli* strain Nissle 1917 in grass pollen-allergic subjects. Int Arch Allergy Immunol. 2014;163:29–35.
43. Lue KH, Sun HL, Lu KH, Ku MS, Sheu JN, Chan CH, et al. A trial of adding *Lactobacillus johnsonii* EM1 to levocetirizine for treatment of perennial allergic rhinitis in children aged 7–12 years. Int J Pediatr Otorhinolaryngol. 2012;76:994–1001.
44. Xiao JZ, Kondo S, Yanagisawa N, Takahashi N, Odamaki T, Iwabuchi N, et al. Effect of probiotic *Bifidobacterium longum* BB536 [corrected] in relieving clinical symptoms and modulating plasma cytokine levels of Japanese cedar pollinosis during the pollen season. A randomized double-blind, placebo-controlled trial. J Investig Allergol Clin Immunol. 2006;16:86–93.
45. Wang MF, Lin HC, Wang YY, Hsu CH. Treatment of perennial allergic rhinitis with lactic acid bacteria. Pediatr Allergy Immunol. 2004;15:152–8.
46. Yonekura S, Okamoto Y, Okawa T, Hisamitsu M, Chazono H, Kobayashi K, et al. Effects of daily intake of *Lactobacillus paracasei* strain KW3110 on Japanese cedar pollinosis. Allergy Asthma Proc. 2009;30:397–405.
47. Wassenberg J, Nutten S, Audran R, Barbier N, Aubert V, Moulin J, et al. Effect of *Lactobacillus paracasei* ST11 on a nasal provocation test with grass pollen in allergic rhinitis. Clin Exp Allergy. 2011;41:565–73.
48. Perrin Y, Nutten S, Audran R, Berger B, Bibiloni R, Wassenberg J, et al. Comparison of two oral probiotic preparations in a randomized crossover trial highlights a potentially beneficial effect of *Lactobacillus paracasei* NCC2461 in patients with allergic rhinitis. Clin Transl Allergy. 2014;4:1.
49. Costa DJ, Marteau P, Amouyal M, Poulsen LK, Hamelmann E, Cazaubiel M, et al. Efficacy and safety of the probiotic *Lactobacillus paracasei* LP-33 in allergic rhinitis: a double-blind, randomized, placebo-controlled trial (GA2LEN study). Eur J Clin Nutr. 2014;68:602–7.

21

Focus on the agents most frequently responsible for perioperative anaphylaxis

E. Di Leo[1], P. Delle Donne[2], G. F. Calogiuri[3], L. Macchia[2] and E. Nettis[2,4*]

Abstract

Adverse reactions (ARs) to drugs administered during general anesthesia may be very severe and life-threatening, with a mortality rate ranging from 3 to 9%. The adverse reactions to drugs may be IgE and non-IgE-mediated. Neuromuscular blocking agents (NMBA) represent the first cause of perioperative reactions during general anesthesia followed by latex, antibiotics, hypnotic agents, opioids, colloids, dyes and antiseptics (chlorhexidine). All these substances (i.e. NMBA, anesthetics, antibiotics, latex devices) may cause severe systemic non-IgE-mediated reactions or fatal anaphylactic events even in the absence of any evident risk factor in the patient's anamnesis. For this reason, in order to minimize perioperative anaphylactic reactions, it is important to have rapid, specific, sensitive in vitro diagnostic tests able to confirm the clinical diagnosis of acute anaphylaxis.

Keywords: Perioperative allergy, Latex, Anaphylaxis, Neuromuscular blocking agents

Background

The potential occurrence of hypersensitivity reactions (IgE-mediated or non-IgE-mediated) is a great concern for anesthesiologists, because adverse reactions (ARs) may be very severe and life-threatening, with a mortality rate ranging from 3 to 9% [1]. Fatal anaphylaxis as well as a great proportion of less severe anaphylactic reactions is caused by drugs and substances related to general anesthesia [2, 3].

The individuation of the culprit agent is very difficult because of the several drugs administered during general anesthesia. Neuromuscular blocking agents (NMBA), latex, antibiotics, induction agents and opiates are the most common substances incriminated in perioperative anaphylaxis [4–6]. Perioperative reactions depend on the underlying mechanism classified in 2 groups: reactions resulting from direct nonspecific mast cell and basophil activation (severe systemic non-IgE-mediated hypersensitivity reactions) and IgE-dependent allergic reactions (IgE-mediated, anaphylaxis) [7].

*Correspondence: ambulatorio.allergologia@uniba.it
[4] Policlinico, Piazza Giulio Cesare, 11, 70124 Bari, Italy
Full list of author information is available at the end of the article

Incidence

The incidence of anaphylaxis is estimated between 1 in 10,000 and 1 in 20,000 anesthetic procedures [2, 3]. However, anaphylactic reactions cannot be clinically distinguished from non-immune mediated reactions which account for 30–40% of hypersensitivity reactions [1, 8].

An IgE-mediated mechanism has been confirmed in 40–70% of cases [9]. Generally reactions resulting from direct histamine release are usually less severe than IgE-mediated reactions [10]. In a recent study on anaphylaxis during general anesthesia, an IgE-mediated cause was identified in 103 patients (64%); NMBA constituted the leading cause (38%) followed by antibiotics (8%), patent blue dye (6%), chlorhexidine (5%) and other agents (7%) [11].

In recent decades perioperative adverse reactions had more attention and the general view is that immediate-type hypersensitivity reactions are largely under reported and causes remain often unknown. In addition, the extremely variable rate of reactions is due to the lack of homogeneity of clinical criteria and diagnostic tests, and the diversity of the populations studied [12].

In case of IgE-mediated perioperative anaphylaxis, NMBA represent the first cause whereas latex is the second responsible allergen, followed by antibiotics [12–15]. About 20% of perioperative anaphylaxis is attributed to latex [16] even if the prevalence of anaphylaxis to latex been declining in the last years due to a highly efficient prevention strategy [11, 17]. Other agents used during general anesthesia are also implied as anaphylaxis causatives or involved in anaphylactic response, such as hypnotic agents, opioids, colloids, dyes, and antiseptics (chlorhexidine) [13]. Non steroidal anti-inflammatory drugs (NSAIDs) and iodinated contrast agents may provoke non allergic anaphylaxis, although also for these drugs IgE-mediated reactions are hypothesized [13].

Neuromuscular blocking agents

NMBA (muscle relaxants) are responsible for 60–70% of anaphylactic episodes during general anesthesia or in the postoperative setting [9, 12], thus representing the most common cause of perioperative reactions in France [8] with an 1:6500 incidence [10]. The NMBAs include: succinylcholine, benzylisoquinolines (atracurium, cisatracurium, doxacurium, mivacurium) and aminosteroids or benzylisoquinolinium-type NMBA: pancuronium, rapacuronium, rocuronium, vecuronium. Hypersensitivity reactions to NMBA may be either IgE or not-IgE mediated in their pathogenesis. An IgE-mediated response is due to the quaternary ammonium (NH4+) structures that represents the main antigenic epitope of NMBAs [18], while the second one is provoked by benzylisoquinolinium-type NMBA (aminosteroids) such as mivacurium, atracurium, and d-tubocurarine that are responsible for non-IgE-mediated hypersensitivity reactions [19]. From 20 to 50% of adverse reactions to NMBAs are considered to result from direct nonspecific mast cell and basophil activation [10]. Histamine release is predominantly found with the use of the d-tubocurarine, atracurium, and mivacurium among the benzylisoquinolines, and rapacuronium among the aminosteroids [20].

Unfortunately, quaternary ammonium groups are ubiquitous epitopes, which are contained in other drugs or disinfectants, so such reactive groups are responsible for cross-reactivity phenomenon with other drugs.

The presence in NMBA of ubiquitous epitopes such as a substituted ammonium group (that are likely the immunodominant determinant recognized by IgE) is responsible for high cross-reactivity among these drugs (most consistently between pancuronium, rocuronium and vecuronium) [21], but cross-reactions also may occur between muscle relaxants and other classes of pharmaceuticals: acetylcholine, choline, morphine, neostigmine, pentolinium and pholcodine [22].

Pholcodine, for instance, is a potentially sensitizing antitussive agent with similar structure to morphine and NMBAs, which was able to induce the production of IgE antibodies cross-reacting with suxamethonium [23]. In addition, Fisher was the first to hypothesize the presence of specific IgE versus natural products containing quaternary ammonium such as foods, cosmetics (tioglycol ammonium), eyedrop preservatives (benzalconium chloride), disinfectants, and industrial materials [24].

In the light of these findings, previous exposure to non-anesthetic drugs or other substances may induce a hidden sensitization to muscle-relaxing agents, resulting in reactions among patients without prior anesthesia.

The commonest triggers of NMBA reactions were found to be the suxamethonium (the most involved), followed by rocuronium, and then in descending order by vecuronium, pancuronium and atracurium [21]. Several studies have been conducted to identify possible risk factors for adverse reactions to muscle relaxants, and to evaluate the predictive value of skin tests with muscle relaxants with discordant conclusions. At present, however, an allergic work upon the implementation of an investigative systematic preoperative screening in the general population for the potential of anaphylaxis from NMBA is not recommended [10].

Natural rubber latex

Latex (*Hevea brasiliensis*) is a long-lasting, resistant and elastic product, which allows to maintain good tactile sensitivity and it protects against diseases transmitted through body fluids, so latex-derived products are largely present in hospital setting (e.g., gloves, catheters, bottles with pierceable septum, tourniquets, AMBU bags, anesthesiological masks, cannulas, drainages, endotracheal tubes, bandages) [7, 25]. Latex represents an important cause of anaphylaxis during anesthesia [26] because it is the second cause of adverse reactions during perioperative period [7, 25, 27]. Multiple surgery procedures in spina bifida patients and professional exposure are associated with an increased frequency of latex allergy. Identification of patients belonging to at risk population, patients already sensitized to latex and medical setting latex-free use, have already allowed to reduce the incidence of perioperative latex adverse reactions. Exposure to latex may occur by contact through skin and mucosae or by inhalation of airborne particles [28]. The risk of developing an allergy to latex is greater for some groups: healthcare workers, children requiring multiple or repetitive surgical and medical procedures (e.g., spina bifida, spinal cord trauma, and urogenital malformations) that need chronic bladder care with repeated insertion of natural rubber latex (NRL) catheters or chronic indwelling catheters [29], housewives or workers occupationally exposed (hairdressers, gardeners, workers in the rubber industry) [30]. Obstetric population appears more prone to develop sensitizations to NRL proteins probably due to repeated contact between latex gloves and mucosal membranes during vaginal examinations or delivery [31].

As latex allergy is suspected by clinical history (symptoms like urticaria or angioedema when skin or mucosa come into contact with manufacts such as balloon, gloves, diving masks, condoms, etc. or during medical examination by latex medical devices), patients have to undergo skin prick test (SPT) and serum-specific IgE tests. SPTs are usually performed with several commercial extracts and with extemporary preparations at various dilutions obtained from high allergens content latex gloves and represents the gold standard in the diagnosis of latex allergy, characterized by high sensitivity and specificity [32].

Serum-specific IgE can be detected through molecular diagnosis by ImmunoCAP/ISAC method (Thermofisher, Uppsala, Sweden) that is able to distinguish between a true sensitization and an asymptomatic cross-reactivity. Latex allergens Hev b 1, Hev b 3, Hev b 5 and Hev b 6 are currently considered markers of genuine latex sensitization [33, 34]. On the other hand, latex-sensitized subjects with a positive serum specific IgE against latex, but negative SPT and without latex-specific symptoms upon contact with latex-containing material, have a profilin sensitization with monosensitization to Hev b 8 [34]. These patients can undergo major surgery in normal surgical setting without any consequences since Hev b 8 represents a marker of asymptomatic latex sensitization [34]. Finally, if latex allergy is strongly suspected and IgE tests gave negative results, a challenge test should be performed by wearing a latex glove to the patient for increasing periods, monitoring for objective signs of an allergic reaction [28].

In sensitized patients, the exposure to NRL proteins can provoke a type I IgE-mediated hypersensitivity reaction and a type IV reaction (not life threatening) responsible for a contact dermatitis that elicits slow-onset eczematous reactions. IgE-mediated reactions may involve various organs and systems, even simultaneously. Clinical manifestations, that occur within a few minutes after contact with NRL proteins, include urticaria, angioedema, conjunctivitis, allergic rhinitis, asthma and anaphylaxis. Immediate reactions, such as anaphylaxis, can be life threatening [28, 35] and may occur after a direct contact with latex, usually gloves, or instruments, or with aerosolization of latex antigen adherent to the cornstarch powder of latex gloves when gloves are donned during operative procedures. The administration of drug through a latex port prior to surgery may cause an intraoperative latex anaphylaxis that is usually also related to the surgical procedure itself [36].

Airborne exposure to latex may also cause a contact dermatitis. It is a non-immune-mediate reaction that appears at the side of contact and cause itching, redness, blisters [35].

Primary prevention is the avoidance of sensitization in at-risk population whereas secondary prevention means avoiding the onset of the allergic reaction in previously sensitized patients by establishing a "latex-free environment" not only in operating rooms, but also in all recovery rooms [37–39]. Several studies performed in different countries demonstrated that using powder-free latex gloves and replacing NRL with another material, make it possible to decrease perioperative latex allergy incidence [40]. Recent findings demonstrate the effectiveness of sublingual immunotherapy in patients with history of latex allergy inducing an effective desensitization to NRL [38, 41].

Antibiotics

Penicillins and cephalosporins are responsible for 70% of perioperative anaphylactic reactions induced by antibiotics [42]. The reactions induced by individual antibiotics are mostly observed after penicillins (0.004–0.015%) and cephalosporins (0.0001–0.1%) [43]. Their frequency has increased over the last 20 years [24]. Currently, allergy to b-lactams represents 12–15% of the perioperative reactions observed in France [44]. The incidence of reactions provoked by these drugs has been increasing due to a widespread use of them for the perioperative antibiotic prophylaxis [45], but also due to the worldwide use of them in the general population. The prevalence of penicillin allergy in the general population varies between 0.7 and 10% [10].

Betalactam antibiotics, vancomycin and quinolones are frequently implicated in adverse reactions during perioperative period representing the third cause of anaphylactic reactions in the surgical patients [46].

Heterogeneous and various mechanisms are involved in adverse drug reactions due to penicillins and other betalactams such as cephalosporins both IgE-mediated and non IgE-mediated in addition to unknown mechanisms.

According to EAACI interest group on drug hypersensitivity, the diagnostic protocol for allergic reactions to b-lactam [47] contemplate dosage of serum IgE for several penicillin determinants [Thermofisher, Sweden, penicilloyl G (c1), penicilloyl V (c2), amoxycilloyl (c6), ampicilloyl (c5) and cefaclor (c7)]. Because beta-lactams specific IgE dosage is generally less sensitive than skin tests, that they represent valuable and safe tools in the diagnostic approach for patients with suspected IgE-mediated beta-lactam allergy [13, 48–50] the investigation methods include in vivo tests, such as SPT and IDT. For SPT the suspected agent can be tested, in addition to the available commercial reagents, such as benzylpenicilloylpoly-L-lysine (PPL) and so-called minor determinants mixture (MDM), including amoxicillin (AX) and ampicillin (AMP) [12, 13].

Provocation tests with b-lactam antibiotics should be performed only in patients with a positive clinical history but negative IgE and skin test investigations [47].

Vancomycin, a glycopeptide antibiotic usually used for treatment of Gram positive resistant organisms and for patients with penicillin allergy, may provoke reactions both IgE-mediated and non IgE-mediated. Typically Vancomycin is responsible for "red man syndrome" consisting in non-IgE-mediated hypersensitivity reactions with flushing, pruritus, an erythematous rash of the head and upper torso, and arterial hypotension. These non-immunologic reactions are associated with a rapid infusion of the drug at the first dose [12, 51]. Sometimes dyspnea, angioedema, and hypotension can occur [12].

Quinolones represent the third most important group of antibiotics involved in perioperative anaphylaxis [46]. They can induce hypersensitivity reactions mediated by IgE and T cells, in addition to non IgE-mediated reactions. IgE-mediated reactions are more common and are severe in over 70% of cases [10]; the most frequent clinical manifestations are anaphylaxis and anaphylactic shock [10]. Diagnostic methods (skin tests or sIgE assays) for quinolones hypersensitivity reactions are not validated, even if in about 50% of patients with quinolones anaphylaxis IgE antibodies were found [52]. Other antibiotics that are often used in the operating room and that may rarely trigger an anaphylactic reaction include clindamycin, gentamicin, and metronidazole. Really, every antibiotic represents a potential cause of anaphylaxis [43].

General anesthetics

Among the barbiturate anesthetics, in the past years, thiopental was in the most frequent agent responsible for anaphylaxis during anesthesia, but in more recent surveys, anaphylaxis from thiopental sodium is only rarely described because of the its less intensive application [12].

Generally, although their frequent application, anaphylaxis from non-barbiturate hypnotics is rare [12].

Propofol is a hypnotic agent that has been associated with anaphylactic reactions [13]. Despite the propofol is formulated in a lipid solution containing 10% soybean oil, 2.25% glycerol, and 1.2% egg lecithin [13], the presence of these components is not related with an increased risk of anaphylactic reactions due to propofol in patients with egg or soy allergy [13]. Immediate reactions involving propofol are most frequently due to an alkyl phenol that bears two isopropyl groups that may act as antigenic epitopes.

Propofol allergy has been diagnosed by skin tests, by sIgE and by histamine-release tests, although propofol can induce also a direct release of histamine concentration-dependent [53].

Yet, benzodiazepines are rarely a cause of immediate hypersensitivity reactions. Among this drug class, midazolam is the main causative agent in the perioperative setting [12, 46], and SPT with the undiluted drug and intradermal test can be performed to investigate about the reaction [46].

Conclusions

In the perioperative period patients are exposed to many substances (i.e., anesthetics, antibiotics, latex devices, blood preparations, heparin, fluids) to ensure maximum safety and best care. All these substances may cause severe systemic non-IgE-mediated reactions or fatal anaphylactic events even in the absence of any evident risk factor in the patient's anamnesis. It is important to keep in mind that is not always possible to detect certainly the culprit agent of a perioperative anaphylaxis because the cause-effect relationship is often difficult to demonstrate. In addition the diagnosis is not easy to make in an anesthetized patient because there are technical objective difficulties to recognize a hypersensitivity reaction in a perioperative setting. Firstly, the patient is unconscious and uncompliant, so anesthetists may only control vital signs and sudden changes in cardiac rate, a drop in blood pressure or a desaturation in pulse-oxymetry is not sufficient to suspect the onset of an immediate type hypersensitivity because such modifications may be associated with other pathologic conditions, i.e., a spontaneous pneumothorax, myocardial infarction or severe arrhythmia, which an anesthetists must consider rapidly.

Muscle relaxants, NRL and antibiotics are the most common anesthetic drugs or substances that may be involved in anaphylaxis.

To prevent successive anaphylaxis events, it is important to document every ARs and, above all, substances and/or drugs used during anesthesia, so that the identification of the causative drug by allergist can be simpler. Once the diagnosis has been made, the patient must be informed about symptoms during the anesthesia, the drugs that have been responsible for the reaction and must be provided with a bracelet or a tag that shows in detail the drugs to which he is allergic.

Prevention is an important component to decrease the incidence of anaphylaxis especially for latex which is the second cause of anaphylactic reactions in perioperative period. Often this is underestimated because when ARs occur, the drugs are considered mainly responsible [30]. Perioperative allergy to latex can be limited if an accurate anamnesis is made about previous adverse reactions to

NRL manufacts and latex-related food, so it is possible to suspect sensitization to latex and to start diagnostic protocols. Avoiding latex exposition in medical settings is the only way to decrease new sensitizations and to reduce incidence of ARs.

In realty, the greatest necessity, in order to minimize perioperative anaphylactic reactions, is to have rapid, specific, sensitive in vitro diagnostic tests able to confirm the clinical diagnosis of acute anaphylaxis.

Authors' contributions

All authors read and approved the final manuscript.

Author details

[1] Unit of Internal Medicine, Section of Allergy and Clinical Immunology, "F. Miulli" Hospital, Acquaviva delle Fonti, BA, Italy. [2] Department of Emergency and Organ Transplantation, School and Chair of Allergology and Clinical Immunology, University of Bari—Aldo Moro, Bari, Italy. [3] Pneumology Department, Sacro Cuore Hospital, Gallipoli, Lecce, Italy. [4] Policlinico, Piazza Giulio Cesare, 11, 70124 Bari, Italy.

Acknowledgements

Writing support for the preparation of this manuscript was provided by Carl Rice, Professor of English, Bari, Italy and by Ippolita Zaza from University of Bari, Italy.

Competing interests

The authors declare that they have no competing interests.

References

1. Caimmi S, Caimmi D, Bernardini R. Perioperative anaphylaxis: epidemiology. Int J Immunopathol Pharmacol. 2011;24(Suppl 3):21–6.
2. Mertes PM, De Blay F. Allergic risk in anesthesia. Presse Med. 2013. https://doi.org/10.1016/j.lpm.2012.04.026.
3. Antunes J, Kochuyt AM. Perioperative allergic reactions: experience in a Flemish referral centre. Allergol Immunopathol (Madr). 2014. https://doi.org/10.1016/j.aller.2013.08.001.
4. Garvey LH. Danish anesthesia allergy centre preliminary results. Acta Anesthesiol Scand. 2001;45:1204–9.
5. Harboe T. Anaphylaxis during anesthesia in Norway: a 6-year single-center follow-up study. Anesthesiology. 2005;102:897–903.
6. Joint Task Force on Practice Parameters. Drug allergy: an updated practice parameter. Ann Allergy Asthma Immunol. 2010;105:259–73.
7. Taylor JS. Latex allergy: diagnosis and management. Dermatol Ther. 2004;17(4):289–301.
8. Dong SW. Hypersensitivity reactions during anesthesia. Results from the ninth French survey (2005–2007). Minerva Anesthesiol. 2012;78(8):868–78.
9. Shrikant M. Anaphylaxis during the perioperative period. Anesth Essays Res. 2012;6(2):124–33.
10. Doña I. Trends in hypersensitivity drug reactions: more drugs, more response patterns, more heterogeneity. J Investig Allergol Clin Immunol. 2014;24(3):143–53.
11. Krishna MT. Multi-centre retrospective analysis of anaphylaxis during general anesthesia in the United Kingdom: aetiology and diagnostic performance of acute serum tryptase. Clin Exp Immunol. 2014;178(2):399–404.
12. Ebo DG. Anaphylaxis during anesthesia: diagnostic approach. Allergy. 2007;62(5):471–87.
13. Galvão VR, Giavina-Bianchi P, Castells M. Perioperative anaphylaxis. Curr Allergy Asthma Rep. 2014;14:452.
14. Castells MC, Horan RH, Ewan PW. Anaphylaxis. In: Holgate ST, Church MK, Lichtenstein LM, editors. Allergy. 2nd ed. London: Mosby; 2001. p. 163–73.
15. Johansson SG. Revised nomenclature for allergy for global use: report of the nomenclature review committee of the World Allergy Organization, October 2003. J Allergy Clin Immunol. 2004;113:832–6.
16. Mertes PM. Reducing the risk of anaphylaxis during anesthesia: guidelines for clinical practice. J Investig Allergol Clin Immunol. 2005;15:91–101.
17. Brockow K. Dilemmas of allergy diagnosis in perioperative anaphylaxis. Allergy. 2014;10:1265–6.
18. Didier A. Role of the quaternary ammonium ion determinants in allergy to muscle relaxants. J Allergy Clin Immunol. 1987;79:578–84.
19. Koppert W. Different patterns of mast cell activation by muscle relaxants in human skin. Anesthesiology. 2001;95:659–67.
20. Doenicke AW. Onset time, endotracheal intubating conditions, and plasma histamine after cis-atracurium and vecuronium administration. Anesth Analg. 1998;87(2):434–8.
21. Bonifazi F, Senna G, Bilò MB. Reazioni allergiche e pseudoallergiche da farmaci. Update Int Congr. 2004;8:583.
22. Garvey LH. Old, new and hidden causes of perioperative hypersensitivity. Curr Pharm Des. 2016;22(45):6814–24.
23. Florvaag E. Prevalence of IgE antibodies to morphine. Relation to the high and low incidences of NMBA anaphylaxis in Norway and Sweden, respectively. Acta Anesthesiol Scand. 2005;49:437–44.
24. Mertes PM, Demoly P. Perioperative anaphylaxis. Immunol Allergy Clin N Am. 2009;29(3):429–51.
25. Mota AN. Perioperative latex hypersensitivity reactions: an integrative literature review. Rev Lat Am Enfermagem. 2012;20(2):411–20.
26. Lieberman P. Anaphylactic reactions during surgical and medical procedures. J Allergy Clin Immunol. 2002;110:64–9.
27. Michalska-Krzanowska G. Anaphylactic reactions during anesthesia and the perioperative period. Anesthesiol Intensiv Ther. 2012;44(2):104–11.
28. Kelly KJ, Sussman G. Latex allergy: where are we now and how did we get there? J Allergy Clin Immunol Pract. 2017;5(5):1212–6.
29. Adriaensens I. Allergic reactions during labour analgesia and caesarean section anesthesia. Int J Obstet Anesth. 2013;22(3):231–42.
30. Nettis E. Type I allergy to natural rubber latex and type IV allergy to rubber chemicals in health care workers with glove-related skin symptoms. Clin Exp Allergy. 2002;32(3):441–7.
31. Nettis E. Sensitization to rubber additives. Allergy. 2001;56(10):1018–20.
32. Gabriel MF. Evaluation and comparison of commercially available latex extracts for skin prick tests. J Investig Allergol Clin Immunol. 2013;23(7):478–86.
33. Cabañes N. Latex allergy: position paper. J Investig Allergol Clin Immunol. 2012;22(5):313–30.
34. Van Kampen V. Evaluation of commercial skin prick test solutions for selected occupational allergens. Allergy. 2013;68(5):651–8.
35. Alenius H. Natural rubber latex allergy. Occup Environ Med. 2002;59(6):419–24.
36. Lieberman P. The diagnosis and management of anaphylaxis practice parameter: 2010 update. J Allergy Clin Immunol. 2010;126:1–42.
37. Mertes PM. Reducing the risk of anaphylaxis during anesthesia: 2011 updated guidelines for clinical practice. J Investig Allergol Clin Immunol. 2011;21(6):442–53.
38. Nettis E, Delle Donne P. Latex immunotherapy: state of the art. Ann Allergy Asthma Immunol. 2012. https://doi.org/10.1016/j.anai.2012.07.004.

39. Luengo O, Cardona V. Component resolved diagnosis: when should it be used? Clin Transl Allergy. 2014. https://doi.org/10.1186/2045-7022-4-28.
40. Bernardini R, Catania P, Caffarelli C. Perioperative latex allergy. Int J Immunopathol Pharmacol. 2011;24(Suppl 3):55–60.
41. Schuler S, Ferrari G, Schmid-Grendelmeier P, Harr T. Microarray-based component-resolved diagnosis of latex allergy: isolated IgE-mediated sensitization to latex profiling Hev b8 may act as confounder. Clin Transl Allergy. 2013;3(1):11.
42. Laxenaire MC. Epidemiology of anesthetic anaphylactoid reactions. Fourth multicenter survey (July 1994–December 1996). Ann Fr Anesth Reanim. 1999;18:796–809.
43. Michalska-Krzanowska G. Anaphylactic reactions during anaesthesia and the perioperative period. Anesthesiol Intensiv Ther. 2012;44(2):104–11.
44. Linda N. Peri-operative anaphylaxis. Br J Clin Pharmacol. 2011;71(5):647–58.
45. Gurrieri C. Allergic reactions during anesthesia at a large United States referral center. Anesth Analg. 2011;113:1202–12.
46. Mertes PM. Anaphylactic and anaphylactoid reactions occurring during anesthesia in France in 1999–2000. Anesthesiology. 2003;99:536–45.
47. Torres MJ. Diagnosis of immediate allergic reactions to beta-lactam antibiotics. Allergy. 2003;58:961–72.
48. Sanz ML. Specific IgE determination in the diagnosis of beta-lactam allergy. J Investig Allergol Clin Immunol. 1996;6:89–93.
49. Garcia JJ. Determination of IgE antibodies to the benzylpenicilloyl determinant: a comparison of the sensitivity and specificity of three radio allergo sorbent test methods. J Clin Lab Anal. 1997;11:251–7.
50. Blanca M. Clinical evaluation of pharmacia CAP system RAST FEIA amoxicilloyl and benzylpenicilloyl in patients with penicillin allergy. Allergy. 2001;56:862–70.
51. Sivagnanam S, Deleu D. Red man syndrome. Crit Care. 2003;7:119–20.
52. Manfredi M. Detection of specific IgE to quinolones. J Allergy Clin Immunol. 2004;113:155–60.
53. Laxenaire MC. Life-threatening anaphylactoid reactions to propofol (Diprivan). Anesthesiology. 1992;77:275–80.

22

Importance of hypersensitivity in adverse reactions to drugs in the elderly

Maria Teresa Ventura[1], Elisa Boni[2], Rosa Cecere[1], Rosalba Buquicchio[1], Gian Franco Calogiuri[3], Irene Martignago[4], Cristoforo Incorvaia[5] and Erminia Ridolo[4*]

Abstract

Background: The use of drugs in the elderly is very extensive because of the frequent occurrence of chronic diseases. Adverse drug reactions (ADRs) commonly occur in geriatric patients receiving multiple therapeutic regimens. In the literature, little attention has been given to ADRs in the elderly, and particularly to allergic reactions.

Objective: The aim of the present study is to provide data on possible inappropriate prescriptions in the elderly in relation to allergic reactions and to identify a list of drugs which are likely inducers of allergic reactions.

Methods: We retrospectively evaluated ADRs in patients referring to Immunoallergy Unit of Hospital Policlinico in Bari on the basis of Beers criteria. Among adverse reactions, hypersensitivity reactions were extracted and a comparison between different age groups was assessed.

Results: Out of 823 patients with ADRs, in 30.6% hypersensitivity drug reactions (HDR) were diagnosed. Data about drug intake, comorbidities and clinical presentation were collected, aiming to identify possible risk factors. An evaluation of drugs most commonly involved was assessed.

Conclusions: HDR are reported to represent 5–10% of all ADRs, while in our study population the prevalence was about 30%. This suggests the need to develop strategies to minimize the incidence of drug allergy in the elderly, as well to reduce the phenomenon of inappropriate prescriptions.

Keywords: Drug allergy, Elderly, Adverse drug reaction, Hypersensitivity drug reaction

Background

The concomitant use of several drugs in the elderly is closely related to the multiple chronic diseases typical of this age. Moreover, polypharmacy determines an increased risk of adverse reactions that can be related to drug–drug or drug-disease interactions [1]. In fact, the percentage of adverse events increases from 13%, in case of concomitant intake of two drugs to 82% in case of intake of 7 or more drugs [2]. Another relevant factor is the alteration in the pharmacokinetics (absorption, distribution, metabolism, excretion) and pharmacodynamics, as well as the changes in the body mass in terms of total body fat and water [3]. Of consequence, the hydrophilic drugs may be overdosed, while lipophilic drugs cannot perform to their full action. Modifications in drug metabolization and excretion, related to liver failure, as well as renal insufficiency should not be neglected [4]. Finally, the decline of the oxidation of cytochrome P450 causes additional problems not only for the consequences of this partial enzyme depletion in terms of drug–drug interactions [5], but also in terms of accumulation of reactive metabolites [6].

From a clinical perspective, adverse drug reactions (ADRs) are often difficult to diagnose and are sometimes mistaken as a new disease and treated with additional medications. Discontinuation of previously prescribed therapy in the elderly is rarely considered. As a result, the older population receives a considerable quantity of doses per day of different pharmacological principles. According to Edwards et al., ADRs are classified as follows: type

*Correspondence: erminia.ridolo@unipr.it
[4] Medicine and Surgery Department, University of Parma, Via Gramsci 14, 43126 Parma, Italy
Full list of author information is available at the end of the article

A (dose-dependent), which are quite frequent, related to the mechanism of action of the molecule, predictable and usually associated with low mortality; type B (bizarre, not dose-dependent), rare and unpredictable with a high mortality, such as hypersensitivity reactions; type C (chronic, dose- and time-dependent), related to the repeated treatment; type D (delayed), rare and generally dose-dependent, occur sometimes following the use (e.g. carcinogenesis); type E (end of use) occur immediately after the suspension; type F (failure), characterized by therapeutic ineffectiveness, dose-dependent and often caused by interactions between drugs [7].

The European Academy of Allergy and Clinical Immunology (EAACI) Nomenclature Task Force introduced a classification of ADRs. The reactions of hypersensitivity to drugs have been divided into two subgroups depending on the genesis of immunological (drug allergy) or non-immunological hypersensitivity (non allergic). Drug allergy is in turn divided into IgE-mediated and non-IgE-mediated [8]. The reactions previously defined pseudoallergic reactions (PAR) and now instead referred to as non allergic [9], that consist of clinical manifestations similar to those induced by allergic reactions, are due to one or more of the following pathogenetic mechanisms: (1) inhibition of cyclooxygenase with reduced production of prostaglandins and production of inflammatory leukotrienes. Responsible drugs are: acetylsalicylic acid (ASA), nonsteroidal anti-inflammatory drugs (NSAIDs), analgesics, barbiturates, antihistamines, sulfonamides, quinine, some local anesthetics, hydrocortisone; (2) direct activation of complement with release of anaphylatoxins able to induce mast cell degranulation. This mechanism is frequent after the administration of iodinated contrast agents, adrenocorticotropic hormone, endovenous anaesthetics, endovenous globulins, plasma substitutes; (3) direct release of histamine due to mast cell instability in predisposed people. Drugs that can provoke this mechanism are morphine, codeine, aminoglycosides, plasma substitutes, antidepressants, sympathomimetics, pesticides; (4) bronchospasm due to the liberation of sulphur dioxide in the course of sulphide therapy or drugs containing sulphites; (5) inhibition of degradation and subsequent accumulation as it occurs following prolonged Angiotensin Converting Enzyme (ACE)-inhibitors assumption. The issue of polypharmacy in the elderly has been reviewed by several authors. Beers et al. [10] in 1991 published an article that contains the "criteria" to be adopted for the management of the therapy in the elderly, in addition to a list of drugs to be avoided at this age. These criteria were then revised by several authors [11–14]. The Beers criteria comprise practical guidelines widely adopted and able to identify inappropriate prescriptions in the elderly. The 2003 update expanded the list of medication and reviewed the comorbidities including cognitive impairment, incontinence and the depressive syndrome associated with Parkinson's disease [14]. Despite the comprehensiveness of Beers's work [10, 12] and the subsequent updates with modifications and implementation of the list of drugs, it should be noted that, while the ADRs of type A and C and interactions are exhaustively included, the hypersensitivity reactions—allergic or non allergic—according to the classification proposed by the EAACI Nomenclature Task Force in 2001, are missing [8, 13].

Methods

The aim of the present study was to evaluate the possibly inappropriate prescriptions in the elderly in relation to allergic reactions and to identify a list of drugs which are potential inducers of allergic reactions to be avoided in the elderly. This is to prevent the risk of IgE- or cell-mediated reactions or potential cross reactions between medications with similar immunological mechanisms. In the study were retrospectively included patients who suffered of drug reactions visited between 2011 and 2012 in the Immunoallergology Unit in Hospital Policlinico in Bari. ADRs were diagnosed on the basis of Beers criteria [10–14]. Diagnosis of hypersensitivity drug reaction (HDR) was made based on the clinical history collected through a questionnaire assessing clinical manifestations, chronology of the symptoms, other medications taken, and the medical background of the patient [15]. The diagnostic process was completed, when indicated, with in vivo and in vitro allergy testing according to EAACI criteria (Table 1) [16]. In case of suspected IgE-dependent reactions to penicillins, cephalosporins, insulin, heparin, contrast media and general and local anesthetics, in vivo tests (skin prick test and/or intradermal test) for the culprit drug were performed if available. Moreover, depending on the drug involved, in vitro tests were performed, including Basophil Activation Test (BAT) (Buhlmann Lab., Basel, Switzerland), specific IgE (CAP system, Thermo Fisher Diagnostic, Uppsala, Sweden), determination of complement factors and circulating immune complexes, measurement of histamine and tryptase in serum (CAP FEIA Thermo Fisher Diagnostic). Drug provocation test with the culprit drug is not a routine test in our Unit, due to age and comorbidities of patients; for the same reason, in case of hypersensitivity reactions to contrast media, provocation test was not performed. An alternative contrast media was indicated with premedication in case of further imaging investigations. An oral challenge test with the various medications was instead performed to find an alternative treatment. In the case of topical medications, the diagnosis was assessed by mean of patch tests [16].

Table 1 Tests for the diagnosis of hypersensitivity to drugs

Type of drug	In vivo tests			In vitro tests	
	Prick test/intradermal test	Patch test	Provocation Test	Specific IgE	Others
Penicillins	+	+	+*	+	
Cephalosporins	+	+	+*	+	
Sulfonamides			+		
Other antibiotics			+		
Aspirin and NSAIDs			+		+
General anesthetics	+		+*		
Local anesthetics	+		+*		
Contrast media	+	+			
Insulin	+			+	
Heparin	+	+	+*		
Immunoglobulins					+
Anticonvulsants			+		

*performed after cutaneous test

With regard to patients with history of HDR, data about gender, smoking habit and use of self-medications was collected. Other clinical data of interest concerned family medical history, atopy history, presence of concomitant diseases (liver diseases, renal failure, cancer, cardiovascular diseases, diabetes, chronic respiratory diseases). Special attention was paid to dose assumption, clinical presentation and severity of HDR, previous reactions to drugs, and current pharmacological regimen. The patients with HDRs were then divided into two subgroups (under 65 and over 65 years) and the data collected were analyzed for each age group.

Statistical analysis

Age, which is a continuous quantitative variable distributed according to Gauss, has been synthesized as mean and standard deviation. Later it was categorized into two classes: above and over 65. This and the other variables object of the analysis that are all qualitative, are summarized as counts and relative percentage. The comparison of the percentages between independent groups was carried out by means of the Chi square test.

Results

From 2011 to 2012, 1782 patients were visited in our Unit. Of them, 823 (mean age 45 $\pm$ 4 years, 543 females and 280 males) were included in the study for suspected ADRs: the diagnosis of ADRs was confirmed in 623 cases (mean age 66 $\pm$ 3). Among patients with ADRs, 421 were females (67.6%) and 202 were males (32.4%). The median time of onset of symptoms was about 10 h after drug intake and in most patients the symptoms were related to pharmacological mechanisms of the drug (e.g. syncope after antihypertensive therapy, diarrhea after use of antibiotics, hypotension due to high dose of diuretic, etc.). In 191 patients (30.6%), 143 females and 48 males, HDR was diagnosed on the basis of clinical manifestations and specific allergy tests; 126 patients (66%) were aged $\geq$ 65 years and 65 (34%) were aged < 65 years. Comorbidities are shown in Fig. 1, they reflected the common distribution in the general population of age-associated diseases. Demographic and medical data of patients who suffered from HDR are reported in Table 2: only 3.9% of geriatric patients had other allergic diseases, compared with 24.6% among younger patients, confirming that there is no correlation between atopy and HDRs in older patients. There were no significant differences between familial history of atopy, smoking habit and alcohol abuse in the two age groups. The prevalence of HDRs was significantly higher in older female patients compared to younger patients (80.15% vs. 64.61%), as well as in the older group concerning multiple chronic therapeutic regimen (86.5% vs 30.7%) and in short course therapies with 3 or more drugs (38% vs 27.6%). With regard to the different clinical presentations of HDRs, as shown in Fig. 2, skin symptoms were the main clinical manifestation of HDRs in both age groups, with urticaria-angioedema syndrome as unique presentation in more than 90% of patients of every age. All immediate reactions appeared within 1–5 h after intake of a drug. On the other hand, non immediate T cell reactions occurred only in 3 patients under the age of 65. Rare manifestations were erythema multiforme, Stevens Johnson syndrome and psoriasis-like eruptions (data not shown). Anaphylactic shock occurred in 7% of patients aged over 65 vs. 1.5% of younger patients. Finally, in Table 3 are listed the drugs responsible for HDRs. Over the age of 65 years ASA and other NSAIDs were the main cause of

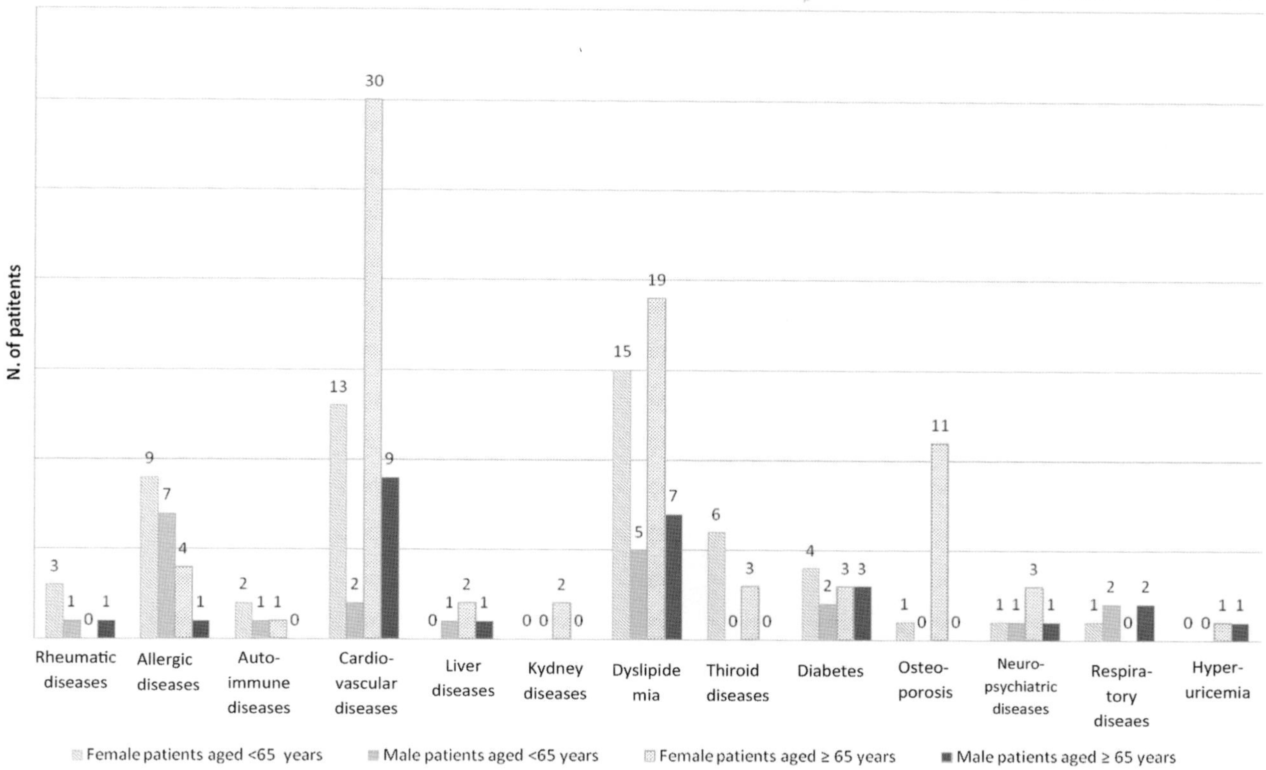

Fig. 1 Comorbidities in patients with hypersensitivity drug reactions

Table 2 Demographic and medical data of patients who suffered from HDR

Feature	Patients aged ≥ 65 year n. (%)	Patients aged < 65 year n. (%)	X^2
Female	101 (80.15%)	42 (64.61%)	0.019
Family history of atopy	0	4 (6.1%)	0.005
Allergic diseases	5 (3.96%)	16 (24.61%)	0.000
Previous ADRs	12 (9.5%)	15 (23.07%)	0.01
Smoker	38 (30.15%)	22 (33.8%)	0.603
Alcohol abuse	19 (15%)	6 (9.23%)	0.256
Multiple chronic drug regimen	109 (86.5%)	20 (30.7%)	0.000
Comorbidities	126 (100%)	6 (9.23%)	0.000
Use of self-medications	31 (24.6%)	22 (33.8%)	0.176
Short course therapy with ≥ 3 drugs	48 (38%)	18 (27.6%)	0.152
Total	126 (100%)	65 (100%)	

drug reactions, followed by antibiotics. Conversely, antibiotics were the first cause of HDR in younger patients and none of them had reactions to ASA or NSAIDs.

Discussion

HDRs, previously called type B or bizarre [17] are not directly related to the drug action but are individual responses in predisposed patients. These reactions are defined as quantitatively and qualitatively abnormal, unpredictable and often dose-independent. Concerning their pathogenesis, they are distinguished between non-immune and immune (or allergic). HDRs are less frequently described in the literature with respect to the ADRs in the elderly. It is well established that only certain drugs or biological agents have the structural characteristics of immunogenicity, being able to trigger

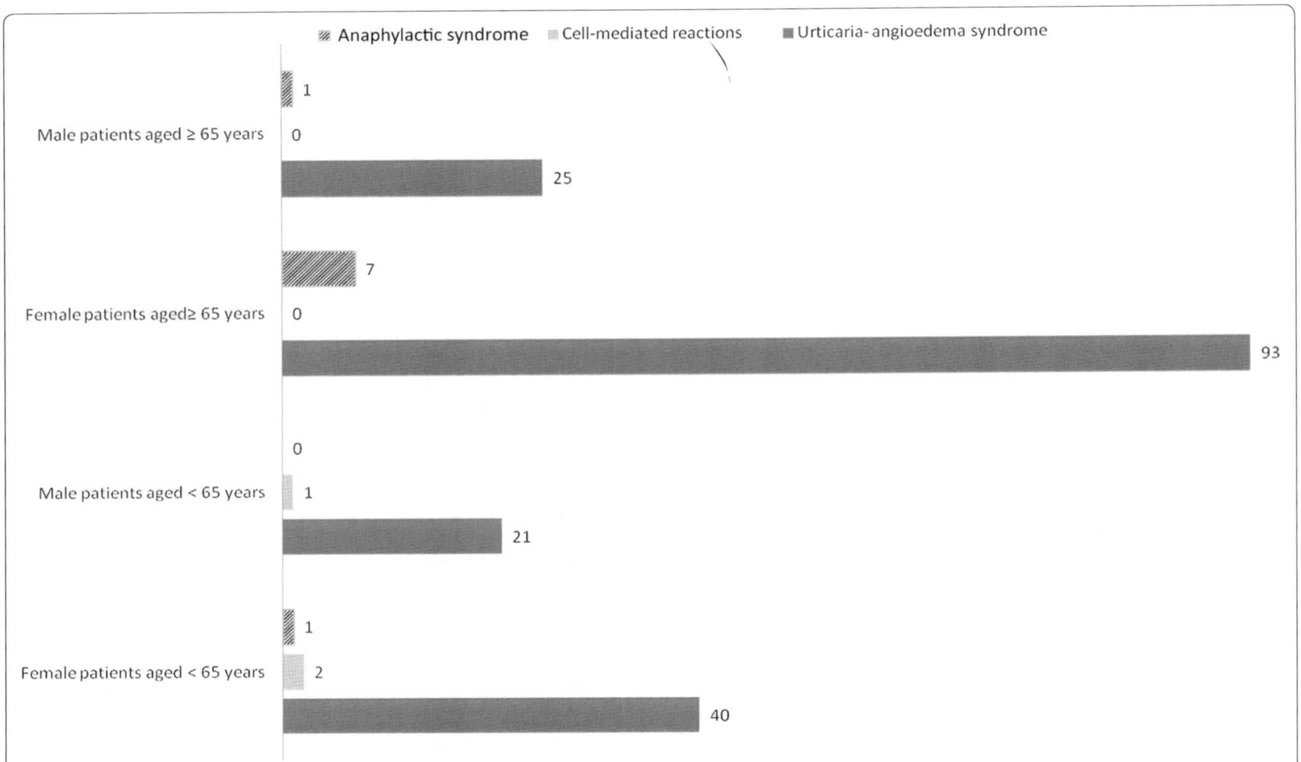

Fig. 2 Clinical manifestation of hypersensitivity drug reactions in different age groups and gender

Table 3 Drugs responsible for HDRs

	Patients aged ≥ 65 year		**Patients aged < 65 year**	
	Females % of pts ≥ 65 (n.)	**Males % of pts ≥ 65 (n.)**	**Females % of pts < 65 (n.)**	**Males % of pts < 65 (n.)**
Antibiotics	33.3 (42)	7.9 (10)	46.1 (30)	23 (15)
NSAIDs	35.7 (45)	7.9 (10)	7.6 (5)	1.5 (1)
Acetylsalicilic acid	11.9 (15)	7.1 (9)	0 (0)	0 (0)
Antihypertensive drugs	1.5 (2)	0 (0)	6.1 (4)	6.1 (4)
Antiacids	4.7 (6)	0 (0)	1.5 (1)	0 (0)
Psicotropic agents	3.1 (4)	0.7 (1)	13.8 (9)	0 (0)
Anesthetics	3.1 (4)	0 (0)	0 (0)	1.5 (1)
Corticosteroids	3.9 (5)	0 (0)	0 (0)	0 (0)
Allopurinol	1.5 (2)	0.7 (1)	0 (0)	0 (0)
Antimycotic	0.7 (1)	1.5 (2)	0 (0)	0 (0)
Contrast media	3.1 (4)	0.7 (1)	0 (0)	0 (0)
Heparin	2.3 (3)	0.7 (1)	0 (0)	1.5 (1)
Statins	1.5 (2)	0.7 (1)	0 (0)	0 (0)
Bone metabolism drugs	1.5 (2)	0 (0)	0 (0)	0 (0)
Drugs for gastrointestinal diseases	1.5 (2)	0 (0)	1.5 (1)	0 (0)
Anticoagulants	0.7 (1)	0 (0)	1.5 (1)	0 (0)
Muscle relaxant	0.7 (1)	0 (0)	1.5 (1)	0 (0)
Plasma expander	0.7 (1)	0 (0)	0 (0)	0 (0)
Iron therapy	0.7 (1)	0 (0)	0 (0)	0 (0)

immunopathological responses. Most drugs or their metabolites, however, have no such immunogenic properties. Therefore, in order to elicit an immune response, a phenomenon of haptenization is necessary. A typical example is provided by β-lactam antibiotics that have high reactivity with carrier proteins, able to induce an IgE-mediated reaction in predisposed patients. Moreover, there are drugs potentially able to induce clinical manifestations similar to allergic reactions, though immunological mechanisms are other than IgE-mediated reaction: ASA and NSAIDs, ACE inhibitors, opioids, iodinated contrast media, antibiotics such as ciprofloxacin and vancomycin, and muscle relaxants with ammonium group. It is known that allopurinol is able to elicit an hypersensitivity syndrome characterized by severe skin involvement, worsening of renal function with fever, leukocytosis and eosinophilia that can be fatal [18]. It recognizes an immunological genesis determined by T lymphocyte clones specific for its metabolite, oxypurinol. Risk factors for the development of this syndrome are represented by an age $\geq$ 65 years, chronic renal insufficiency, concomitant treatment with thiazide diuretics and intermittent therapy with allopurinol [19, 20]. HDRs represent 5–10% of all adverse reactions to drugs [21], but as they are unpredictable and potentially lethal, they represent the most important kind of adverse reactions both in youth and elderly. In our study population the rate of HDRs was 30%, that is much higher than previously reported, presumably due to the fact that in our area many patients affected by ADRs are not referred to specialist's evaluation. Risk factors related to patients are female gender, previous reactions to medications, genetic factors such as familiarity for drug allergy, association with particular MHC antigens, acetylator phenotype, and a personal history of atopy [22]. Other risk factors comprise concomitant diseases such as viral infections, chronic liver disease or chronic renal failure [23]. Moreover, renal failure not clinically apparent may result in an increased risk of ADRs, especially in water-soluble drugs, such as insulin and glibenclamide [4, 24]. According to Beyth, the risk is correlated with the number of drugs taken and with the number of pathologies, as well as with the nutritional status and with alterations of pharmacodynamics and pharmacokinetics of the molecule involved [25]. In the present study we observed that gender as well as multiple therapeutic regimens are risk factors in older age for HDRs, with an higher rate than patients aged under 65 years. Smoking habit, alcohol abuse and personal and familiar history of atopy did not differ between younger and older subjects. Atopy and previous reactions to drugs do not seem to represent risk factors in the elderly, while we observed a positive association with multiple drugs intake. This offers confirmation to previous observations about the lack of association of atopy and HDRs [26], although this could be influenced by the severity of reactions in atopic subjects [27]. The main clinical manifestation according to our data is skin involvement, as previously described in a study conducted on a cohort of 2644 subjects. In that study, after allergy testing HDRs were diagnosed in 2.1% of cases; 96% of symptoms were cutaneous (urticaria, angioedema, erythema, Steven Johnson syndrome, and psoriasis-like reactions). It was also observed that the peak of HDRs dramatically decreases in the eighth decade of life, with significant prevalence in females (80%). In the same study, comparing the two groups of patients (elderly and aged < 65 years), the family history and personal history of atopy was similar, comorbidities and multiple treatment regimen were instead a peculiarity of the elderly [26]. Some authors have found that HDRs are less frequent and less severe in children and in elderly, probably due to immaturity and involution of the immune system typical of these periods of life [28]. This is in contrast with our data that shows that anaphylactic shock is more frequent in > 65 years aged than in younger patients. In addition, in the present study antibiotics, medications for cardiovascular disease, NSAIDs and ASA were the drugs most frequently responsible for HDRs in the elderly. We observed that ASA and NSAIDs are the main factors of drug reactions in > 65 years aged while antibiotics are the main factor in < 65 years aged patients. Some chronic degenerative diseases such as atherosclerosis are favored by inflammatory phenomena that tend to induce chronic vascular endothelial lesions typical of this disease. A common mechanism appears to contribute to atherosclerosis and atopy [29]. The activation of perivascular mast cells promotes atherosclerosis by the release of inflammatory cytokines that contribute to the activation and chemotaxis of macrophages, which incorporate the excess fats becoming "foam cells" (fatty cells) and generate the atherosclerotic plaque [30]. Similarly, it is believed that leukotrienes play an important role in promoting atherosclerosis. A genetic variant of the 5-lipoxygenase has been associated both with asthma and atherosclerosis [31]. In turn, the inflammatory cytokines released by mast-cells and macrophages in the genesis of the atherosclerotic plaque can form the protein component to which the hapten drug can bind, even in absence of albumin, the production of which by the liver is always reduced in the elderly [32]. A recent study has also highlighted that the increased DNA methylation predisposes the elderly to respiratory allergic diseases, but could also predispose to HDRs [33]. The misuse of complementary and alternative medicine and polypharmacy during different degenerative diseases afflicting the elderly is another risk factor for the development of drug allergy [34]. A recent retrospective survey on 161 hospitalized patients (mean age 63 years) who had an HDR to medications during their hospital stay suggested that the administration of proton pump inhibitors (PPI), used in 83% of hospitalized patients, could favor the occurrence of HDRs, especially to NSAIDs. In fact, with the suppression of gastric acid, PPIs increase the persistence of labile proteins able to bind stably to other drugs taken by oral route, thus preventing the complete denaturing of the other drugs [35]. Similarly, in a case report a patient aged 60 years developed generalized urticaria immediately after a second course of therapy with diclofenac and PPI, the latter having been used previously for gastroesophageal reflux. The authors postulated that allergy to diclofenac could have been favored by suppression of gastric acid and confirmed it on a murine model of sensitization [36]. Considering the extensive use of PPIs as gastroprotective drugs in older patients treated with low dose ASA as a preventive therapy of myocardial ischemia, one could speculate that PPI might represent a co-factor in HDRs to ASA. In conclusion, the purpose of this study was to find data able to suggest the basis to develop strategies to minimize the incidence of HDRs in the elderly, as the Beers criteria have served to reduce significantly the phenomenon of inappropriate prescriptions in this time of life. According to the results, the comorbidity and proinflammatory status of the immune system, typical of the elderly, such as metabolic disorders, cardiovascular diseases, and osteoporosis may favor the onset of HDRs. In these patients not only beta-lactam antibiotics, able to elicit IgE-mediated responses, but also drugs that are able to elicit non IgE or cell-mediated drug reaction, as ASA, NSAIDs, ACE inhibitors or cyclooxygenase and bradykinin inhibitors have to be administered with caution in older patients. At the same time, in order to re-evaluate the issue of HDRs in the elderly and to establish shared parameters about the administration of drugs at risk of reactions, responsible for anaphylaxis or urticaria-angioedema syndrome, the incidence of HDRs in geriatric age and the risk factors for this type of reactions should be estimated. Based on adequate data, guidelines for the management of HDRs in the elderly should be issued.

Abbreviations

ADR: adverse drug reaction; HDR: hypersensitivity drug reaction; NSAID: non steroidal anti-inflammatory drugs; ASA: acetylsalicylic acid; BAT: basophil activation test; ACE: angiotensin converting enzyme.

Authors' contributions

VMT, CR, EB, ER wrote and coordinated the draft of the manuscript. BR, CI, IM, CI, GFC carried out the bibliographic search, contributed to the draft of the manuscript and made substantial contribution to the revision of the article. All authors read and approved the final manuscript.

Author details

[1] Department of Interdisciplinary Medicine, University of Bari, Bari, Italy. [2] S.O.S.Allergy, ASL, Alessandria, Italy. [3] Pneumology Department, Ospedale Sacro Cuore Gallipoli (Lecce), Lecce, Italy. [4] Medicine and Surgery Department, University of Parma, Via Gramsci 14, 43126 Parma, Italy. [5] Cardiac/Pulmonary Rehabilitation, ASST Pini/CTO, Milan, Italy.

Funding

No sources of funding were used to conduct this study or prepare this manuscript.

References

1. Onder G, Pedone C, Landi F. Adverse drug reactions as a cause of hospital admissions: results of Italian Group of Pharmacoepidemiology in the Elderly (GIFA). J Am Geriatr Soc. 2002;50(12):33–52.
2. Goldberg RM, Mabee J, Chan L, Wong S. Drug-drug and drug-disease interactions in the emergency department: analysis of a high-risk population. Am J Emerg Med. 1996;14(5):447–50.
3. Meyer BR. Clinical Pharmacology and ageing. In: Grimley Evans J, Franklin Williams T, Lynn Beattie B, Michael J-P, Wilcock G, editors. Textbook of geriatric medicine. 2nd ed. Oxford: Oxford University Press; 2003. p. 127–36.
4. Corsonello A, Pedone C, Corica F. Concealed renal failure and adverse drug reactions in older patients with type 2 diabetes mellitus. J Gerontol A Biol Sci Med Sci. 2005;60(9):1147–51.
5. Gallagher P, Barry P, O'Mahony D. Inappropriate prescribing in the elderly. Am J Emerg Med. 2007;14:447–50.
6. Knowles SR, Uetrecht J, Shear NH. Idiosyncratic drug reactions: the reactive metabolite syndromes. Lancet. 2000;35:1587–91.
7. Edwards IR, Aronson JK. Adverse drug reactions: definitions, diagnosis, and management. Lancet. 2000;356:1255–97.
8. Johansson SG, Hourihane JOB, et al. Position paper. A revised nomenclature for allergy. An EAACI position statement from the EAACI nomenclature task force. Allergy. 2001;56:813–24.
9. Farnam K, Chang C, Teuber S, Gershwin ME. Nonallergic drug hypersensitivity reactions. Int Arch Allergy Immunol. 2012;159:327–45.
10. Beers MH, Ouslander JG, Rollingher I. Explicit criteria for determining inappropriate medication use in nursing home residents. Arch Intern Med. 1991;151(9):1825–32.
11. Stuck AE, Beers MH, Steiner A. Inappropriate medication use in community residing older persons. Arch Intern Med. 1994;154(19):2195–200.
12. Beers MH. Explicit criteria for determining potentially inappropriate medication use by the elderly, An update. Arch Intern Med. 1997;157(14):1531–6.
13. Zhan C, Sangl J, Bierman AS, Miller MR, Friedman B, Wickizer SW, Meyer GS. Potentially inappropriate medication use in the community-dwelling elderly: findings from the 1996 Medical Expenditure Panel Survey. JAMA. 2001;286(28):2823–9.
14. Fick DM, Cooper JW, Wade W. Updating the Beers criteria for potentially inappropriate medication use in older adults—results of a US consensus Panel of experts. Arch Intern Med. 2003;163:2716–24.
15. Demoly P, Kropf R, Bircher A, Pichler WJ. Drug hypersensitivity: questionnaire. EAACI interest group on drug hypersensitivity. Allergy. 1999;54(9):999–1003.
16. Ventura MT, Sanapo F, Calogiuri GF, Satriano F. Anaphylaxis induced by intramuscular betamethasone disodium phosphate: reflections on a clinical case. Int J Immunopathol Pharmacol. 2007;20:387–91.
17. Rawlins MD, Thompson JW. Pathogenesis of adverse drug reactions. In: Davies DM, editor. Textbook of adverse drug reactions. Oxford: Oxford University Press; 1977. p. 10–45.
18. Gutiérrez-Macías A, Lizarralde-Palacios E, Martínez-Odriozola P, Miguel-De la Villa F. Fatal allopurinol hypersensitivity syndrome after treatment of asymptomatic hyperuricemia. BMJ. 2005;331:623–4.
19. Lee HY, Ariyasinghe JT, Thirumoorthy T. Allopurinol hypersensitivity syndrome: a preventable severe cutaneous adverse reaction? Singap Med J. 2008;49:384–7.

20. Yun J, Mattsson J, Schnyder K, Fontana S, Largiader CR, Pichler WJ, Yerly D. Allopurinol hypersensitivity is primarily mediated by dose dependent oxypurinol—specific T-cell response. Clin Exp Allergy. 2013;43(11):1246–55.
21. Demoly P, Bousquet J. Epidemiology of drug allergy. Curr Opin Allergy Clin Immunol. 2001;1:305–10.
22. Guglielmi L, Guglielmi P, Demoly P. Drug hypersensitivity: epidemiology and risk factors. Curr Pharm Des. 2006;12:3309–12.
23. Ventura MT, Muratore L, Calogiuri GF, et al. Allergic and pseudoallergic reactions induced by glucorticoids: a review. Curr Pharm Des. 2003;9:1956–64.
24. Turnheim K. When drug therapy gets old: pharmacokinetics and pharmacodynamics in the elderly. Exp Gerontol. 2003;38:843–53.
25. Beyth RJ, Shorr RI. Epidemiology of adverse drug reactions in the elderly by drug class. Drugs Aging. 1999;14(3):231–9.
26. Ventura MT, Laddaga R, Cavallera P, Pugliese P, Tummolo R, Buquicchio R, Pierucci P, Passalacqua G. Adverse drug reactions as the cause of emergency department admission: focus on the elderly. Immunopharmacol Immunotoxicol. 2010;32:426–9.
27. Haddi C, Charpin D, Tofforeau M, Kulling G, Lanteaume A, Kleisbauer JP. Atopy and systemic reactions to drugs. Allergy. 1990;45:236–9.
28. Barranco P, Lopez-Serrano MC. General and epidemiological aspects of allergic drug reactions. Clin Exp Allergy. 1998;28(4):61–2.
29. Kovanen PT. Mast cells in atherogenesis: actions and reactions. Curr Atheroscler Rep. 2009;11:214.
30. Jala VR, Haribabu B. Leukotrienes and atherosclerosis: new roles for old mediators. Trends Immunol. 2004;25:315–22.
31. Dwyer JH, Allayee H, Dwyer KM, Fan J, Wu H, Mar R, Lusis AJ, Mehrabian M. Arachidonate 5-lipoxygenase promoter genotype, dietary arachidonic acid and atherosclerosis. N Engl J Med. 2004;350:29–37.
32. Brooks BM, Thomas AL, Coleman JW. Benzylpenicillin differentially conjugates to IFNγ, TNFα, IL-1β, IL-4 and IL-13 but selectively reduces IFNγ activity. Clin Exp Immunol. 2003;131:268–74.
33. Sordillo JE, Lange NE, Tarantini L, Bollati V, Zanobetti A, Sparrow D, Vokonas P, Schwartz J, Baccarelli A, Demeo D, Litonjua AA. Allergen sensitization is associated with increased DNA methylation in older men. Int Arch Allergy Immunol. 2013;161:37–43.
34. Ventura MT, Viola M, Calogiuri GF, Gaeta F, Pesole O, Romano A. Hypersensitivity reactions to complementary and alternative medicine products. Curr Pharm Des. 2006;12:3393–9.
35. Ramirez E, Cabana R, Laserna LS, Fiandor A, Tong H, Prior N, Calderon O, Medrano N, Boblea I, Frias J, Quirce S. Proton pump inhibitors are associated with hypersensitivity reactions to drugs in hospitalized patients: a case control need in a retrospective cohort study. Clin Exp Allergy. 2013;43:344–52.
36. Riemer AB, Gruber S, Pali-Scholl I, Kinaciyan T, Untersmayr E, Jensen-Jarolim E. Suppression of gastric acid increases the risk of developing immunoglobulin E-mediated drug hypersensitivity: human diclofenac sensitization and a murine sensitization. Clin Exp Allergy. 2010;40:486–93.

Markers of atopic dermatitis, allergic rhinitis and bronchial asthma in pediatric patients: correlation with filaggrin, eosinophil major basic protein and immunoglobulin E

Zafar Rasheed[1*], Khaled Zedan[2], Ghada Bin Saif[3], Ragaa H. Salama[1], Tarek Salem[1], Ahmed A. Ahmed[4], Alaa Abd El-Moniem[5], Maha Elkholy[5], Ahmad A. Al Robaee[6] and Abdullateef A. Alzolibani[6]

Abstract

Background: Allergic reactions have been implicated as contributions in a number of atopic disorders, including atopic dermatitis (AD), allergic rhinitis (AR) and bronchial asthma (BA). However, the potential for filaggrin protein, eosinophil major basic protein (MBP) and immunoglobulin E (IgE) to elicit allergic response or to contribute to atopic disorders remains largely unexplored in pediatric patients. This study was undertaken to investigate the status and contribution of filaggrin protein, eosinophil MBP and total IgE in pediatric patients with AD, AR and BA.

Methods: Sera from 395 pediatric patients of AD, AR or BA with varying levels of disease activity according to the disease activity index and 410 age-matched non-atopic healthy controls were evaluated for serum levels of atopic markers, including filaggrin, eosinophil MBP and IgE.

Results: Serum analysis showed that filaggrin levels were remarkably high in pediatric patients with AD, followed by BA and AR, whereas its levels were low in non-atopic pediatric controls. Eosinophil MBP levels in sera of atopic patients were significantly high as compared with their respective controls, but its levels were highest in AR patients, followed by AD and BA. Total IgE in sera of AD patients was markedly high, followed by AR and BA patients, whereas its levels were low in non-atopic pediatric controls. Interestingly, not only was an increased number of subjects positive for filaggrin protein, eosinophil MBP or total IgE, but also their levels were statistically significantly higher among those atopic patients whose disease activity scores were higher as compared with atopic patients with lower disease activity scores.

Conclusions: These findings strongly support a role of filaggrin protein, eosinophil MBP and IgE in the onset of allergic reactions in pediatric patients with AD, AR and BA. The data suggest that filaggrin, eosinophil MBP or IgE might be useful in evaluating the progression of AD, AR or BA and in elucidating the mechanisms involved in the pathogenesis of these pediatric disorders.

Keywords: Atopic disorders, Pediatric patients, Atopic dermatitis, Allergic rhinitis, Bronchial asthma, Filaggrin, Eosinophil MBP, IgE

*Correspondence: zafarrasheed@qumed.edu.sa
[1] Department of Medical Biochemistry, College of Medicine, Qassim University, P.O. Box 6655, Buraidah 51452, Saudi Arabia
Full list of author information is available at the end of the article

Introduction

The atopic disorders of childhood involve mainly atopic dermatitis (AD), allergic rhinitis (AR), and bronchial asthma (BA). These atopic disorders share a common pathogenesis, being mediated by immunoglobulin E (IgE) [1]. Frequency of these atopic disorders is on the rise and now it reached up to 20% worldwide [2]. The concept of the atopic march was developed to describe the progression of atopic disorders from AD to AR in infants or from AD to BA in children [3]. It is also reported that the onset of atopic disorders can be occurred due to a personal or familial propensity to produce sensitization or IgE antibodies in response to the environmental triggers [1, 2]. Not only environmental triggers, heritability also plays an important role in the onset of these atopic disorders in 71–84% AD patients, 33–91% AR patients and 35–95% BA patients [4, 5].

Many of the key structural proteins in the outer most layer of the epidermis involved cornification, which are encoded in a locus on chromosome 1q21, which is basically an epidermal differentiation complex (EDC) [6]. The genes found within this locus, encode for filaggrin, a key member of the EDC [6–8]. The filaggrin has now been considered as a major predisposing gene for various atopic disorders, which resulted in a major paradigm in the dermatology and allergy research [8]. Many studies pointed out an association of filaggrin gene with different atopic disorders. More specifically, mutations in the filaggrin gene have been reported to have an association with various atopic/allergic disorders [5–8]. Investigators reported that there is a strong and consistent association between filaggrin mutations and development of AD [9]. Some studies also noticed an association between filaggrin mutations with atopic sensitization in AR or BA [8, 9]. Allergic disorders are characterized by an IgE-mediated reaction as a consequence of the exposure to a specific allergen. Thus, allergen-specific IgE (sIgE) production are considered to be the hallmark of allergy [10]. Moreover, studies have also pointing out a clear association between serum IgE levels with AD or BA patients [10, 11]. Reports have also shown that children with very high serum IgE levels are at risk for anaphylactic reactions and for the occurrence of more severe AD [10]. The eosinophil major basic protein (MBP), a constituent of the eosinophil secondary granule, is implicated in cytotoxicity and mediation of allergic disorders such as asthma and the level of eosinophil MBP was reported to be high in biological fluids from patients with asthma and other eosinophil-associated disorders [12].

Even through allergic reactions have been implicated in the pathogenesis of pediatric AD, AR or BA, the potential of atopic markers such as filaggrin protein and eosinophil MBP in eliciting a pathogenic response and in contributing in the pathogenesis of these atopic disorders remains largely unexplored. In view of these, the present study was hypothesized that overproduction of filaggrin protein, eosinophil MBP and total IgE in the serum of different atopic pediatric patients may be involved in the contribution of atopic/allergic disorders. To assess this hypothesis, the levels of filaggrin protein, eosinophil MBP and total IgE were determined in the sera of pediatric patients with AD, AR and BA and their levels were compared with non-allergic pediatric controls. Our results not only support a role of filaggrin protein, eosinophil MBP and total IgE in atopic disorders, but also suggest that filaggrin, eosinophil MBP and total IgE may be important in the evaluation and in the elucidation of the mechanisms of pediatric AD, AR and BA.

Subjects and methods

Human subjects

This is a prospective case–control study, which enrolled atopic children with BA, AR and AD who were diagnosed according to recent guidelines described by Global Initiatives for Asthma (GINA) for BA [13], Allergic Rhinitis and its Impact on Asthma (ARIA) for AR [14] and SCORAD index for AD [15]. The study was carried out in accordance with the Code of Ethics of the World Medical Association (Declaration of Helsinki as revised in Tokyo 2004) for humans and was approved by Ethical Committee of College of Medicine, QU and study protocol was approved by the National Plan for Science, Technology and Innovation of KSA (NSTIP # 11-BIO1459-09). Informed consent from parents of all studied children was taken before samples collection. All studied atopic children were consecutively recruited from Outpatient Clinics affiliated to Qassim University (pediatric and dermatology clinics) during 1 year duration. A total of 395 allergic children, 202 males (51.1%), 193 females (48.9%), with a mean age of 6.7 years (±1.27) were enrolled in the study. Also the study included 410 age and sex matched children who were free of any atopic disease and were used as controls. Out of 395 atopic patients, 130 patients were AD (age 1.43±1.36), 120 AR patients (age 4.21±1.72) and 145 were BA (age 7.42±1.46). These atopic patients were further divided into two groups based on their severity scores as described previously [13–15]. Specifically, BA patients were divided into mild-moderate persistent BA and severe persistent BA on the basis of clinical features described by GINA [13], whereas AR patients were also divided into mild-moderate persistent AR and severe persistent AR on the basis of visual analog scale (VAS) as described previously [14]. In the same ways, patients with AD were also divided into mild-moderate AD and severe AD on the basis of SCORAD index [15]. Venous blood from all studied patients and controls were taken and sera were stored in − 80 °C until analyzed.

Measurement of filaggrin protein, eosinophil major basic protein and immunoglobulin E in atopic patients

Levels of filaggrin, eosinophil MBP and total IgE were measured in the serum samples of all tested atopic patients and their levels were compared with their respective non-atopic healthy controls' sera. Serum filaggrin levels were measured by specific human filaggrin sandwich ELISA in accordance with the manufacturers' instructions (cat. # SEJ103Hu, Cloud-Clone Corp., Hubei, PRC.). Whereas, serum eosinophil MBP levels were measured by human eosinophil MBP specific sandwich ELISAs (cat. # SEB650Hu) according to their manufacturers' instructions (Cloud-Clone Corp., Hubei, PRC). Whereas, total IgE serum levels were measured by human IgE specific sandwich ELISA (cat. # 20783–72876, GenWay Biotech, CA, USA).

Statistical analysis

All statistical analysis was carried out by Graph Pad Prism version 5.0 (Graph Pad Software Inc., San Diego, CA, USA). One-way ANOVA of variance followed by Tukey–Kramer multiple comparisons test, or Two-way ANOVA of variance followed by Bonferroni comparisons test. $p < 0.05$ was considered significant. Results are expressed as the mean ± SEM unless stated otherwise.

Results

Filaggrin in different atopic disorders

In this study, we determined the serum levels of filaggrin in pediatric patients with different atopic disorders (n = 395) and their levels were compared with their respective non-atopic healthy pediatric controls (n = 410). The data showed filaggrin levels were significantly increased in different atopic patients when compared its levels in non-atopic healthy pediatric controls ($p < 0.0001$). The average serum filaggrin levels (± SEM) in all studied atopic subjects and non-atopic healthy controls were 7.20 ± 0.10 and 3.21 ± 0.13 ng/ml, respectively (Fig. 1a). Specifically, the average filaggrin levels (± SEM) in the patients sera with AD (n = 130), AR (n = 120), BA (n = 145) and their respective non-atopic controls (n = 410) were 9.36 ± 0.87, 6.50 ± 0.36, 8.50 ± 0.32 and 3.21 ± 0.13 ng/ml, respectively (Fig. 1b–d). Results pointed that among all tested atopic pediatric patients, AD patients contained highest filaggrin levels followed by BA and AR patients (Fig. 1).

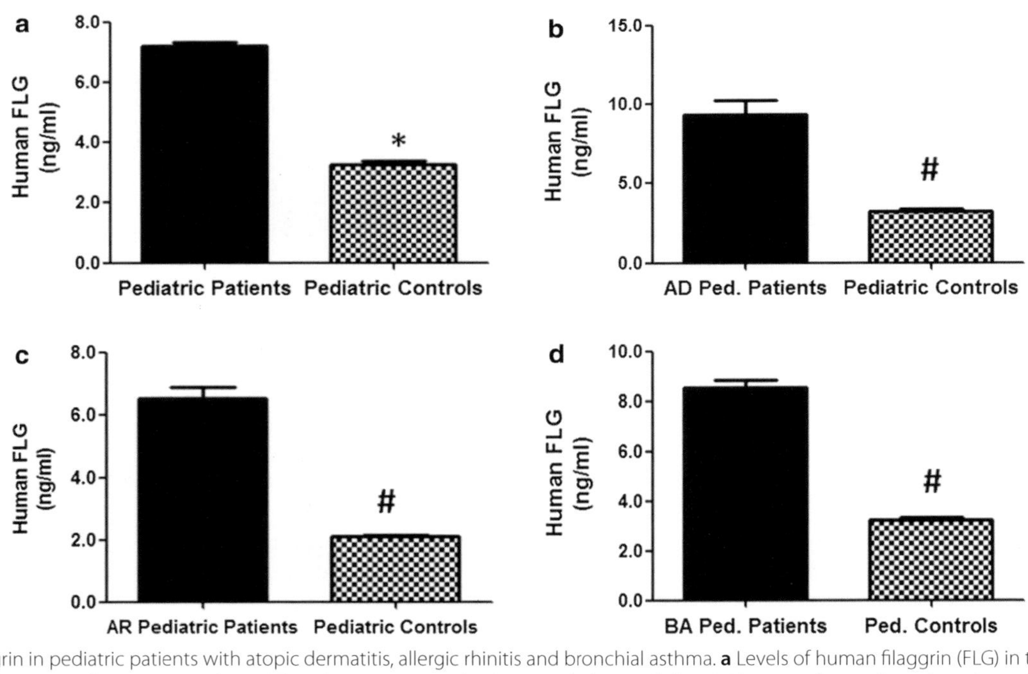

Fig. 1 Filaggrin in pediatric patients with atopic dermatitis, allergic rhinitis and bronchial asthma. **a** Levels of human filaggrin (FLG) in the sera of all studied atopic pediatric patients (n = 395) and non-atopic pediatric controls (n = 410). *$p < 0.01$ versus all tested atopic patients. **b** Levels of human FLG in the patients' sera of atopic dermatitis pediatric patients (AD Ped. Patients; n = 130) and non-atopic pediatric controls (n = 410). $^{\#}p < 0.001$ versus AD Ped. Patients. **c** Levels of human FLG in the patients' sera of allergic rhinitis pediatric patients (AR pediatric patients; n = 120) and non-atopic pediatric controls (n = 410). $^{\#}p < 0.001$ versus AR pediatric patients. **d** Levels of human FLG in the patients' sera of bronchial asthma pediatric patients (BA Ped. Patients; n = 145) and non-atopic pediatric controls (n = 410). $^{\#}p < 0.01$ versus AR Ped. Patients

Eosinophil major basic protein in different atopic disorders

The serum levels of eosinophil MBP in patients with different atopic disorders (n = 395) were found to be highly significantly higher as compared with respective non-atopic healthy pediatric controls (n = 410) (p < 0.001). The average eosinophil MBP levels (± SEM) in all studied atopic subjects and non-atopic controls were 10.99 ± 0.27 and 5.54 ± 0.21 ng/ml, respectively (Fig. 2a). Importantly, the average eosinophil MBP levels (± SEM) in the patients' sera with AD (n = 130), AR (n = 120) and BA (n = 145) were 11.97 ± 1.86, 14.39 ± 0.92 and 8.86 ± 0.77 ng/ml, respectively (Fig. 2b–d). These results not only showed the higher eosinophil MBP levels in all tested atopic patients but also pointed out that among all atopic pediatric patients, AR patients contained highest filaggrin levels followed by AD and BA patients (Fig. 2).

Total immunoglobulin E in different atopic disorders

The serum levels of total IgE in patients with different atopic disorders (n = 395) were found to be significantly higher as compared with respective non-atopic healthy pediatric controls (n = 410) (p < 0.001). The average IgE levels (± SEM) in all studied atopic subjects and non-atopic controls were 72.66 ± 5.38 ng/ml and 45.95 ± 2.05 ng/ml, respectively (Fig. 3a). Specifically, the average IgE levels (± SEM) in the patients sera with AD (n = 130), AR (n = 120) and BA (n = 145) were 96.19 ± 21.3 ng/ml, 82.17 ± 6.50 ng/ml and 60.58 ± 6.56 ng/ml, respectively (Fig. 3b–d). These results not only demonstrated significant higher levels of total IgE levels in these atopic patients, but also determined that pediatric patients with AD had highest total IgE level, followed by AR and BA patients (Fig. 3b–d).

Severity-related increase of filaggrin, eosinophil major basic protein and total immunoglobulin E in different atopic disorders

To provide further support to our hypothesis and to assess the protein levels of filaggrin, eosinophil MBP and total IgE in atopic subjects, patients with AD, AR and BA were divided into different groups based on their severity scores. The average human filaggrin (±) SEM in patients' sera with mild-moderate AD (n = 97), severe AD (n = 33), mild-moderate persistent AR (n = 83), severe persistent AR (n = 37), mild-moderate persistent BA (n = 93) and severe persistent BA (n = 52) was 6.58 ± 0.71, 12.14 ± 1.08, 4.69 ± 0.15, 8.31 ± 0.69, 6.68 ± 0.24 and 10.32 ± 0.51 ng/ml, respectively (Fig. 4a).

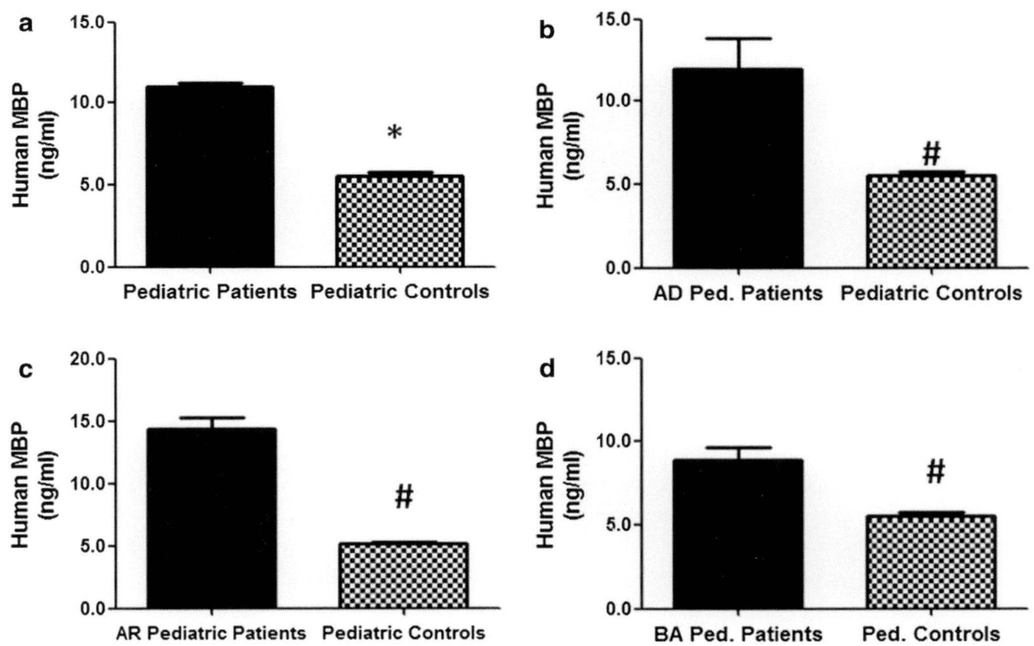

Fig. 2 Eosinophil major basic protein in pediatric patients with atopic dermatitis, allergic rhinitis and bronchial asthma. **a** Levels of eosinophil major basic protein (MBP) in the sera of all studied atopic pediatric patients (n = 395) and non-atopic pediatric controls (n = 410). *p < 0.001 versus all tested atopic patients. **b** Levels of eosinophil MBP in the patients' sera of atopic dermatitis pediatric patients (AD Ped. Patients; n = 130) and non-atopic pediatric controls (n = 410). #p < 0.001 versus AD Ped. Patients. **c** Levels of eosinophil MBP in the patients' sera of allergic rhinitis pediatric patients (AR pediatric patients; n = 120) and non-atopic pediatric controls (n = 410). #p < 0.0001 versus AR pediatric patients. **d** Levels of eosinophil MBP in the patients' sera of bronchial asthma pediatric patients (BA Ped. Patients; n = 145) and non-atopic pediatric controls (n = 410). #p < 0.001 versus AR Ped. Patients

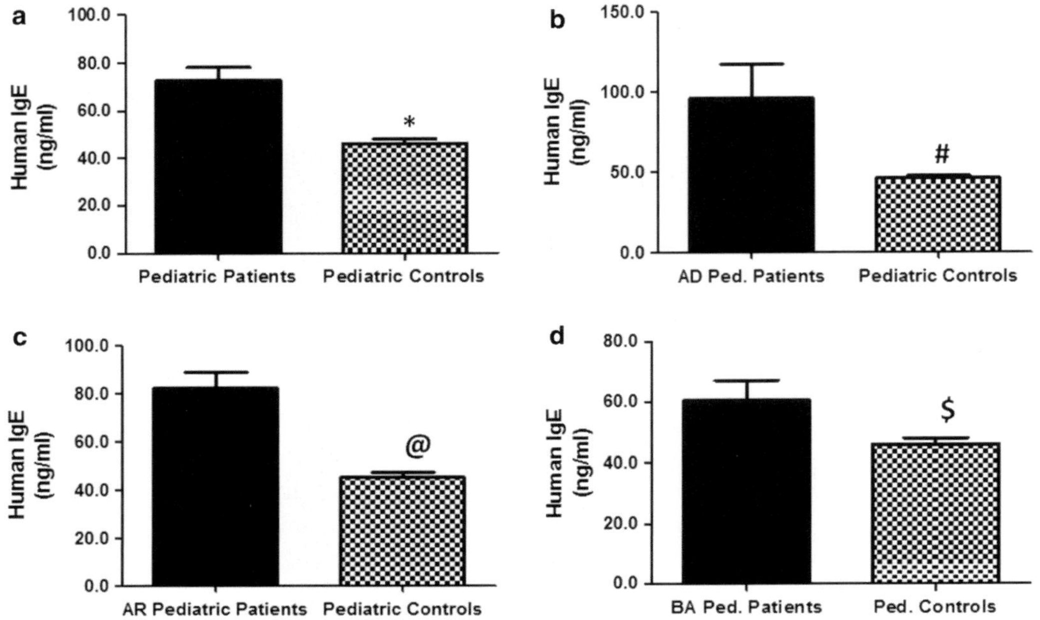

Fig. 3 Immunoglobulin E in pediatric patients with atopic dermatitis, allergic rhinitis and bronchial asthma. **a** Levels of human immunoglobulin E (Human IgE) in the sera of all studied atopic pediatric patients (n = 395) and non-atopic pediatric controls (n = 410). *p < 0.01 versus all tested atopic patients. **b** Levels of human IgE in the patients' sera of atopic dermatitis pediatric patients (AD Ped. Patients; n = 130) and non-atopic pediatric controls (n = 410). #p < 0.001 versus AD Ped. Patients. **c** Levels of human IgE in the patients' sera of allergic rhinitis pediatric patients (AR pediatric patients; n = 120) and non-atopic pediatric controls (n = 410). @p < 0.01 versus AR pediatric patients. **d** Levels of human IgE in the patients' sera of bronchial asthma pediatric patients (BA Ped. Patients; n = 145) and non-atopic pediatric controls (n = 410). $p < 0.05 versus AR Ped. Patients

Whereas, the average human eosinophil MBP (±) SEM in patients' sera with mild-moderate AD (n = 97), severe AD (n = 33), mild-moderate persistent AR (n = 83), severe persistent AR (n = 37), mild-moderate persistent BA (n = 93) and severe persistent BA (n = 52) was 9.60 ± 1.96, 14.34 ± 1.21, 11.47 ± 0.81, 17.31 ± 1.31, 7.41 ± 0.62 and 10.31 ± 0.82 ng/ml, respectively (Fig. 4b). The average human total IgE (±) SEM in patients' sera with mild-moderate AD (n = 97), severe AD (n = 33), mild-moderate persistent AR (n = 83), severe persistent AR (n = 37), mild-moderate persistent BA (n = 93) and severe persistent BA (n = 52) was 67.18 ± 10.31, 125.21 ± 40.31, 66.97 ± 8.31, 97.37 ± 5.19, 40.93 ± 7.82 and 80.23 ± 5.25 ng/ml, respectively (Fig. 4c). These results demonstrated that filaggrin protein, eosinophil MBP or total IgE were significantly increased in the serum of patients with severe atopic disorders when compared with mild-moderate patients ($p < 0.05$).

Discussion

This study demonstrated the role of filaggrin protein, eosinophil major basic protein and immunoglobulin E in the pathogenesis of pediatric patients with atopic dermatitis, allergic rhinitis and bronchial asthma. The filaggrin is a key structural protein required for the normal biogenesis and physiology of the stratum corneum [16]. It is now well documented that genetic variants of filaggrin was found in up to 50% of AD patients, which enhanced our understanding on the role of filaggrin, not only in the skin barrier defect or AD pathogenesis but also in the subsequent progression of an atopic march [17]. The atopic march concept describes the progression of atopic disorders from AD to AR in infants and from AD to BA in childhood [3, 17]. The mutations in filaggrin gene have now been considered as a major risk factor for AD onset especially in pediatric patients [18]. Furthermore, not only in AD patients, filaggrin gene mutations have also been reported in patients with AR and BA [19, 20]. Importantly, it has also been shown that almost 50% of all severe cases of eczema may have at least one mutated filaggrin gene [20–23]. Truncation mutations R501X and 2284del4 are considered to be the most common mutations among the white population especially a population from the Tayside and Dumfries of Scotland [21, 22]. In addition, the barrier defect has also seen in filaggrin null which carriers also appears to lead to increased asthma susceptibility and exacerbations. Filaggrin deficiency is one of the top genome-wide genetic determinants of asthma, along with the variants found that regulate ORMDL3 expression [20–23]. In view of these, the

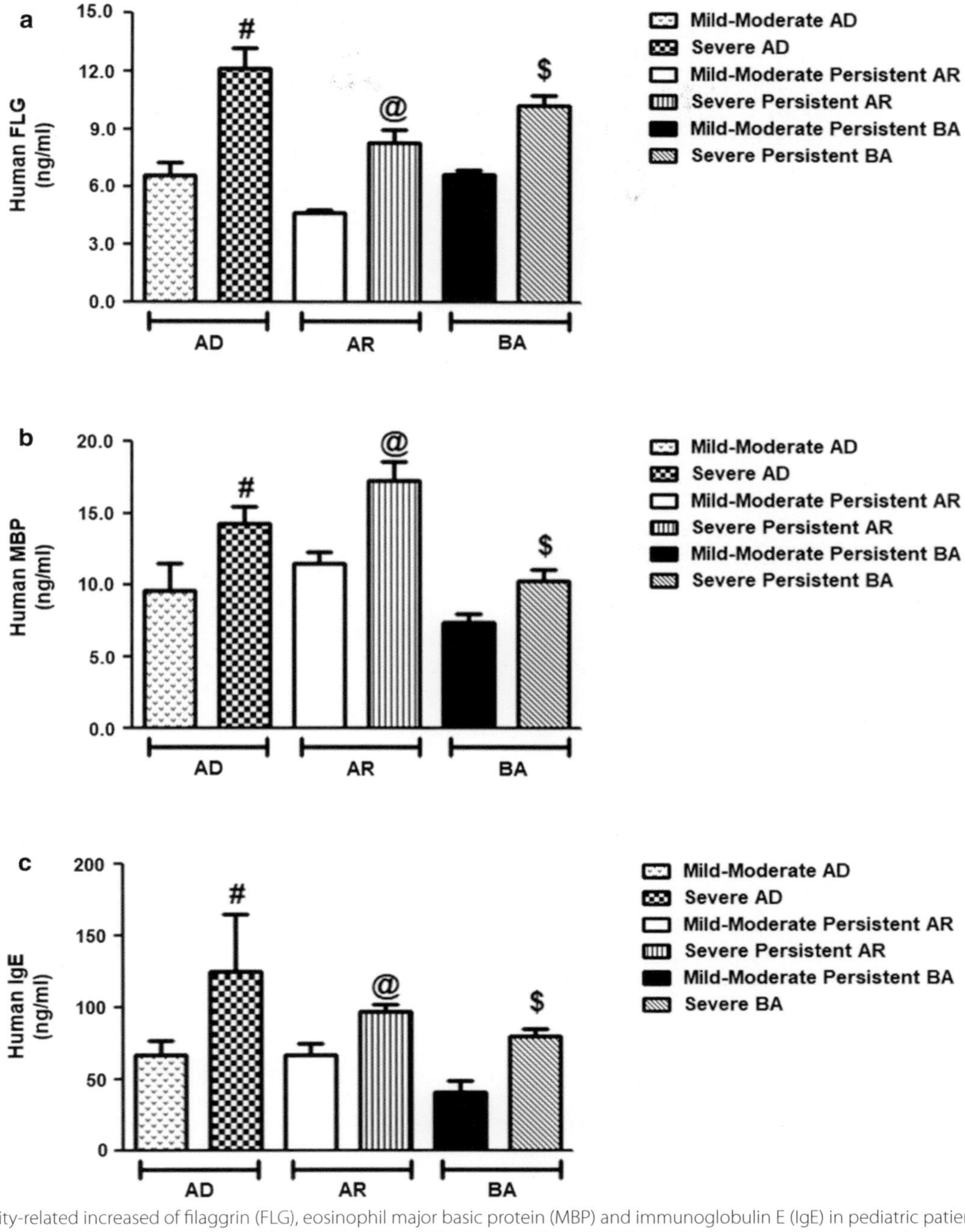

Fig. 4 Severity-related increased of filaggrin (FLG), eosinophil major basic protein (MBP) and immunoglobulin E (IgE) in pediatric patients with atopic dermatitis (AD), allergic rhinitis (AR) and bronchial asthma (BA). **a** Levels of human FLG protein in mild-moderate AD patients' sera (n = 97), severe AD patients' sera (n = 33), mild-moderate persistent AR (n = 93), severe persistent AR (n = 52), mild-moderate persistent BA (n = 83), severe persistent AR (n = 37). $^{\#}p < 0.05$ versus mild-moderate AD; $^{@}p < 0.05$ versus mild-moderate AR; $^{\$}p < 0.05$ versus mild-moderate BA. **b** Levels of human MBP in mild-moderate AD patients' sera (n = 97), severe AD patients' sera (n = 33), mild-moderate persistent AR (n = 93), severe persistent AR (n = 52), mild-moderate persistent BA (n = 83), severe persistent AR (n = 37). $^{\#}p < 0.05$ versus mild-moderate AD; $^{@}p < 0.05$ versus mild-moderate AR; $^{\$}p < 0.05$ versus mild-moderate BA. **c** Levels of human IgE in mild-moderate AD patients' sera (n = 97), severe AD patients' sera (n = 33), mild-moderate persistent AR (n = 93), severe persistent AR (n = 52), mild-moderate persistent BA (n = 83), severe persistent AR (n = 37). $^{\#}p < 0.05$ versus mild-moderate AD; $^{@}p < 0.05$ versus mild/moderate AR; $^{\$}p < 0.05$ versus mild-moderate BA

present study was hypothesized to investigate whether mutations in filaggrin gene also effect on its protein level in the serum of BA and other allergic disorders. To the best of our knowledge, the present study for the very first time showed elevated serum levels of filaggrin protein, not only in AD and BA pediatric patients but also in patients with AR. Specifically, the data from the present study show that the filaggrin in the serum of these pediatric patients was significantly increased as compared with their non-atopic healthy pediatric controls. Not only have these, data also pointed out that filaggrin levels were markedly increased in children with AD, followed by BA and AR patients. An increased of serum levels of filaggrin in these atopic patients not only suggesting its dysfunctionality at protein level, but also indicates its potential role in the pathogenesis and/or progression of these atopic disorders.

Increased of filaggrin gene mutations has previously been detected in AD, AR and BA, but the significance of serum levels of filaggrin protein in the initiation and development explaining the mechanism of these atopic disorders remains largely unexplored. In this study, when the AD, AR or BA patients were divided into two groups (mild-moderate and severe) based on their severity scores [13–15], both groups showed higher serum levels of filaggrin protein than were observed in healthy controls, but the levels were much greater in the severe patients groups, suggesting the involvement of filaggrin protein in ongoing atopic disorders. These findings strongly support the role of filaggrin protein in the pathogenesis of AD, AR or BA and in the subsequent progression along with the atopic march. Our results not only further support the potential role of filaggrin protein in these atopic disorders, but also suggest that targeting serum levels of filaggrin may be useful in predicting the severity status of atopic disorders in pediatric patients.

Eosinophils are well known for their vital role in allergic inflammatory processes and the eosinophil major basic protein is the most abundant constituent of the eosinophil secondary granules [24]. Evidences from previous studies have shown that the eosinophil and its granular proteins might be assumed to mediate the hypersensitivity disorders [24]. In this study, the serum levels of eosinophil MBP were determined in different atopic pediatric patients and were found to be significantly high as compared with their controls. Moreover, our results also pointed out that out of all tested atopic patients, eosinophil MBP levels were found to be highest in AR patients, followed by AD and BA. In a line with our results, a previous study on tissue damage has shown that MBP has direct association with eosinophil infiltration in BA pediatric patients [24]. In addition, activated eosinophils and depositions of eosinophil granular proteins were found in AD skin biopsies [25]. Furthermore, studies have also reported higher levels of MBP in biological fluids of asthmatic patients [26]. All these studies supported our findings and clearly suggesting a direct role of eosinophil MBP in pediatric patients with atopic disorders. To further validate our central hypothesis that initiation of AD, AR or BA may be mediated by increased eosinophil's MBP, serum eosinophil's MBP was determined in mild-moderate atopic patients and their results were compared with severe atopic patients. Our novel results showed marked increased of eosinophil's MBP in severe atopic patients as compared with mild-moderate atopic patients. Increased levels of eosinophil's MBP in severe patients with AD, AR or BA, suggesting another important potential mechanism involved in the pathogenesis and/or progression of these atopic disorders.

Atopic disorders in pediatric patients can be a familial or familial propensity, which involved in the production of IgE antibodies and its associated sensitization in response to various known or unknown factors particularly environmental triggers, which linked with atopic march especially in pediatric patients [27]. The IgE sensitization and severity of atopic disorders have been well connected with each other, particularly in AD progression and BA persistence [28]. It is important to point out that it is reported that many patients with allergic disorders have elevated levels of total IgE [28–32]; however, there is no specific cutoff value that discriminates patients with allergic disorders from those without, and there is considerable overlap. Thus, total IgE by itself is rarely adequate to diagnose allergic disorders. Studies have shown that adults with IgE greater than 66 IU/ml have a 37-fold greater risk of having allergen-specific IgE antibodies to aeroallergens compared with those patients with the lowest levels of total IgE [29]. In one study, school-aged children had a mean IgE level of 51 IU/ml. Children with both AD and asthma had mean IgE levels of 985 IU/ml; those with asthma alone, 305 IU/ml; those with eczema alone, 273 IU/ml, and those with AR, 171 IU/ml [30]. Using a total serum IgE level of 100 IU/ml to discriminate allergic from non-allergic patients, the sensitivity was 78% for patients with asthma and 60% for AR, but 20% of patients were misclassified [32]. Although there is no specific cut off value of total IgE for atopic disorders but it's abnormally is well reported, therefore it assumes to be a useful biomarker for the diagnosis of AD, AR or BA in addition with other atopic markers as defined here. In the current study, we found that higher levels of total IgE in different atopic disorders as compared with their respective non-atopic pediatric controls. Most importantly, our data also pointed out that out of all studied atopic disorders in children, total IgE levels were highest in AD patients, followed by AR and BA. The enhanced total IgE levels observed in atopic patients in this study drew our attention to evaluate its levels in different atopic subjects with varying disease severity. Our data clearly showed that the total IgE levels were significantly higher in the group of patients with high disease severity scores as compared with mild-moderate disease groups of AD, AR or BA pediatric patients. The increased of serum levels of total IgE in severe atopic patients suggest that IgE levels in the serum of these subjects are associated with increased disease activity in these atopic patients. These results are well supported by previous findings, showed that eczema patients with IgE antibodies against common environmental allergens were at higher risk for the development/progression of atopic disorders especially in pediatric patients [33, 34]. The increased levels of IgE observed in the patients with AD, AR or BA in the present study, together with significant increases of filaggrin protein and eosinophil MBP, provide strong evidences of their involvement in these disorders and clearly indicating that filaggrin protein, eosinophil MBP and total IgE are useful in evaluating of AD, AR or BA disease activity, and would therefore be helpful for predicting the progression of these atopic disorders in pediatric patients.

Conclusions

Our data clearly show that the levels of filaggrin protein, eosinophil MBP and total IgE were increased in pediatric patients with atopic dermatitis, allergic rhinitis and bronchial asthma. These results conclude that serum levels of filaggrin, eosinophil MBP and total IgE might be useful in the diagnosis of these atopic disorders in pediatric patients. Longitudinal studies in atopic pediatric patients are necessary to invent novel agents that can antagonize or modify the effects of filaggrin, eosinophil MBP or total IgE on the atopic march, thereby we can better treat, prevent or control these atopic disorders especially in pediatric patients.

Authors' contributions

AAAZ, KZ, GBS, AAEM, ME, AAAR participated in study design, coordination, sample collection and were responsible for obtaining patients written consents. RHS, AAA, TS carried out experimentation, statistical analysis and data interpretation. ZR has consulted for data interpretation and manuscript drafting. All authors read and approved the final manuscript.

Author details

[1] Department of Medical Biochemistry, College of Medicine, Qassim University, P.O. Box 6655, Buraidah 51452, Saudi Arabia. [2] Department of Pediatrics, College of Medicine, Qassim University, Buraidah, Saudi Arabia. [3] Department of Dermatology, College of Medicine, King Saud University, Riyadh, Saudi Arabia. [4] Research Center, College of Medicine, Qassim University, Buraidah, Saudi Arabia. [5] Department of Medicine, College of Medicine, Qassim University, Buraidah, Saudi Arabia. [6] Department of Dermatology, College of Medicine, Qassim University, Buraidah, Saudi Arabia.

Acknowledgements

The authors thank Mr. Casimero A. Victoria (senior laboratory technologist) for help in experimentation.

Funding

This work was supported by the grant from National Plan for Science, Technology and Innovation of KSA (NSTIP # 11-BIO1459-09).

References

1. Moreno MA. JAMA pediatrics patient page. Atopic diseases in children. JAMA Pediatr. 2016;170:96.
2. Spergel JM. Epidemiology of atopic dermatitis and atopic march in children. Immunol Allergy Clin North Am. 2010;30:269–80.
3. Spergel JM, Paller AS. Atopic dermatitis and the atopic march. J Allergy ClinImmunol. 2003;112:S118–27.
4. Gupta J, Johansson E, Bernstein JA, Chakraborty R, Khurana Hershey GK, Rothenberg ME, Mersha TB. Resolving the etiology of atopic disorders by using genetic analysis of racial ancestry. J Allergy ClinImmunol. 2016;138:676–99.
5. Thyssen JP, Linneberg A, Johansen JD, Carlsen BC, Zachariae C, Meldgaard M, Szecsi PB, Stender S, Menné T. Atopic diseases by filaggrin mutations and birth year. Allergy. 2012;67:705–8.
6. Mischke D, Korge BP, Marenholz I, Volz A, Ziegler A. Genes encoding structural proteins of epidermal cornification and S100 calcium-binding proteins form a gene complex ("epidermal differentiation complex") on human chromosome 1q21. J Invest Dermatol. 1996;106:989–92.
7. Al-Shobaili HA, Ahmed AA, Alnomair N, Alobead ZA, Rasheed Z. Molecular genetic of atopic dermatitis: an update. Int J Health Sci. 2016;10:96–120.
8. Sandilands A, Sutherland C, Irvine AD, McLean WH. Filaggrin in the frontline: role in skin barrier function and disease. J Cell Sci. 2009;122:1285–94.
9. Batchelor JM, Grindlay DJ, Williams HC. What's new in atopic eczema? An analysis of systematic reviews published in 2008 and 2009. Clin Exp Dermatol. 2010;35:823–7.
10. Laske N, Bunikowski R, Niggemann B. Extraordinarily high serum IgE levels and consequences for atopic phenotypes. Ann Allergy Asthma Immunol. 2003;91:202.
11. Zedan K, Rasheed Z, Farouk Y, Alzolibani AA, Bin Saif G, Ismail HA, Al Robaee AA. Immunoglobulin e, interleukin-18 and interleukin-12 in patients with atopic dermatitis: correlation with disease activity. J Clin Diagn Res. 2015;9:WC01–5.
12. Bystrom J, Garcia RC, Hakansson L, Karawajczyk M, Moberg L, Soukka J, Venge P. Eosinophil cationic protein is stored in, but not produced by peripheral blood neutrophils. Clin Exp Allergy. 2002;32:1082–91.
13. Koshak EA. Classification of asthma according to revised 2006 GINA: evolution from severity to control. Ann Thorac Med. 2007;2:45–46.
14. Bousquet PJ, Combescure C, Neukirch F, Klossek JM, Mechin H, Daures JP. Visual analog scales can assess the severity of rhinitis graded according to ARIA guidelines. Allergy. 2007;62:367–72.
15. Oranje AP, Glazenburg EJ, Wolkerstorfer A, de Waard-van der Spek FB. Waard-van der Spek FB. Practical issues on interpretation of scoring atopic dermatitis: the SCORAD index, objective SCORAD and the three-item severity score. Br J Dermatol. 2007;157:645–8.
16. McAleer MA, Irvine AD. The multifunctional role of filaggrin in allergic skin disease. J Allergy ClinImmunol. 2013;131:280–91.
17. Marenholz I, Nickel R, Rüschendorf F, Schulz F, Esparza-Gordillo J, et al. Filaggrin loss-of- function mutations predispose to phenotypes involved in the atopic march. J Allergy Clin Immunol. 2006;118:866–71.

18. Stemmler S, Parwez Q, Petrasch-Parwez E, Epplen JT, Hoffjan S. Two common loss-of-function mutations within the filaggrin gene predispose for early onset of atopic dermatitis. J Invest Dermatol. 2007;127:722–4.
19. Bantz SK, Zhu Z, Zhen T. The atopic march: progression from atopic dermatitis to allergic rhinitis and asthma. J Clin Cell Immunol. 2014;5(2):202.
20. Ying S, Meng Q, Corrigan CJ, Lee TH. Lack of filaggrin expression in the human bronchial mucosa. J Allergy ClinImmunol. 2006;118:1386–8.
21. Basu K, Palmer CN, Lipworth BJ, McLean WH, Terron-Kwiatkowski A, Zhao Y, Liao H, Smith FJ, Mitra A, Mukhopadhyay S. Filaggrin null mutations are associated with increased asthma exacerbations in children and young adults. Allergy. 2008;63:1211–7.
22. Palmer CN, Ismail T, Lee SP, Terron-Kwiatkowski A, Zhao Y, Liao H, Smith FJ, McLean WH, Mukhopadhyay S. Filaggrin null mutations are associated with increased asthma severity in children and young adults. J Allergy Clin Immunol. 2007;120:64–8.
23. Henderson J, Northstone K, Lee SP, Liao H, Zhao Y, Pembrey M, Mukhopadhyay S, Smith GD, Palmer CN, McLean WH, Irvine AD. The burden of disease associated with filaggrin mutations: a population-based, longitudinal birth cohort study. J Allergy Clin Immunol. 2008;121(872–7):e9.
24. Acharya KR, Ackerman SJ. Eosinophil granule proteins: form and function. J Biol Chem. 2014;289:17406–15.
25. Bruijnzeel PL, Rihs S, Betz S. Eosinophilic granulocytes and their significance in allergic diseases. Schweiz Med Wochenschr. 1992;122:173–80.
26. Wassom DL, Loegering DA, Solley GO, Moore SB, Schooley RT, Fauci AS, Gleich GJ. Elevated serum levels of the eosinophil granule major basic-protein in patients with eosinophilia. J Clin Invest. 1981;67:651–61.
27. Johansson SG, Bieber T, Dahl R, Friedmann PS, Lanier BQ, et al. Revised nomenclature for allergy for global use: report of the Nomenclature Review Committee of the World Allergy Organization, October 2003. J Allergy Clin Immunol. 2004;113:832–6.
28. Wuthrich B, Schmid-Grendelmeier P. Natural course of AEDS. Allergy. 2002;57:267–8.
29. Omenaas E, Bakke P, Elsayed S, Hanoa R, Gulsvik A. Total and specific serum IgE levels in adults: relationship to sex, age and environmental factors. Clin Exp Allergy. 1994;24:530–9.
30. Wittig HJ, Belloit J, De Fillippi I, Royal G. Age-related serum immunoglobulin E levels in healthy subjects and in patients with allergic disease. J Allergy Clin Immunol. 1980;66:305–13.
31. Stone KD, Prussin C, Metcalfe DD. IgE, mast cells, basophils, and eosinophils. J Allergy Clin Immunol. 2010;125:S73–80.
32. Klink M, Cline MG, Halonen M, Burrows B. Problems in defining normal limits for serum IgE. J Allergy Clin Immunol. 1990;85:440–4.
33. Novembre E, Cianferoni A, Lombardi E, Bernardini R, Pucci N, Vierucci A. Natural history of "intrinsic" atopic dermatitis. Allergy. 2001;56:452–3.
34. Mavroudi A, Karagiannidou A, Xinias I, Cassimos D, Karantaglis N, Farmaki E, Imvrios G, Fotoulaki M, Eboriadou M, Tsanakas J. Assessment of IgE-mediated food allergies in children with atopic dermatitis. Allergol Immunopathol (Madr). 2017;45:77–81.

Permissions

All chapters in this book were first published in CMA, by BioMed Central; hereby published with permission under the Creative Commons Attribution License or equivalent. Every chapter published in this book has been scrutinized by our experts. Their significance has been extensively debated. The topics covered herein carry significant findings which will fuel the growth of the discipline. They may even be implemented as practical applications or may be referred to as a beginning point for another development.

The contributors of this book come from diverse backgrounds, making this book a truly international effort. This book will bring forth new frontiers with its revolutionizing research information and detailed analysis of the nascent developments around the world.

We would like to thank all the contributing authors for lending their expertise to make the book truly unique. They have played a crucial role in the development of this book. Without their invaluable contributions this book wouldn't have been possible. They have made vital efforts to compile up to date information on the varied aspects of this subject to make this book a valuable addition to the collection of many professionals and students.

This book was conceptualized with the vision of imparting up-to-date information and advanced data in this field. To ensure the same, a matchless editorial board was set up. Every individual on the board went through rigorous rounds of assessment to prove their worth. After which they invested a large part of their time researching and compiling the most relevant data for our readers.

The editorial board has been involved in producing this book since its inception. They have spent rigorous hours researching and exploring the diverse topics which have resulted in the successful publishing of this book. They have passed on their knowledge of decades through this book. To expedite this challenging task, the publisher supported the team at every step. A small team of assistant editors was also appointed to further simplify the editing procedure and attain best results for the readers.

Apart from the editorial board, the designing team has also invested a significant amount of their time in understanding the subject and creating the most relevant covers. They scrutinized every image to scout for the most suitable representation of the subject and create an appropriate cover for the book.

The publishing team has been an ardent support to the editorial, designing and production team. Their endless efforts to recruit the best for this project, has resulted in the accomplishment of this book. They are a veteran in the field of academics and their pool of knowledge is as vast as their experience in printing. Their expertise and guidance has proved useful at every step. Their uncompromising quality standards have made this book an exceptional effort. Their encouragement from time to time has been an inspiration for everyone.

The publisher and the editorial board hope that this book will prove to be a valuable piece of knowledge for researchers, students, practitioners and scholars across the globe.

List of Contributors

G. Walter Canonica
Respiratory and Allergy Clinic, DIMI-Department of Internal Medicine, University of Genoa, IRCCS Aou San Martino, Largo Rosanna Benzi 10, 16132 Genoa, Italy

Massimo Triggiani
Division of Allergy and Clinical Immunology, University of Salerno, Salerno, Italy

GianEnrico Senna
Allergy Unit, University Hospital Verona, Verona, Italy

M. S. Magnoni F. Arpinelli and A. Rizzi
Medical and Scientific Department, GlaxoSmithKline, Verona, Italy

M. Caminati and G. Senna
Asthma Center and Allergy Unit, Verona University Hospital, Verona, Italy

G. W. Canonica
Personalized Medicine Asthma & Allergy Clinic, Humanitas University-Research Hospital, Rozzano, Milano, Italy

A. Linneberg
Research Centre for Prevention and Health, The Capital Region of Denmark, Copenhagen, Denmark
Department of Clinical Experimental Research, Rigshospitalet, Copenhagen, Denmark
Department of Clinical Medicine, Faculty of Health and Medical Sciences, University of Copenhagen, Copenhagen, Denmark

K. Dam Petersen
Department of Business and Management, Faculty of Social Sciences, Aalborg University, Aalborg, Denmark

J. Hahn-Pedersen, E. Hammerby and N. Serup-Hansen
ALK, Hørsholm, Denmark

N. Boxall
MAPI, London, UK

Paola Lucia Minciullo and Stefania Isola
School and Division of Allergy and Clinical Immunology, Department of Clinical and Experimental Medicine, University Hospital "G. Martino", Messina, Italy

Sebastiano Gangemi
School and Division of Allergy and Clinical Immunology, Department of Clinical and Experimental Medicine, University Hospital "G. Martino", Messina, Italy
Institute of Applied Sciences and Intelligent Systems (ISASI), Messina Unit, Messina, Italy

Antonio Cascio
Department of Health Promotion Sciences and Mother and Child Care "G. D'Alessandro", University of Palermo, Palermo, Italy

Gianfranco Calogiuri
Pneumology and Allergy Department, Hospital Sacro Cuore, Gallipoli, Lecce, Italy

Elisabetta Di Leo
Section of Allergy and Clinical Immunology, Unit of Internal Medicine-"F. Miulli" Hospital, Acquaviva delle Fonti, Bari, Italy

Lavjay Butani
Department of Pediatrics, University of California Davis School of Medicine, Sacramento, USA

Stefano Pizzimenti
Allergy Outpatients' Clinic, ASL-TO3, Ospedale Civile "E. Agnelli", Pinerolo, Turin, Italy

Cristoforo Incorvaia
ASST Specialistic Center Gaetano Pini/CTO, Milan, Italy

Luigi Macchia and Eustachio Nettis
Section of Allergy and Clinical Immunology, Department of Internal Medicine and Infectious Diseases, University of Bari Medical School, Bari, Italy

Carina Gabriela Uasuf, Caterina Di Sano, Elisabetta Pace and Mark Gjomarkaj
Allergy Diseases Center "Prof. G. Bonsignore", Institute of Biomedicine and Molecular Immunology "A. Monroy"(IBIM)-National Research Council (CNR), Palermo, Italy

Danilo Villalta and Maria Elisabetta Conte
Allergy and Clinical Immunology Unit, A.O "S. Maria degli Angeli di Pordenone", Pordenone, Italy

Maria Barrale, Vincenzo Cantisano and Ignazio Brusca
Clinical Pathology, Allergy Unit, Buccheri La Ferla Hospital, Palermo, Italy

Sebastiano Gangemi
School and Division of Allergy and Clinical Immunology, Department of Clinical and Experimental Medicine, University of Messina, Messina, Italy

Ilaria Massaro
Cell Therapy and Transfusion Medicine, Azienda Ospedaliero Universitaria Careggi, Florence, Largo Brambilla 1, 50134 Florence, Italy

Oliviero Rossi
Allergy Unit, Azienda Ospedaliero Universitaria Careggi, Florence, Florence, Italy

Cristoforo Incorvaia
Cardiac Pulmonary Rehabilitation, Centro Specialistico Gaetano Pini CTO, Milan, Italy

Carlo Lombardi
Allergy and Pneumology Departmental Unit, Fondazione Poliambulanza Hospital, Brescia, Italy

Tomás Chivato
Decanato. Facultad de Medicina, Facultad de Medicina Universidad CEU San Pablo. Grupo Hospitales HM, Avda. Montepríncipe s/n, Boadilla del Monte, 28668 Madrid, Spain

Pedro Álvarez-Calderón
Hospital Clínico Universitario de Santiago, La Coruña, Spain

Carmen Panizo
Hospital Ntra Sra del Prado, Toledo, Spain

Ricardo Abengozar
Hospital Virgen del Valle, Toledo, Spain

César Alías
Clínica Corachán, Barcelona, Spain

Ali Al-Baech and José Arias-Irigoyen
Private Office, Huelva, Spain

M. José Caballero
Clínica ASISA, Córdoba, Spain

Lluis Conill
Hospital Can Misses, Ibiza, Spain

Silvia de Miguel
Policlínico Salud 4, Madrid, Spain

Rafael Laguna
Private Office, Madrid, Spain

Joan Martínez-Benazet
Hospital Ntra Sra de Meritxell, Escaldes-Engordany, Andorra

Francisco Matoses
Hospital General, Valencia, Spain

Jose Camilo Martínez-Alonso
Hospital Virgen de la Concha, Zamora, Spain

Lourdes Mendizábal
Clínica Virgen de Fátima, Seville, Spain

Celsa Pérez-Carral
Hospital Comarcal da Costa, Lugo, Spain

Carlos Puerto
Private Office, Asturias, Spain

Joan Serra-Batllés
Hospital de Vic, Barcelona, Spain

Adolfo Vélez
Hospital San Juan de Dios, León, Spain

Jonathan Vicente
Hospital General, Soria, Spain

Fernando de la Torre
ALK-Abelló, S.A, Madrid, Spain

Fabrizio De Luca, Laura Michelina Losappio, Corrado Mirone, Jan Walter Schroeder, Maria Gloria Aversano, Joseph Scibilia and Elide Anna Pastorello
Department of Allergology and Immunology, Ospedale Metropolitano Niguarda Ca' Granda, Piazza Ospedale Maggiore, 3, 20162 Milan, Italy

Antonella Citterio
Department of Burn/Intensive Care, Ospedale Metropolitano Niguarda Ca' Granda, Milan, Italy

Manuela Capone, Laura Maggi, Veronica Santarlasci, Maria Caterina Rossi, Alessio Mazzoni, Gianni Montaini, Francesco Liotta, Enrico Maggi, Marie Pierre Piccinni, Sergio Romagnani and Lorenzo Cosmi
Department of Experimental and Clinical Medicine and DENOTHE Center, University of Florence, 50134 Florence, Italy

Francesco Annunziato
Department of Experimental and Clinical Medicine and DENOTHE Center, University of Florence, 50134 Florence, Italy

Department of Internal Medicine, University of Florence, Viale

Rolando Cimaz
Anna Meyer Children's Hospital and University of Florence, 50134, Florence, Italy

Matteo Ramazzotti
Dept. of Biomedical Experimental and Clinical Sciences "Mario Serio", University of Florence, 50134 Florence, Italy

Giusi Barra
Dept. of Clinical & Experimental Medicine, Second University of Naples, 80131 Naples, Italy

Raffaele De Palma
Dept. of Clinical & Experimental Medicine, Second University of Naples, 80131 Naples, Italy
Institute of Protein Biochemistry, CNR, 80131, Naples, Italy

Pieraccini
Department of Internal Medicine, University of Florence, Viale

Donatella Macchia
SS Allergology and Clinical Immunology, S. Giovanni di Dio Hospital, Florence, Italy

Giovanni Melioli
Respiratory Diseases and Allergy, University of Genoa, IRCCS AOU S. Martino-IST, Genoa, Italy

Valerio Pravettoni and Marta Piantanida
Allergology and Immunology Unit, IRCCS Ca' Granda, Osp. Maggiore Policlinico, Milan, Italy

Eleonora Nucera and Domenico Schiavino
Servizio di Allergologia, Policlinico Gemelli, Rome, Italy

Marco Caminati
Allergy Unit, Verona University and General Hospital, Verona, Italy

Corrado Campochiaro and Mona-Rita Yacoub
Department of Allergy and Clinical Immunology, IRCCS San Raffaele Hospital, Milan, Italy

Roberto Paganelli
Department of Medicine and Science of Ageing, G. d'Annunzio University, Chieti, Italy

Mario Di Gioacchino
Unit of Allergy and Immunotoxicology, CeSi, "G. d'Annunzio" University Foundation, Chieti, Italy

Erminia Ridolo and Irene Martignago
Medicine and Surgery Department, University of Parma, Via Gramsci 14, 43126 Parma, Italy

Anti Rogkakou and Giovanni Passalacqua
Allergy and Respiratory Diseases Clinic, DIMI, University of Genoa, IRCCS AOU San Martino-IST, Genoa, Italy

Maria Teresa Ventura
Department of Interdisciplinary Medicine, University of Bari, Bari, Italy

Cristoforo Incorvaia
Cardiac/Pulmonary Rehabilitation, ASST Pini/CTO, Milan, Italy

Gabriele Di Lorenzo
Dipartimento BioMedico di Medicina Interna e Specialistica (Di.Bi.M.I.S), Università di Palermo, Palermo, Italy

Erminia Ridolo, Valerie Melli, Gianluigi De' Angelis and Irene Martignago
Department of Clinical and Experimental Medicine, University of Parma, via Gramsci, 14, 43100 Parma, Italy

Adam Tobias Fox and George du Toit
Division of Asthma, Allergy and Lung Biology, Guy's and St. Thomas' NHS Foundation Trust, London SE1 7EH, UK

Ru-Xin Foong
Division of Asthma, Allergy and Lung Biology, Guy's and St. Thomas' NHS Foundation Trust, London SE1 7EH, UK
Institute of Child Health, University College of London, London, UK

Graham Roberts
University of Southampton and National Institute for Health Research Respiratory Biomedical Research Unit, Southampton and David Hide Centre, Southampton, UK

Gennaro Tartarisco and Giovanni Pioggia
Messina Unit, National Research Council of Italy (CNR)-Institute of Applied Science and Intelligent System (ISASI), Messina, Italy

Alessandro Tonacci and Lucia Billeci
Pisa Unit, National Research Council of Italy (CNR)-Institute of Clinical Physiology (IFC), Pisa, Italy

Paola Lucia Minciullo and Sebastiano Gangemi
School and Division of Allergy and Clinical Immunology, Department of Clinical and Experimental Medicine, University Hospital "G. Martino", Messina, Italy

Cristoforo Incorvaia
Cardiac/Pulmonary Rehabilitation, ASST PINI/CTO, Via Bignami 1, Milan, Italy

Marie-Pierre Piccinni, Letizia Lombardelli, Federica Logiodice, Ornela Kullolli, Paola Parronchi and Sergio Romagnani
Center of Excellence for Research, Transfer and High Education DENOTHE of the University of Florence, Florence, Italy
Department of Experimental and Clinical Medicine, University of Florence, Largo Brambilla 3, 50134 Florence, Italy

M. Russo and A. Salzillo
Department of Pulmonology, Haematology and Oncology. Division of Pneumology and Allergology, High Speciality "A. Cardarelli" Hospital, Naples, Italy

G. Liccardi
Department of Pulmonology, Haematology and Oncology. Division of Pneumology and Allergology, High Speciality "A. Cardarelli" Hospital, Naples, Italy
Postgraduate School of Respiratory Medicine. Department of Experimental Medicine and Surgery, University of Rome "Tor Vergata", Rome, Italy

L. Calzetta and P. Rogliani
Postgraduate School of Respiratory Medicine. Department of Experimental Medicine and Surgery, University of Rome "Tor Vergata", Rome, Italy
Department of Experimental Medicine and Surgery, University of Rome Tor Vergata, Rome, Italy

G. Baldi
Respiratory Medicine Unit, ASL (District 66), Salerno, Italy

A. Berra
Respiratory Allergy Unit, G. Da Procida Hospital, Salerno, Italy

L. Billeri
Department of Laboratory Medicine, University Hospital Padova, Padua, Italy

M. Caminati
Asthma Center and Allergy Unit, Verona University and General Hospital, Verona, Italy

P. Capano
Unit of Pulmonary Immunology and Respiratory Diseases Ospedale "Santa Maria Della Speranza", Battipaglia, Salerno, Italy

E. Carpentieri
Division of Pneumology, "Santa Maria Novella" Hospital, Galatina, Lecce, Italy

A. Ciccarelli
Allergy Unit, Loreto Crispi Hospital, Naples, Italy

M. A. Crivellaro
Unit of Allergy and Occupational Medicine, University Hospital Padova, Padua, Italy

M. Cutajar
Allergy Center, Division of Internal Medicine, Ospedali Riuniti Penisola Sorrentina, Sorrento, Naples, Italy

M. D'Amato and A. Stanziola
Department of Respiratory Disease, "Federico II" University – AO "Dei Colli", Naples, Italy

I. Folletti and G. Paolocci
Department of Medicine, Section of Occupational Medicine, Respiratory Diseases and Toxicology, Terni Hospital, University of Perugia, Perugia, Italy

F. Gani
Allergy Unit, S. Luigi Gonzaga Hospital, Orbassano, Turin, Italy

D. Gargano
Allergy Unit, High Speciality "San Giuseppe Moscati" Hospital, Avellino, Italy

D. Giannattasio
Respiratory Physiopathology and Allergy, High Speciality Center, "Mauro Scarlato" Hospital, Scafati, Salerno, Italy

M. Giovannini
Pulmonary Diseases Department, Mirandola Hospital, Modena, Italy

C. Lombardi
Departmental Unit of Allergy, Clinical Immunology and Respiratory Diseases, Fondazione Poliambulanza, Brescia, Italy

M. Lo Schiavo, C. Montera and R. Pio
Allergy and Clinical Immunology, "G. Fucito" Hospital, S. Giovanni di Dio e Ruggi D'Aragona University Hospital, Salerno, Italy

F. Madonna
Allergy Unit, ASL (Sanitary District n°12), Caserta, Italy

M. Maniscalco
Pulmonary Rehabilitation Unit, ICS Maugeri, Telese Terme, Benevento, Italy

A. Meriggi
Allergy and Immunology Unit, Fondazione "Salvatore Maugeri", Institut of Research and Care, Scientific Institute of Pavia, Pavia, Italy

C. Micucci
Division of Pneumology and Allergology Hospital "Carlo Urbani", Jesi, Ancona, Italy

M. Milanese
Division of Pneumology, S. Corona Hospital, Pietra Ligure, Savona, Italy

R. Parente
Division of Allergy and Clinical Immunology, University of Salerno, Salerno, Italy

A. Pedicini
Division of Internal Medicine and Allergy, Fatebenefratelli Hospital, Benevento, Italy

F. Puggioni
Respiratory Diseases Department- IRCCS Humanitas Research and Clinical Center, Rozzano, Milan, Italy

P. Scavalli
Unit of Respiratory Physiopathology, Allergy and Occupational Medicine, ASL Viterbo, Viterbo, Italy

N. Scichilone
Biomedical Department of Specialistic and Internal Medicine, University of Palermo, Palermo, Italy

B. Sposato
Pneumology Unit, Azienda Ospedaliera "Misericordia", Grosseto, Italy

G. Steinhilber
Division of Pneumology, Spedali Civili Brescia, Brescia, Italy

A. Vatrella
Department of Medicine and Surgery, University of Salerno, Fisciano, Italy

G. Passalacqua
Allergy and Respiratory Diseases, Policlinico San Martino, University of Genoa, Genoa, Italy

Diomira Magliacane
Division Allergy and Clinical Immunology, Department of Medicine ASL Salerno, "Santa Maria della Speranza" Hospital, Battipaglia, Salerno, Italy

Giovanni Florio
Division Allergy and Clinical Immunology, Department of Medicine ASL Salerno, "Santa Maria della Speranza" Hospital, Battipaglia, Salerno, Italy
Postgraduate Program in Allergy and Clinical Immunology-University of Naples Federico II, Naples, Italy

Vincenzo Patella
Division Allergy and Clinical Immunology, Department of Medicine ASL Salerno, "Santa Maria della Speranza" Hospital, Battipaglia, Salerno, Italy
Postgraduate Program in Allergy and Clinical Immunology-University of Naples Federico II, Naples, Italy
Air Pollution and Climate Change Task Force of the Italian Society of Allergology, Asthma and Clinical Immunology (SIAAIC), Milan, Italy

Arturo Genovese
Postgraduate Program in Allergy and Clinical Immunology-University of Naples Federico II, Naples, Italy
Air Pollution and Climate Change Task Force of the Italian Society of Allergology, Asthma and Clinical Immunology (SIAAIC), Milan, Italy

Maria Angiola Crivellaro
Air Pollution and Climate Change Task Force of the Italian Society of Allergology, Asthma and Clinical Immunology (SIAAIC), Milan, Italy
Department of Cardiac, Thoracic and Vascular Sciences, University of Padua, Padua, Italy

Daniela Di Bartolomeo
Air Pollution and Climate Change Task Force of the Italian Society of Allergology, Asthma and Clinical Immunology (SIAAIC), Milan, Italy
Association of International Culture, Athena of Paestum, Capaccio-Paestum, Salerno, Italy

Mario Palmieri
Air Pollution and Climate Change Task Force of the Italian Society of Allergology, Asthma and Clinical Immunology (SIAAIC), Milan, Italy
Former Primary of Unit of Pediatry, Hospital of Eboli, Salerno, Italy

Amedeo Postiglione
Air Pollution and Climate Change Task Force of the Italian Society of Allergology, Asthma and Clinical Immunology (SIAAIC), Milan, Italy
International Court of the Environment Foundation (ICEF), Rome, Italy

Erminia Ridolo
Air Pollution and Climate Change Task Force of the Italian Society of Allergology, Asthma and Clinical Immunology (SIAAIC), Milan, Italy
Department of Medicine and Surgery, University of Parma, Parma, Italy

Cristina Scaletti
Air Pollution and Climate Change Task Force of the Italian Society of Allergology, Asthma and Clinical Immunology (SIAAIC), Milan, Italy
Unit of Internal Medicine, Department of Experimental and Clinical Medicine, University of Florence, Florence, Italy

Maria Teresa Ventura
Air Pollution and Climate Change Task Force of the Italian Society of Allergology, Asthma and Clinical Immunology (SIAAIC), Milan, Italy
Department of Interdisciplinary Medicine, University of Bari, Bari, Italy

Anna Zollo
Air Pollution and Climate Change Task Force of the Italian Society of Allergology, Asthma and Clinical Immunology (SIAAIC), Milan, Italy
Department of Studies and Researches, Movimento Ecologista Europeo FareAmbiente, Rome, Italy

Ada Giuliano
Laboratory of Environmental Analysis, Department of Public Health, ASL Salerno, Salerno, Italy

Boaz Palterer, Gianfranco Vitiello, Alessia Carraresi, Maria Grazia Giudizi, Daniele Cammelli and Paola Parronchi
Experimental and Clinical Medicine Department, University of Florence, Largo Brambilla 3, 50134 Florence, Italy

Filippo Fassio
SOC Allergologia e Immunologica Clinica, Azienda USL Toscana Centro, Nuovo Ospedale S. Giovanni di Dio, Via di Torregalli, 3, 50143 Florence, Italy

Fabio Guagnini
Allergy Therapeutics Italia, via IV Novembre 76, 20019 Settimo Milanese, Milan, Italy

E. Di Leo
Unit of Internal Medicine, Section of Allergy and Clinical Immunology, "F. Miulli" Hospital, Acquaviva delle Fonti, BA, Italy

P. Delle Donne and L. Macchia
Department of Emergency and Organ Transplantation, School and Chair of Allergology and Clinical Immunology, University of Bari—Aldo Moro, Bari, Italy

E. Nettis
Department of Emergency and Organ Transplantation, School and Chair of Allergology and Clinical Immunology, University of Bari—Aldo Moro, Bari, Italy
Policlinico, Piazza Giulio Cesare, 11, 70124 Bari, Italy

G. F. Calogiuri
Pneumology Department, Sacro Cuore Hospital, Gallipoli, Lecce, Italy

Maria Teresa Ventura, Rosa Cecere and Rosalba Buquicchio
Department of Interdisciplinary Medicine, University of Bari, Bari, Italy

Elisa Boni
S.O.S.Allergy, ASL, Alessandria, Italy

Gian Franco Calogiuri
Pneumology Department, Ospedale Sacro Cuore Gallipoli (Lecce), Lecce, Italy

Irene Martignago and Erminia Ridolo
Medicine and Surgery Department, University of Parma, Via Gramsci 14, 43126 Parma, Italy

Cristoforo Incorvaia
Cardiac/Pulmonary Rehabilitation, ASST Pini/CTO, Milan, Italy

Zafar Rasheed, Ragaa H. Salama and Tarek Salem
Department of Medical Biochemistry, College of Medicine, Qassim University, Buraidah 51452, Saudi Arabia

Khaled Zedan
Department of Pediatrics, College of Medicine, Qassim University, Buraidah, Saudi Arabia

Ghada Bin Saif
Department of Dermatology, College of Medicine, King Saud University, Riyadh, Saudi Arabia

Ahmed A. Ahmed
Research Center, College of Medicine, Qassim University, Buraidah, Saudi Arabia

Alaa Abd El-Moniem and Maha Elkholy
Department of Medicine, College of Medicine, Qassim University, Buraidah, Saudi Arabia

Ahmad A. Al Robaee and Abdullateef A. Alzolibani
Department of Dermatology, College of Medicine, Qassim University, Buraidah, Saudi Arabia

Index